Physical Activity and Rehabilitation in Life-threatening Illness

This book is a comprehensive summary of the recommendations for best practice, and current evidence, for physical activity and rehabilitation of functional deficits in individuals with end-stage diseases. While advances in technology have afforded us the opportunity to live longer lives, it has also demanded an expansion of focus of medical interventions towards palliative care to enhance the quality of life.

Exercise and healthcare professionals must strive to broaden their perspectives to provide for the unique needs of these individuals, and to successfully engage with them, to achieve the most positive outcomes throughout the entire continuum of care. Healthcare providers play a critical role in advocating for care to allow individuals to remain physically active for as long as possible, even in the face of declining health. Finally, due to the increasing and progressively emergent healthcare utilization required by these individuals, a significant cost burden is experienced by healthcare systems, patients, families, and payers. There is evidence of substantial protective effects of physical activity, prevention, safety, and rehabilitative procedures to reduce hospital readmissions, reduce length of stay, and assist in avoiding unwarranted or unnecessary diagnostic tests or procedures.

Physical activity has been proven to have a substantial impact and protective effects on virtually all medical conditions. During curative management, but especially during transitional phases to palliative care, other strategies need enhanced consideration to complement the existing plan of care and help to improve patient's quality of life. Ideally, physical medicine would be at the forefront of allowing individuals to live their best life until the very end.

Physical Activity and Rehabilitation in Life-threatening Illness is key reading for academics and policy makers in physical activity, international exercise, wellness and rehabilitation, and related disciplines, as well as research-focused clinicians in settings where patients with advanced illness are frequently encountered.

Amy J. Litterini PT, DPT is an Associate Clinical Professor in the Doctor of Physical Therapy Program at the University of New England in Portland, Maine, USA. Her clinical career has focused on adult rehabilitation, with an interest in advanced cancer survivorship. She is a certified patient navigator by the Harold P. Freeman Patient Navigation Institute and a certified hospice volunteer with Compassus Hospice. Amy served in governance positions in the American Physical Therapy Association's Academy of Oncologic Physical Therapy and the Oncologic Specialty Council of the American Board of Physical Therapy Specialists.

Christopher M. Wilson PT, DPT, DScPT is an Assistant Professor in the Physical Therapy Program in the School of Health Sciences at Oakland University, Rochester, MI, USA and the Residency Program Director for the Beaumont Health Oncology Residency, Troy, MI, USA. He is the Vice President of the Academy of Oncologic Physical Therapy of the American Physical Therapy Association and served as the Hospice Palliative Care Coordinator for the oncology subgroup of the World Confederation for Physical Therapy (now World Physiotherapy).

Routledge Research in Physical Activity and Health

The *Routledge Research in Physical Activity and Health* series offers a multi-disciplinary forum for cutting-edge research in the broad area of physical activity, exercise and health. Showcasing the work of emerging and established scholars working in areas ranging from physiology and chronic disease, psychology and mental health to physical activity and health promotion and socio-economic and cultural aspects of physical activity participation, the series is an important channel for groundbreaking research in physical activity and health.

Physical Activity and the Gastro-Intestinal Tract
Responses in Health and Disease
Roy J. Shephard

Technology in Physical Activity and Health Promotion
Edited by Zan Gao

Physical Activity and the Abdominal Viscera
Responses in Health and Disease
Roy J. Shephard

Obesity
A Kinesiologist's Perspective
Roy J. Shephard

The Politics of Physical Activity
Joe Piggin

Physical Activity and Rehabilitation in Life-threatening Illness
Amy J. Litterini and Christopher M. Wilson

For more information about this series, please visit: https://www.routledge.com/sport/series/RRPAH

Physical Activity and Rehabilitation in Life-threatening Illness

Amy J. Litterini and
Christopher M. Wilson

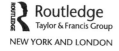
Routledge
Taylor & Francis Group

NEW YORK AND LONDON

First published 2021
by Routledge
52 Vanderbilt Avenue, New York, NY 10017

and by Routledge
2 Park Square, Milton Park, Abingdon, Oxon, OX14 4RN

Routledge is an imprint of the Taylor & Francis Group, an informa business

© 2021 Taylor & Francis

Library of Congress Cataloging-in-Publication Data
A catalog record for this title has been requested

ISBN: 978-0-367-90256-8 (hbk)
ISBN: 978-0-367-71063-7 (pbk)
ISBN: 978-1-003-02504-7 (ebk)

Typeset in Baskerville
by codeMantra

To Reyna Colombo for a quarter century of mentorship, support, and friendship – Chris

To my husband Vince for his ongoing support, and to each of my patients over the years who taught me what I know today – Amy

Contents

Figures

Tables

Boxes

Contributors

Developmental Editor:

Richard Briggs PT, MA

Principal Consultant, Hospice Physical Therapy Associates, Chico, CA, USA, and Founding Chair of the Hospice and Palliative Care Special Interest Group of the Academy of Oncologic Physical Therapy

Line Editor:

Danielle Black, BS, SPT

Graduate Assistant, Oakland University, Rochester, MI, USA

Contributors:

Kendra D. Koch, PhD

Research Associate, Autism and Neurodevelopment Disability, Fellow, Institute for Collaborative Health Research and Practice, Steve Hicks School of Social Work, The University of Texas at Austin, Austin, TX, USA

Jeannette Q. Lee, PT, PhD

Associate Professor, University of California San Francisco/ San Francisco State University Graduate Program in Physical Therapy, San Francisco, CA

Selected Illustrations:

Paul Mangiafico, PT, DPT

Physical Therapist, graduate, University of New England Doctor of Physical Therapy Program, Portland, ME, USA

Foreword

Richard Briggs PT, MA
Founding Chair of the Hospice and Palliative Care Special Interest
Group of the American Physical Therapy Association

Congratulations. You have in your hands the first textbook addressing activity and rehabilitation practices with people living with life threatening illness, as they move towards the end of their life. This body of information reflects over 50 years of hospice care development that began at St. Christopher's Hospice in London, England. It offers a broad range of possibilities in clinical, administrative, and health policy practice.

I have had the privilege of knowing the authors as professional colleagues, enjoyed observing their growth as subject matter experts in hospice and palliative care, and as clinicians and faculty over many years. It was my honor to be invited to review this work and write this note of introduction. My clinical practice for the past 40 years focused in this specialty area and began when none of this information had been developed, much less published.

My initial response during the experience of reviewing this manuscript was that there is now an enormous amount of collective knowledge that can be applied to rehabilitation practice in end-of-life care. In fact, I imagined a possible reaction one might feel as a care provider during educational training or as a clinician relatively new to practice, trying to internalize all that is in this volume on end-of-life care. **Fear not**. There are several approaches that might be helpful.

First, one must consider that rehabilitation, by its nature, is a palliative and not a curative endeavor. From the early work of restorative aides following World War I, our professions have worked to maximize physical and functional recovery after injury or onset of disease. While in some cases full recovery is possible, most often there is some residual limitation. If we follow a patient over a lifetime, there will be successive bouts or conditions to be addressed, as well as the eventual life-threatening condition that will bring the decline at end of life. We can apply our knowledge and experience in all of these circumstances.

Second, understand that your education and training has already established a solid foundation for this area of practice with your previously learned evaluative and treatment skills. Use this text as a resource to expand your offerings in clinical application. Perhaps draw only one or two new concepts from a single chapter, and apply it to your current practice. How did that work out? What might you do differently next time? What did you learn? Try this using one topic or chapter at a time. Developing a more advanced practice in any area, especially end-of-life care, is a career path and lifelong process. I recall in my last week before retirement as a clinician still observing and learning new things.

Another process that might be helpful is to share these new ideas with your colleagues as a point of discussion or through in-service and inter-professional learning. There are clinical aspects, but also the psychological, emotional, and spiritual dimensions that arise in the process of caring for and accompanying the dying. By talking about the many aspects of this challenging care, we mature and develop not only our professional but also our personal selves.

Lastly, be gentle with yourself. Your willingness to undertake learning and practice around end-of-life care already demonstrates a level of compassion. We recognize we cannot cure and most often not even slow the natural processes that occur during the decline at the end of life. But, we can help people maintain a sense of dignity and choice, if not control, as they and their caregivers travel this path together. A wise person once advised me, "they may not remember what you did, and they may not remember what you said, but they will remember how you made them feel."

Textbooks such as this need to be kept close at hand and this one will age well. There are chapters that you may refer to regularly as you develop and refine your clinical and organizational practice. Part I, Chapters 1–7, offers an overview of clinical philosophy, explains various care roles, and describes how hospice and palliative care teams function. Part II, Chapters 8–16, will be most useful to revisit when specific clinical conditions or diagnoses present and you seek specific symptom management and treatment approaches. Part III, Chapters 17–20, provides standardized tests, measures, and interventions useful when working in end-of-life care. Part IV covers education, policy, and regulatory information, and looks to what the future might potentially hold. Part V has samples of forms and documentation that facilitate care. Every practitioner will find valuable and transformational ideas throughout this book.

In closing, I would offer that as you begin learning and developing your practice, recognize that despite all of the knowledge you glean from this text, when you step into the clinic with your next client, you will be at the vanguard of end-of-life practice. There is much still to be learned, as this specialty area of practice is in the nascent and earliest stages of development in most environments. I invite you to share your knowledge, experience, and advocacy as we continue to advance professional practice for those who entrust us with their care.

– Rich

Part I

Core Concepts in Life-threatening Illness

1 Palliative Care for Adults

Christopher M. Wilson and Amy J. Litterini

Introduction

Medical and therapeutic professionals providing care for those with a life-threatening illness using physical activity interventions is a relatively new and not well-understood concept. It often seems counterintuitive that physical activity and rehabilitative interventions would be applied to a patient with a terminal illness; however, there is a growing body of evidence that these interventions, when properly applied via skilled professionals, can improve a person's remaining quality of life, safety, and comfort. Palliative care (PC) is the holistic, compassionate, interdisciplinary proactive approach to help relieve suffering and distress at or near the end of life (EoL). Therapists have a unique skill set and knowledge base to assist these individuals to improve, maintain, or slow the decline of their symptoms, functional limitations, or participation restrictions, but only when there is a clear understanding by all members of the team as to the therapist's contribution to the team.

Terminal Illness and Physical Activity: Oxymoron or Best Practice?

Illness and dying are part of life. Every individual, no matter how healthy, how rich, or how safety conscious, will inevitably face serious illness or death. In modern society, death and serious illness have been progressively medicalized. This is logical, as those with life-threatening illnesses increasingly seek medical attention to slow down or manage the disease as it progresses and to help control its symptoms. In the authors' experience, those living with a life-threatening illness become less amenable to pursuing medical care as they approach death; this occurs concurrently with the decreasing effectiveness of the medical treatments and interventions. This results in a paradox between terminally ill individuals becoming more reluctant to pursue medical care and concurrently feeling the need for medical care as their health issues are less controllable, culminating in increasing fear of loss of independence and not being able to remain at home or near the EoL. In a study of 606 Canadian participants examining their preferred location of living in the last months of life, 74% preferred to spend this time at home. Conversely, only 16% of people preferred to spend their last months in a hospital and only 10% of people preferred a long-term care setting (i.e. nursing home or rehab facility). Overall, 52% of people passed away in their preferred location, but only 40% of people who preferred to die at home achieved this goal.[1] This striking fact may be a key consideration in providing compassionate, individualized, proactive care, especially as physical activity and physical functioning are closely related to residing at home.[2]

This societal dilemma, although it takes many forms globally, highlights a key role for exercise, physical activity, and rehabilitation professionals. The untapped knowledge base, skill set, and professional integration of these professionals (including, but not limited to, physical therapists/physiotherapists, occupational therapists, exercise physiologists, kinesiologists, athletic and personal trainers, rehabilitation nurses, recreation therapists, and massage therapists) is an evolving component of care in life-threatening illness. As this group of professionals is diverse, with a variety of knowledge bases and scopes of practice, it would be unwieldy to list these professions each time they are referenced in this text. For the sake of clarity, the term *therapists* will be used within this text to describe this group of professionals, although the authors recognize that this term does not fully capture the individual unique value, skills, professional credentials, and perspectives of these varied caring professionals. The term *therapist* may also be additionally applicable to this population because *therapy* connotes thoughts of counseling, healing, and support, in addition to the medical use of the term. It is likely a better approach than utilizing a term like *rehabilitation professional* as many of these individuals will not be able to *rehabilitate*, to recover function, in light of their disease process. In addition, as there is much discussion on the use of the term *patient* with individuals facing life-threatening illness, especially near death due to the medical connotations, use of this term will be minimized unless talking specifically within the context of a medical procedure, hospitalization, or any other healthcare-related topic.

Although somewhat counterintuitive, physical activity concepts can have quite an impact on and be beneficial for those with an incurable, life-limiting illness. The term *prehabilitation* is defined by Silver and Baima[3] as

> "A process on the continuum of care that occurs between the time of cancer diagnosis and the beginning of acute treatment, includes physical and psychological assessments that establish a baseline functional level, identifies impairments, and provides targeted interventions that improve a patient's health to reduce the incidence and the severity of current and future impairments."

Although Silver and Baima were only discussing prehabilitation within the context of cancer care and did not specifically focus on advanced life-limiting disease, the core concepts still apply. Prehabilitation intends to build up the person's body and mind in anticipation of future physiological insults – in this case a physiologic insult that may ultimately take the person's life. To further clarify this approach to prehabilitation, a more descriptive term of *palliative prehabilitation* is best utilized. In palliative prehabilitation, the optimum opportunity to strengthen and optimize functional capacity is prior to the onset of a life-altering symptom burden. This timeframe is critical to optimize the quality of life (QoL) when symptoms do begin to impact function and participation in order to optimize remaining QoL and participation in life's rich experiences (Figure 1.1).

Physical activity has been long associated with improving strength, endurance, and functional capacity. More recently, physical activity and rehabilitation interventions have been described to maintain or slow the decline of dysfunction during a progressive disease process.[4-7] When this process requires the skills of a highly trained professional, it is termed *skilled maintenance*. Without this interventional approach, the person's physical and functional status would be expected to decline at an increased rate (Figure 1.2).

Physical activity may not always require the skill of a highly trained professional and can be carried out by the individual, their family members, or caregivers. In general, the skills of a therapist may be needed in the presence of medical instability to ensure safety or to accomplish a task that would be otherwise not achievable without the specialized skills and training of this therapist.[8] These physical activity interventions should always strive to align with the individual's care goals, optimizing quality of life, and within the context of the greater PC philosophy.[9]

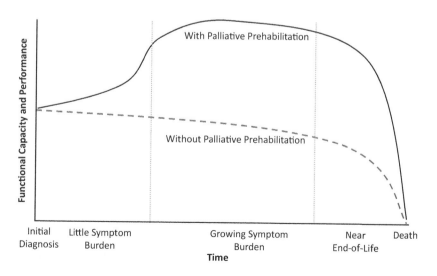

Figure 1.1 Palliative Prehabilitation.

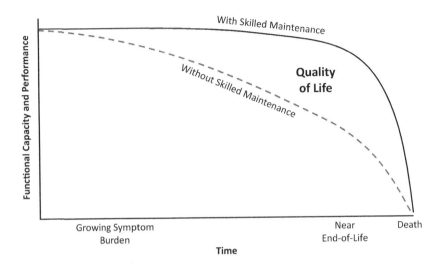

Figure 1.2 Skilled Maintenance.

History of Hospice and Palliative Care

Although people have been dying as long as humankind has existed, it is only within the last century or so that societies have made an organized, concerted effort to systematically ease suffering, anxiety, and the trauma of an advancing disease process and death. Before the 20th century, many of these efforts initially were facilitated through religious institutions that developed and organized homes for the "incurably ill."[10] Oftentimes these homes were intended for those who were poor or did not have family to care for them near death. The first organized hospice was St Christopher's in London, England, where care was provided to those with a terminal illness in 1967.[10] Dame Cicely Saunders is most often credited with the establishment of the modern hospice movement. She described and popularized many care concepts that are now inseparable from PC and hospice care philosophies. These include the concept of Total Pain (entailing domains of *physical, emotional, social,* and *spiritual distress* described further in Chapter 17), proactive pain control via appropriate opioid use, and increasing the emphasis on supporting and collaborating with families and caregivers.[11] Another landmark moment for caring for those facing death was in 1969 when Elisabeth Kubler-Ross published the book entitled *On Death and Dying.*[12] She described five stages that terminally ill individuals encounter when progressing through the dying process - denial, anger, bargaining, depression, and acceptance. This book, and its subsequent public attention, further accelerated the hospice movement and care of the individual facing death. In 1982, the United States federal government established the Medicare Hospice Benefit to provide appropriate care for individuals facing death and reduce healthcare costs. This further solidified the unique needs and care provision for those facing imminent death.

Hospice and end-of-life care is one component of the larger care philosophy of PC. The growth of PC has been increasing over the past few decades. In 2013, Lynch, Connor, and Clark[13] mapped PC growth across the globe. Lynch et al. noted, "In 2011, 136 of the world's 234 countries (58%) had one or more hospice-palliative care services established, an increase of 21 countries (9%) from 2006." Lynch also noted that nations demonstrating the most growth in PC activity or institutions were located in the global regions of *Africa*, the *Middle East*, and the *Americas/Caribbean*. As an example of this overall growth within nations, in the United States, the Center to Advance Palliative Care (www.capc.org) reported that, "The rise in prevalence of palliative care in U.S. hospitals has been steady over the last 16 years. In 2000, less than one-quarter of U.S. hospitals (658) had a palliative care program, compared to three quarters (1,831) in 2016."[14] Despite this growth, there are still some locales that are not demonstrating integration or growth of PC due to barriers in policy, education, medication availability, and implementation.[15] In these locales where PC is inconsistent or nonexistent, therapists may best serve their terminally ill clients by providing and supporting basic PC concepts within their individual scopes of practice, in addition to their professional expertise as therapists.

Overview of Palliative Care, Chronic Disease, and End-of-Life Care

As most therapists are not consistently integrated into the care of those with an advancing illness, clarification of key terms is important. Some laypersons may misunderstand that the terms hospice and PC do not mean the same thing; adding further to the confusion, these terms may vary between nations as well. In 2010, Radbruch[16] discussed the consequences of a lack of clear distinction between the terms hospice and PC among European nations. He argued that this lack of clear terminology has impaired development of international standards and has hindered research efforts in this area. This lack of clear and universal terminology among nations can be attributed to differences in language or different terms for similar care services (i.e. hospice, hospice care, continuing care, end-of-life care, supportive care, comfort care). An additional example is in several nations (i.e. United Kingdom, Australia, Canada), a hospice may be referred to as a physical location where end-of-life care is provided. Conversely, in the United States, hospice is defined as a holistic care approach when a person is certified to have less than six months of expected life. In the United States, hospice care is often defined by the Medicare Hospice health insurance benefit, as opposed to a location or a building.

The term palliative care is well defined by the World Health Organization (WHO) as

> "...an approach that improves the quality of life of patients and their families facing the problem associated with life-threatening illness, through the prevention and relief of suffering by means of early identification and impeccable assessment and treatment of pain and other problems, [of a] physical, psychosocial and spiritual [nature]."[17]

Palliative care:

- provides relief from pain and other distressing symptoms;
- affirms life and regards dying as a normal process;
- intends neither to hasten nor postpone death;
- integrates the psychological and spiritual aspects of patient care;
- offers a support system to help patients live as actively as possible until death;
- offers a support system to help the family cope during the patient's illness and in their bereavement;
- uses a team approach to address the needs of patients and their families, including bereavement counseling, if indicated;
- will enhance quality of life, and may also positively influence the course of illness;
- is applicable early in the course of illness, in conjunction with other therapies that are intended to prolong life, such as chemotherapy or radiation therapy, and includes those investigations needed to better understand and manage distressing clinical complications

PC is often perceived as a transition from active care to end-of-life care (often known as hospice care in the United States and some other nations); however, PC also includes patients with life-threatening illness not imminently dying but in physical decline that need support services similar to end-of-life care.[18]

The WHO estimated that over 40 million people require PC each year and only 14% of people who require PC actually receive it. This results in unnecessary suffering and distress at the end stages of life.[19] A challenge for PC practitioners is the wide diversity of people who would benefit from PC.[19] Figure 1.3 highlights the breadth of diagnostic categories that may be encountered or are beneficial during PC.

In addition to these major diagnostic categories, the WHO reminds us that there are other diagnoses that benefit from PC, "including kidney failure, chronic liver disease, multiple sclerosis, Parkinson's disease, rheumatoid arthritis, neurological disease, dementia, congenital anomalies and drug-resistant tuberculosis."[19] This can present a very unique challenge to therapists and physical activity professionals, as not only do they have to be experts in exercise, activity, and rehabilitation concepts, they must be able to speak fluently and understand aspects of a wide diversity of diagnoses and clinical practice models. This requires a PC therapist to consider themselves a 'jack of

Palliative Care Needs by Diagnostic Category

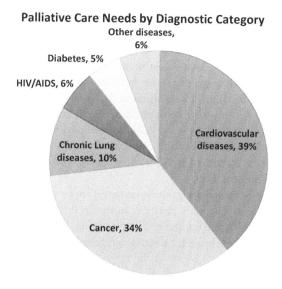

Figure 1.3 Distribution of Palliative Care Needs by Diagnosis.

all trades' and as the proverb goes, with this approach is the risk of mastery of none of the trades without a concerted effort. In reality, this 'jack of all trades' philosophy is, in essence, mastery of PC at a specialist level.

Depending on their individual practice setting and the amount of interaction the professionals may have with persons with terminal illness, PC education is necessary at three different target levels.[15] At the most basic level, all health professionals should have basic PC training in care concepts and best practices. For individuals who routinely work with individuals with life-threatening illness, intermediate training should occur, including education on pain control, communication skills, preventing health crises, and avoiding unwarranted or unnecessary tests. Finally, for PC specialists who solely work with persons with a life-threatening illness, advanced training or certifications are necessary to provide optimum care for those who require advanced symptom management and care navigation needs.

Patient/Family Centered Care and the Biopsychosocial Model

As an individual's disease process advances, they tend to do less well in the traditional 'curative' medical model, where some care providers do not closely monitor or address a patient's social and psychological domains of health. In early stage disease, although not recommended, this superficial care may be passable, as the patient's disease may not be substantially affecting these domains of health. One of the initial efforts to describe this much-needed approach was the biopsychosocial model. In 1977, Engel introduced the biopsychosocial model as a novel way of approaching healthcare. In the biopsychosocial model, information such as social and psychological aspects are provided the same consideration as other medical and physiological issues during healthcare provision.[20] This initial foray into incorporating all aspects of the patient was a revolutionary way of approaching healthcare and complimented the emerging hospice and PC movement. More recently, the term patient/family centered care integrated the biopsychosocial model by incorporating the patient preferences, family situation, and the patient's unique contextual factors, barriers, and facilitators, to strive for medical care that meets the needs of the person at that exact time and life situation.

A key outcome of the patient/family centered care model is to establish the patient and the family as equal partners in the healthcare delivery system.[21] One example of this is during patient interviewing, instead of just collecting data to make a medical choice for the patient, Smith et al.[22] describes four key habits during a subjective history: (1) Invest in the patient's life and outcomes from the beginning; (2) Strive to elicit the patient's perspective during the interview; (3) Demonstrate empathy; and (4) Invest again at the end of the interview by assuring that all information was covered and understood and achievable next steps are established. These broad approaches and healthcare evolutions set the framework for the overall PC approach.

Key Components of Palliative Care Practice

Within the PC philosophy there are a variety of clinical and programmatic goals that provide opportunities for therapists to best support individuals and provide coordinated client-centered care. Each patient has individual health, psychosocial, life circumstances, and goals; these are highly individualized and time dependent.

Death with Dignity and the Concept of a Good Death

A key outcome of PC and quality end-of-life care is the concept of a good death. Upon first consideration, the terms *good* and *death* seem to be diametrically opposed; however, when circumstances are carefully arranged by a coordinated, trained team, a person can pass away with dignity and peace in the location and manner of their choosing. A good death, although still emotionally challenging, can be an enriching, meaningful life milestone and a celebration of a person's life. Oftentimes, a good death is described as being surrounded by loved ones, in a comfortable location of the person's choosing, free of pain or distress, and being able to reflect on a life well spent without regrets. As can be imagined, circumstances of a good death are a highly individualized concept, and early, frequent, and in-depth discussions should ensue around this topic.

Clarifying Current and Future Goals of Care

A key role of PC is clarification of the current care goals within the context of an increasingly uncertain and variable disease trajectory. Although asking individuals with a terminal illness directly what their goals are would seem to make sense, it may not always elicit a realistic or fully thought-out response. One of the most important roles of the PC team is deep, reflective discussions with the person and the family. As this approach requires a clear and easy to understand discussion about the realities of the medical condition, PC providers involved are often physicians, physician assistants, or nurse practitioners. These individuals receive advanced training in merging life goals and aspirational hopes with the reality of a worsening disease process to establish an achievable plan.

"Hope is not a plan." – Dr. Atul Gawande[23]

One of the key ways that these care discussions ensue is through advance care planning (ACP) discussions. Many nations and jurisdictions have some form of ACP and means to document it. Rietjens et al.[24] executed a Delphi study with the aim of developing a consensus definition of ACP and provide recommendations for its application. Experts from Europe (n = 82), North America (n = 16), and Australia (n = 16) established the definition of ACP as "the ability to enable individuals to define goals and preferences for future medical treatment and care, to discuss these goals and preferences with family and health-care providers, and to record and review these preferences if appropriate."[24] Three key recommendations were made: (1) Adapting ACP as indicated by the individual's readiness; (2) Modifying or targeting the content of an ACP as the disease worsens; (3) Using a non-physician facilitator to assist with the ACP process.[24]

A term closely tied to ACP is an advance care directive or advance directive. This document is completed by an individual to describe and detail their wishes in certain situations, should their health condition advance rapidly or they become unable to communicate their wishes. The 109 experts in the Rietjens[24] study recommended, "Advance care directives need both a structured format to enable easy identification of specific goals and preferences in emergency situations, and an open-text format so individuals can describe their values, goals, and preferences." The experts also recommended that the advance care directive be stored within a health system's medical record and the decisions outlined (i.e. DNR and who is a surrogate decision-maker) should be legally binding.[24] Initially the ACP process was mainly intended to facilitate completion of an advance care directive; however, this reflective process has evolved into an entire approach to facilitating conversations and clarifying care goals in advance of a disease process (see Appendix 1).[24]

Interdisciplinary Care

As an individual's disease process and symptoms worsen, the number of care team providers assisting with a component of care increases, which also compounds the challenges of communication and competing priorities. Illustrative of this is the case of a 75-year-old male admitted to the hospital who was diagnosed with Stage IV Lung Cancer three months prior. Metastatic disease was found in his spine, brain, and both of his femurs. His direct care team might include a thoracic surgeon, medical oncologist, radiation oncologist, physical therapist, nurse navigator, dietician/nutrition specialist, occupational therapist, pulmonologist, neurologist, physical medicine and rehabilitation specialist (physiatrist), orthopedic physician, spiritual care professional, social worker, and his primary care physician. Each of these professionals has their own perspective and eager skill set to best 'help' the patient. As communication among these several busy professionals is challenging, let alone each of these individuals clearly understanding and integrating the patient's goals, a key role of the PC team is to be the advocate and voice for the patient's goals to the rest of the care team. This may be accomplished by convening an interdisciplinary team meeting, which may or may not always include the patient and family. Depending on the institution, this may occur regularly (i.e. daily or weekly) or on an ad hoc basis. Care coordination may also occur formally through medical chart documentation or orders, or informally via conversations between individual providers. If a therapist does not embrace or perceive the value of working closely with the interdisciplinary team, providing care for those with a life-threatening illness may not be a positive and sustainable practice setting.

Ethics and Ethical Discussions

Traditionally, in therapists' clinical practice, ethical dilemmas with life and death consequences are uncommon, yet these are regular topics of discussion in PC situations. One of the benefits of early, proactive ACP and advance care directives is that all parties are clearly aware of the person's wishes in a variety of life-threatening health situations. If an advance care directive is not completed or a health issue worsens rapidly before one could be completed, the healthcare team has to attempt to learn the individual's wishes second-hand or even guess.

HW was an 83-year-old male with advanced dementia who resided in a memory care unit. He had not documented his wishes via ACP prior to losing the ability to be legally competent for decision-making. His wife passed away two years earlier and he had four children who lived in the area. During a meal, HW severely aspirated his food and went into respiratory distress. In the absence of a DNR, HW's respiratory tract was cleared and he was intubated, after several minutes of unconsciousness, by emergency medical professionals. He was rushed to the local hospital via ambulance. Despite his advanced dementia and perilous health situation, two siblings thought that their father would have wanted continued life-sustaining measures while the other two siblings felt it was time for nature to take its course. While the siblings argued, HW was admitted to the intensive care unit where he received several invasive procedures until the medical care team was able to achieve family consensus to let HW pass away several days later.

In cases where care team members disagree on a course of action or additional expert opinions would be valuable, many health systems have an ethics team, which can be consulted by anyone, including non-healthcare team members. In rare cases, legal guardianship or a court advocate might be appointed to progress through decision-making. By this time, the peace and dignity of a good death are often out of reach, and physical and emotional distress has already occurred.

Balancing Quality of Life and Expert Symptom Control with Curative Treatments

QoL is defined by the World Health Organization as

> "...an individual's perception of their position in life in the context of the culture and value systems in which they live and in relation to their goals, expectations, standards and concerns. It is a broad ranging concept affected in a complex way by the person's physical health, psychological state, personal beliefs, social relationships and their relationship to salient features of their environment."[25]

All palliative and hospice care is focused on optimizing the remaining quality of life. PC practitioners and care team members receive advanced training in evidence-based best practices as it relates to pain control, including the use of opioids and other pharmacologic and non-pharmacologic measures. As therapists often have skills and interventions to directly impact improving QoL and treating the causes of or the symptoms of pain, their role in this area is important but underutilized.[9]

At some point in the person's disease process, curative or restorative treatments such as surgery, chemotherapy, radiation therapy, or overly vigorous rehabilitation may be detrimental to a person's quality of life. Some interventions may even shorten the life of a person with a terminal illness. The PC team is intended to look at the big picture, incorporate the patient's current goals, medical reality, and life circumstances and advocate for the patient, even if it means to advocate for cessation of futile "curative" treatments. This role often requires expert communication skills, professional confidence, and a strong grasp of the research evidence related to this person's complex medical issues.

Anticipating and Mitigating Future Issues

Finally, within PC, reducing or mitigating avoidable medical events should be the focus of the care team, even if these events might be unlikely. As was mentioned earlier, individuals prefer not to spend their remaining days in the hospital or receiving unnecessary medical or surgical treatments. The interdisciplinary care team should collaboratively consider what foreseeable emergent events may occur and work to provide the resources that will reduce the chance of these occurrences. In the absence of these proactive and preventative interventions, the individual and family may feel that they need to call emergency services which subsequently may result in avoidable readmission or institutionalization. It should be noted that the majority of hospital readmissions in PC may be unavoidable, as they were found to be related to disease progression or a new diagnosis.[26] See Table 1.1 for some examples of possible health issues and what may be provided by the PC team to mitigate these issues.

Disease Stages and Categorizations

Therapists who practice clinically in only one setting (e.g. community exercise facility, outpatient/ambulatory, acute hospital, hospice) often only have the opportunity to work with a patient for a condensed point in time. For these therapists, it is important to consider and understand the life and disease trajectory of an individual facing life-threatening illness. For therapists who work with an individual who is newly diagnosed with a disease, it may not be immediately apparent to consider the progressively advancing trajectory that will ultimately lead to death. Conversely, for a hospice therapist faced with a very

Table 1.1 Health Issues that May Require Readmission and Interventions to Address Them

Health Issue	Sample Interventions
Uncontrolled pain crisis (aka breakthrough pain)	Convenient availability of stronger pain medications. Education in meditation, guided imagery, or other non-pharmacologic measures.
Fall at home	Provision of more advanced assistive devices (i.e. walkers, wheelchairs), modifying ADL to avoid risky movement patterns and home modifications
Inappropriate or premature discharge home	Provision of family/caregiver training and provision of education on safety concerns and consequences of discharge home
Referrals not made for discharge needs	Frequent review and update of discharge plan including facilitation of referrals
Lack of finances/ resources to complete care at home	Proactive clarification of plan and provision of appropriate resources, items
Unexpected dyspnea	Educate on breathing techniques (pursed lip breathing, diaphragmatic breathing, airway clearance techniques) and adequate emergency inhalers (i.e. albuterol nebulizer)
New weakness, gait or mobility disturbance	Educate and provide alternative means to complete ADL (i.e. bedpan or bedside commode if unable to walk to bathroom)

ill and distraught individual, it may be challenging to consider that it may only have been a few weeks or months ago that this person was planning their next holiday, exercising regularly, and thinking about what their lives would entail years and decades from now. Once considered, these dramatic changes will help the therapist to understand the individual's recent life journey. It may make it more understandable when this person may have unrealistic goals related to their prognosis or exhibit seemingly 'irrational' behavior. In general, within each progressive disease process, individuals will encounter each of these stages, but depending on the type of disease and when the diagnosis is made, stages may be longer or shorter.

In order to best synthesize these abstract and arbitrary stages, they will be detailed utilizing a patient case and discussing his physical, psychosocial, functional, and emotional states. Although specific therapist interventions and procedures will not be detailed in order to focus on the progressive disease stages, readers are encouraged to consider how, where, and which of the therapist's skills would be beneficial in each of the stages. See Figure 1.4 for the depiction and overview of these stages.

Stage 0 – Pre-Diagnosis Prevention, Wellness, and Health Promotion

Until diagnosed with a life-threatening disease or disorder, all individuals have the opportunity to make health and lifestyle changes as they relate to reducing disease risk. It is not a novel concept that inadvisable health behaviors lead to shorter and less active lives, with increased chronic disease. Cardiovascular risk factors include behaviors such as unhealthy diet, unfavorable cholesterol/lipid

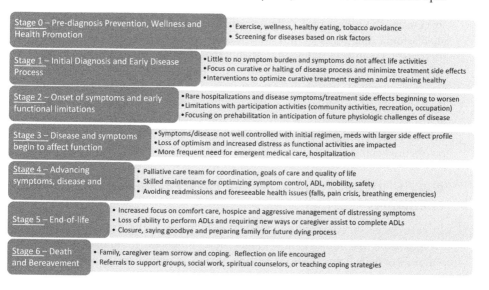

Figure 1.4 Stages of Disease Processes.

profile, sedentary lifestyle, obesity, and tobacco/nicotine/alcohol use, all of which directly contribute to increased risk of morbidity and mortality.[27] There is a growing body of research further establishing the relationship between physical inactivity and cancer risk.[28] Regardless of disease risk, aging is the condition that will affect all individuals, and with it comes the predictable age-related changes which exercise and healthy behaviors can proactively mitigate.

Patient Case: TS was a 45-year-old gentleman living in the Midwest region of the United States. He had two children in their early twenties who lived out of state. He was divorced and lived with his long-term girlfriend. He enjoyed his work fabricating machine parts in a tool and dye shop. Recreationally, he enjoyed hunting, fishing, and prided himself on being a hockey player when he was younger. He had no significant medical history and although he had a body mass index of 28, he perceived himself to be in good active health.

Stage 1 – Initial Diagnosis and Early Disease Process

Once diagnosed with progressive disease or incurable illness, symptoms may be minimal or well controlled. Outpatient medical care may be infrequent and hospitalizations are rare. This individual may be able to carry out normal daily personal and community tasks with little to no difficulty. A medication or structured treatment regimen is likely to be initiated in order to halt or slow the disease process or to minimize symptoms.

Patient Case: During work one day, TS experienced a seizure. He was rushed by ambulance to the nearest emergency room, as he had no history of seizures. In the emergency room, medication was administered to reduce the chance of future seizures, especially within the light of the unknown etiology of the first seizure. A computerized tomography scan revealed a space-occupying mass in TS's brain which was ultimately revealed to be a glioblastoma multiforme (GBM). TS was admitted to the hospital and was prescribed a course of radiation to shrink the tumor in order to facilitate future surgical excision. He was able to return home after a one-week hospital stay but was not cleared to drive or return to work due to the seizure. Other than slight balance impairments and right lower extremity weakness, TS was able to participate fully in life activities but was distraught by his limitation in driving and working, as his independence and role as a family provider was an essential component of his personal identity.

Stage 2 – Onset of Symptoms and Early Functional Limitations

In early stage diagnosis, the individual is living with the disease, but the symptoms are beginning to affect higher-level functioning and instrumental activities of daily living (ADL). The individual may require more medications or more aggressive medications with a more substantial side-effect profile. Surgical or medical procedures may be required to address the disease or symptoms. Some hospitalizations may be necessary.

Patient Case: TS completed his neoadjuvant radiation treatment to reduce the tumor burden of his GBM and was scheduled for surgery. The external beam radiation had taken a toll on his endurance and strength. He felt like he was having more 'senior moments' of forgetfulness but was still overall optimistic about his health. His family had been providing exceptional support, with his girlfriend and neighbors driving him to doctor appointments and errands. He was taking one to two naps during the day due to his fatigue but still was able to participate actively in recreational activities without significant difficulty. He was looking forward to removing the tumor to reduce the psychological burden of having it inside his head.

Stage 3 – Disease and Symptoms Begin to Impact Function

As the disease process advances, symptoms affect the individual's daily routine and function. Hospitalizations may be necessary and tests, procedures, and surgeries become more frequent. The person may experience adverse effects such as infections, falls, or other peripheral health challenges. In the authors' experience, PC practitioners have stated that this is the stage where they would like to begin to work closely with the individual to help with early stage disease management, discuss advance directives, or assist with logistics in completing necessary health appointments. An important role for PC practitioners is to provide or facilitate psychosocial and emotional support, as in this stage the individual and family will likely be receiving progressively more negative news about their condition and its impact on the person's life.

Patient Case: TS completed the excisional surgery of the GBM. After surgery he required an intensive care unit stay for approximately one week and remained in the hospital for another two weeks. After surgery, his right leg strength was initially graded as a 3-/5 (able to move partially against gravity but could not hold against gravity) as measured via manual muscle testing. Both arms and his left leg were weak as well and he was unable to walk after surgery. He also had cognitive and speech impairments. After a 13-day inpatient rehabilitation stay, he was able to return home with the use of a cane. Once home, it took another three weeks to be able to walk up and down the block of his neighborhood. After microbiology testing, the surgical pathology report indicated that the tumor margins were not clear and tumor cells remained in the brain. In addition, he was no longer a candidate for surgical excision and would begin a regimen of chemotherapy and an additional course of radiation.

Stage 4 – Advancing Symptoms, Disease, and Physical Limitations

In this stage, the patients are most likely to benefit from the consultative and coordination services of the PC team. This patient will likely experience several adverse events, including two to three hospital readmissions in the year; incidents such as falls or uncontrolled symptoms may also be experienced.

Emotionally and psychologically, the patient and family may become more fearful of the decreasing likelihood of a curative outcome (or continued disease stability), resulting in increased distress. The patient's functional and physical performance status may be significantly impaired.

Patient Case: Despite the ongoing chemotherapy and radiation, TS's GBM has advanced and he is now only performing household activities with difficulty. He has difficulty concentrating on normal daily tasks and progressive lower extremity weakness has resulted in two falls. Each of these falls resulted in increased anxiety and decreased confidence in performing functional activities and therefore he began to walk less. He and his longtime girlfriend chose to get married and it was discussed that a component of this decision was related to his increasingly poor prognosis.

Stage 5 – End of Life

During EoL, care provision may occur at home, in a hospice unit, a nursing or long-term care facility, or a hospital. Individuals were more likely to pass away at home if there were multidisciplinary home PC services and if the person preferred death at home.[2] Additional factors for death at home included having cancer versus other diagnoses, receiving early PC, not living alone, having a caregiver, and the caregiver's coping skills.[2] In this stage, the emphasis is on aggressive symptom control (pain, dyspnea), maintaining dignity and safety, and engagement in life's remaining activities.

Patient Case: With the evidence of the limited effectiveness of radiation and chemotherapy, TS and his family chose to stop treatments and focus on getting his affairs in order and spend time at home with his family. His neurological symptoms worsened and he had enrolled in at-home hospice care. His mobility, communication, and cognitive status deteriorated and he spent most of his time in his recliner chair or bed. He spent his remaining days in the comfort of his own home surrounded by his family and being cared for by qualified, dedicated hospice providers in relative comfort.

Stage 6 – Death and Bereavement

In the final stage, the family and caregivers will be dealing with the emotions and life changes of acute loss. At this stage in the process it is important to offer, and if indicated, provide coping strategies or counseling services. This may include recommendations for support groups, spiritual professional consultation, social work, or a bereavement counselor.

Summary

Support for the person and family facing a life-threatening illness is a critical step in addressing the often-predictable events that occur near the EoL. Therapists have the opportunity to employ their skills in preparing for and mitigating the side effects of this process; however, they are not consistently integrated into the care team. Prehabilitation before the onset of substantial symptoms and skilled maintenance to slow or stop the onset of functional loss have the opportunity to optimize the QoL of the person and their family. Integration into the PC team and thorough knowledge will help the therapist employ their skills to facilitate QoL and achieve a good death.

References

1 Burge F, Lawson B, Johnston G, Asada Y, McIntyre PF, Flowerdew G. Preferred and actual location of death: What factors enable a preferred home death? *J Palliat Med.* 2015;18(12):1054–1059.

2 Costa V, Earle CC, Esplen MJ, et al. The determinants of home and nursing home death: A systematic review and meta-analysis. *BMC Palliat Care.* 2016;15(1):8. doi:10.1186/s12904-016-0077-8.

3 Silver J, Baima J. Cancer prehabilitation: An opportunity to decrease treatment-related morbidity, increase cancer treatment options, and improve physical and psychological health outcomes. *Am J Phys Med Rehabil.* 2013;92(8):715–727. doi:10.1097/PHM.0b013e31829b4afe.

4 Jensen W, Bialy L, Ketels G, Baumann FT, Bokemeyer C, Oechsle K. Physical exercise and therapy in terminally ill cancer patients: A retrospective feasibility analysis. *Support Care Cancer.* 2014;22(5):1261–1268.

5 Jensen W, Baumann FT, Stein A, et al. Exercise training in patients with advanced gastrointestinal cancer undergoing palliative chemotherapy: A pilot study. *Support Care Cancer.* 2014;22(7):1797–1806.

6 Oldervoll LM, Loge JH, Lydersen S, et al. Physical exercise for cancer patients with advanced disease: A randomized controlled trial. *Oncologist.* 2011;16(11):1649–1657.

7 Buss T, de Walden-Gałuszko K, Modlińska A, Osowicka M, Lichodziejewska-Niemierko M, Janiszewska J. Kinesitherapy alleviates fatigue in terminal hospice cancer patients—an experimental, controlled study. *Support Care Cancer.* 2010;18(6):743–749.

8 Wilson CM, Mueller K, Briggs R. Physical therapists' contribution to the hospice and palliative care interdisciplinary team. *J Hosp Palliat Nurs.* 2017;19(6):588–596. doi:10.1097/NJH.0000000000000394.

9 Wilson CM, Stiller CH, Doherty DJ, Thompson KA. The role of physical therapists within hospice and palliative care in the United States and Canada. *Am J Hosp Palliat Med.* 2017;34(1):34–41. doi:10.1177/1049909115604668.

10 Lutz S. The history of hospice and palliative care. *Curr Probl Cancer.* 2011;35(6):304–309.

11 Clark D. Total pain: The work of Cicely Saunders and the hospice movement. *Am Pain Soc Bull.* 2000;10(4):13–15.

12 Kubler-Ross E. *On Death and Dying.* London, England: Macmillan; 1969.

13 Lynch T, Connor S, Clark D. Mapping levels of palliative care development: A global update. *J Pain Symptom Manage.* 2013;45(6):1094–1106. doi:10.1016/j.jpainsymman.2012.05.011.

14 Center to Advance Palliative Care. Palliative care continues its annual growth trend, according to latest center to advance palliative care analysis. Center to Advance Palliative Care website. https://www.capc.org/about/press-media/press-releases/2018-2-28/palliative-care-continues-its-annual-growth-trend-according-latest-center-advance-palliative-care-analysis/Updated2018.Accessed August 21, 2020.

15 Connor SR, Sepulveda Bermedo MC. *Global Atlas of Palliative Care at the End of Life*. Geneva, Switzerland: World Health Organization; 2014.

16 Radbruch L, Payne S. White paper on standards and norms for hospice and palliative care in Europe: Part 1. *Eur J Palliat Care*. 2009;16(6):278–289.

17 World Health Organization. WHO definition of palliative care. https://www. who.int/cancer/palliative/definition/en/. Accessed August 21, 2020.

18 Lynn J, Adamson DM. *Living Well at the End of Life: Adapting Health Care to Serious Chronic Illness in Old Age*. Santa Monica, CA: RAND Corporation; 2003.

19 World Health Organization. Palliative Care: Key facts. https://www.who.int/ news-room/fact-sheets/detail/palliative-care. World Health Organization website. Updated August 5, 2020. Accessed August 21, 2020.

20 Engel GL. The need for a new medical model: A challenge for biomedicine. *Science*. 1977;196(4286):129–136.

21 Institute for Patient- and Family-Centered Care. What is patient family centered care? https://www.ipfcc.org/about/pfcc.html. Institute for Patient- and Family-Centered Care website. Accessed August 21, 2020.

22 Smith RC, Fortin AH, Dwamena F, Frankel RM. An evidence-based patient-centered method makes the biopsychosocial model scientific. *Patient Educ Couns*. 2013;91(3):265–270.

23 Breslow JM. Dr. Atul Gawande: "Hope is not a plan" when doctors, patients talk death. https://www.pbs.org/wgbh/frontline/article/dr-atul-gawande-hope-is-not-a-plan-when-doctors-patients-talk-death/. Updated February 10, 2015. Accessed August 21, 2020.

24 Rietjens JA, Sudore RL, Connolly M, et al. Definition and recommendations for advance care planning: An international consensus supported by the European Association for Palliative care. *Lancet Oncol*. 2017;18(9):e543–e551.

25 World Health Organization. WHOQOL: Measuring quality of life. World Health Organization website. https://www.who.int/healthinfo/survey/ whoqol-qualityoflife/en/. Publication date unknown. Accessed August 21, 2020.

26 Grim RD, Mcelwain D, Hartmann R, Hudak M, Young S. Evaluating causes for unplanned hospital readmissions of palliative care patients. *Am J Hosp Palliat Med*. 2010;27(8):526–531. doi:10.1177/1049909110368528.

27 American Heart Association. Understand your risks to prevent a heart attack. https://www.heart.org/en/health-topics/heart-attack/understand-your-risks-to-prevent-a-heart-attack. Updated 2016. Accessed August 21, 2020.

28 Patel AV, Friedenreich CM, Moore SC, et al. American College of Sports Medicine roundtable report on physical activity, sedentary behavior, and cancer prevention and control. *Med Sci Sports Exerc*. 2019;51(11):2391–2402.

2 Palliative Care Philosophy for Children and Adolescents

Kendra D. Koch

Introduction

Pediatric palliative care (PPC) seeks to prevent and relieve suffering in children and adolescents in medical, psychosocial, and spiritual domains while considering the social context and needs of the family. PPC differs from adult palliative care in key areas, including: a child's trajectory of illnesses; access to concurrent care; incorporating parental decision-making; provision of primary caregiving; the family context; and population/diagnostic considerations. As with adult palliative care, providers to children with life-limiting and life-threatening illness are often interdisciplinary, and include not only palliative care physicians, nurses, or social workers but also pediatricians and pediatric therapists. This approach broadens the reach of palliative care philosophies and skills, which are still difficult to access for many seriously ill children and their families. Although not standard of care yet, palliative care activities, including care coordination and promoting medical care within the home, often benefit children with serious illness greatly by providing continuous and consistent care. Skills associated with PPC include identifying, assessing, and treating pain and other distressing symptoms, while focusing on concise and accessible communication between provider, parent, and child. This approach will facilitate a strong therapeutic relationship, and optimize information exchange to assist parents and adolescents in lifespan decision-making.

PPC

PPC is a medical practice that seeks to prevent and relieve suffering while meeting gaps in care for children and adolescents facing serious illness or death.[1] PPC is not just a service or specialty but an interdisciplinary practice and philosophy that seeks to provide services that address medical, social-emotional, and spiritual needs for the child and the child's family. Palliative care addresses these three domains both during illness and after the child's death, if it occurs.[2] Children who receive palliative care services are generally at critical points in their care, at the end of life, or need life-sustaining interventions (i.e. tracheostomy, ventilation); however, some children who have life-limiting or life-threatening illness may receive palliative care services before a crisis occurs. Some children with life-threatening illnesses may receive primary and lifespan care that makes daily use of palliative care philosophies including emphasizing relational and shared decision-making, quality of life (QoL), social context and family, and burden versus benefit of treatment.

PPC as an integrated practice is relatively new, when compared to adult palliative care, and is increasingly recognized as a standard of care for children and adolescents with life-limiting (no realistic hope of cure) and life-threatening illness (where cure may be possible).[3] The World Health Organization (WHO) characterizes palliative care for children and adolescents as follows:

- The active total care of the child's body, mind, and spirit, and also involves giving support to the family.
- Beginning when illness is diagnosed, and continuing regardless of whether or not a child receives treatment directed at the disease.
- Requiring evaluation by providers to alleviate a child's physical, psychological, and social distress.
- Requiring a broad multidisciplinary approach that includes the family and makes use of available community resources; it can be successfully implemented even if resources are limited.
- It is provided in tertiary care facilities, in community health centers, and in children's homes.[4]

Palliative Care Education Needed across Disciplines

Depending on the discipline, healthcare professionals can complete fellowships and differing levels of certification or licensure in palliative care practice. However, even when healthcare disciplines do not have a palliative care concentration, it is important that all members of a child's healthcare team have a working and applicable knowledge of palliative care skills and philosophy. Currently, many children and families do not have access to consultation with a PPC team. Promoting palliative care knowledge and practice across healthcare disciplines increases access to appropriate care and may decrease the disparities that occur from lack of access. As expertise in physical function can be key to supporting daily activities, managing pain and other problem symptoms, engaging with the community, completing self-care and hygiene, and supporting QoL, it is especially vital that professionals who provide rehabilitative services employ palliative care philosophy and skills in their practice.

Differences in Adult and Pediatric Palliative Care

Although pediatric and adult palliative care are closely related in philosophy, palliative care for children has several key differences that may affect provider assessment and practice.

Trajectory of Illness

When compared to adults with serious illness, the trajectory of illness of many children and adolescents may be less predictable; this may be the result of a relatively good health status before traumatic injury or onset of disease, an undefined disease process, or difficulty with diagnosing a disease. This can make decisions difficult for healthcare providers, including when to refer to palliative care services; which treatments to recommend; what types of anticipatory guidance to offer; and when to make recommendations for the child to enter hospice care. It is not unusual for children to go back and forth between receiving palliative care services and not receiving palliative care services, and in some cases from being enrolled in hospice services (indicating that the child may die within the next six months), and disenrolled in hospice services when the child recovers function or hits a "plateau," causing their health decline to stop or slow radically.[5-7]

Concurrent Care

Before 2010 (before the Affordable Care Act was enacted), in the United States healthcare professionals and families of children with life-limiting illnesses were often forced to choose between curative care (including physical therapy and other rehabilitative procedures), or palliative care or hospice. Although it may be dependent on the payer or insurance plan associated with the payment for the child's medical care, parents of children in the United States are now generally given the option of their child receiving concurrent care.[8] Having the choice of pursuing concurrent care affects children's access to physical therapy and other rehabilitative therapy services. Having concurrent palliative and curative care services also means that discussions about decision-making and goal setting may be more complex, requiring options and a conversational framework that consider the patient and family's goals for cure *and* comfort.[9]

Parent Decision-Making

Unlike adult palliative care, where the wishes of the ill adult are elicited, or the adult's closest relative is asked to make decisions on their behalf (often a spouse or partner, or in the case of very elderly people, siblings, or adult children), PPC decisions (and all pediatric medical decisions) are most often made by parents on behalf of their children. Although older children and adolescents may be educated about treatment or therapeutic options, and even asked to assent or agree to treatment, consent to treatment is given by parents. This surrogate decision-making may create complex communication and ethical challenges for providers.[9,10] In addition to pediatric-specific considerations found later in this chapter, decision-making considerations are also discussed in Chapter 1 and Appendix 1.

Primary Caregiving

Parents are not only the primary decision-makers for their children but also the primary caregivers. In pediatrics especially, mothers traditionally have performed most caregiving for ill children. The toll of caregiving that extends beyond those roles expected of parents of typical children can be exhausting and overwhelming for parents. Parents with primary caregiver status may have a specialized and more thorough understanding of the illness' impact, the child's physical functioning, pain/symptoms, and other child needs. Healthcare professionals may gain a better understanding of the child-patient by acknowledging and attending to the special understanding of parent caregivers.[11] For additional discussions on caregiver considerations, refer to Chapter 5.

Family Context

Children exist in the context of families. Family members' health, mental health, access to financial resources, social support, and inter-family dynamics can all affect the well-being of the ill child. When healthcare providers support the family, they are supporting the child. Knowing the strengths and challenges of families may allow healthcare providers to complete more accurate assessments, plan accessible and appropriate goals, and obtain needed resources and support for both the family and the ill child.[12,13]

Populations

Although PPC is most often associated with cancer, in the United States cancer accounts for only 0.5% of deaths in infants and less than 9% of deaths in children.[3] Likewise, in Canada more infant and child deaths are associated with congenital diseases (22.1%) or diseases of the central nervous system (39.1%).[3] A large number of deaths in childhood and adolescence is due to external reasons, like car accidents or violence (see Chapters 10 and 16).[3] Population characteristics are also of interest as the death of an adult, especially older adults, is often thought of as "expected" unlike the death of a child, which can be harder for families to accept.[10]

Children with Medical Complexity

Due to advances in treatment and technology, children with medical complexity (CMC), also known as *children with complex chronic conditions* (CCC), many of whom would have died in infancy or childhood even one or two decades ago, are living into adolescence, and commonly even into adulthood. Research shows that deaths of CCC have recently declined in adolescence and increased in adulthood, highlighting the need for models of care that allow for a more seamless transition from pediatric to adult care and services in all disciplines, so that young adults with medical complexity from diseases of childhood or congenital conditions might have continuity of care and palliative care support throughout their lifespan.[3,14,15]

Supporting Children with Medical Complexity with Integrated Palliative Care

Historically, palliative care practices have been tied more to life-limiting diagnoses and less to chronic diseases.[3] For instance, palliative care would have been provided more often for a poor prognosis in cancer than to serving children with cerebral palsy who might live well into adulthood. However, increasingly, developments in treatment and technology have led to prolonged lifespans for CCC, who in the not-so-distant-past would likely have died in infancy or childhood.[15–17] To respond to this longer lifespan, palliative care has sometimes acted as a "safety net" for CMC, addressing decision-making, while considering QoL, pain, and the goals and values of the child and family.[2]

Especially in pediatrics, palliative care is not a stand-alone philosophy or practice. It is often used concurrently with curative or maintenance treatment.[9] This approach, within the context of an uncertain trajectory in many pediatric diseases as well as the higher number of CCC who may (and should) receive palliative care services, children and families may be best supported by a more integrated and comprehensive framework for care. In *Children with Medical Complexity: An Emerging Population for Clinical and Research Initiatives*, Cohen et al.[15] present a framework that is intended to characterize CMC. It also provides a lens through which healthcare providers might examine their practice to evaluate whether or not they are committing to holistic and comprehensive care for CMC. Cohen et al.'s[15] framework includes: (1) needs; (2) chronic conditions; (3) functional limitations; and (4) healthcare utilization (see Figure 2.1). Although the purview of each medical discipline is different, all disciplines can identify these four domains during care provision with CMC, and ensure that within their own scope of practice, they address them.

Addressing these domains within practice will contain aspects of all pediatric medical care integrated with palliative care practice, including the following.

Care Coordination

Wherever pediatric patients receive care, providers should strive for optimal care coordination. A recent large study of parents with CMC ranked care coordination as one of the two most difficult areas for parent caregivers.[18] In complex pediatric populations, poor communication between services and providers creates the greatest challenges for parents.[19] Leaders in palliative care practice suggest that primary objectives for practitioners addressing care coordination from a palliative care perspective might be: (1) collaborating with specialists and other healthcare providers; (2) identifying resources and

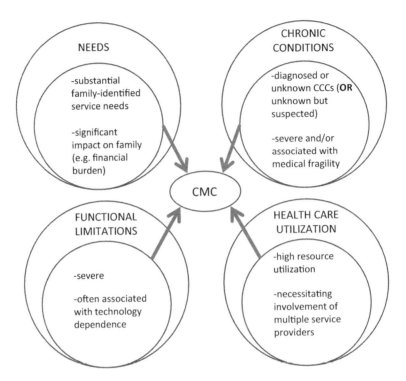

Figure 2.1 Cohen's Framework for Children with Medical Complexity. Modified from Cohen E, Kuo D, Agrawal R, et al. Children with medical complexity: An emerging population for clinical research initiatives. *Pediatrics.* 2011;127(3):529–538.[15]

partnering with community programs; (3) identifying financial resources and payment mechanisms; and (4) partnering with school programs.[1] Care coordination has been associated with reduced parental stress and increased caregiver satisfaction.[18,20,21]

In theory, many of these needs should be met through a pediatric *medical home* (see Chapter 5). A medical home is a primary practice with six foundational characteristics: (1) each patient has an adequately trained personal physician with whom they have a therapeutic relationship; (2) the physician leads a team which, together, is responsible for meeting the needs of the patient; (3) the physician and the team meet needs in a way that responds to the comprehensive needs of the whole child; (4) care is coordinated and integrated across all elements of the healthcare system including subspecialty care, hospitals, home health agencies, nursing homes, and community (care is also presented in a manner that ensures that patients receive care that is culturally and linguistically appropriate); (5) quality and safety are addressed; and (6) enhanced access to care allows for open scheduling, expanded hours, and open avenues of communication among patients, their physician, parents, and practice staff.[22] In addition, the American Academy of Pediatrics contends that medical home care should be "accessible, continuous, comprehensive, family centered, coordinated, compassionate, and culturally effective."[23]

In practice, often palliative care services have acted as a *de facto* medical home to provide more comprehensive care to children and families who are with pediatricians who do not have the resources or knowledge to provide CMC with adequate care.[24] More recently, medical home practices have been formed that attempt to provide comprehensive care to CMC as part of primary practice and usual care. In these practices, palliative care is treated not as a specialty but as an integrated and emerging practice built on family centeredness, whole family care, and QoL.[25]

The medical home approach has a special relationship with rehabilitative services in that many prescriptions and referrals for rehabilitative services come from the pediatrician in the child's medical home. This relationship may be enhanced by an ongoing conversation between therapists and medical providers who may gain much-needed information on symptoms and function from therapy providers who have access to more consistent exposure to the ill child during times of crisis and relative wellness. Consistent reporting and conversation with primary healthcare providers offer a benefit to ill children and families and may also support a more robust and shared decision-making process for families.

Condition-Related Pain and Distress Symptoms

The well-being of the ill child affects the well-being of their family, including parents and siblings. Parents especially find their child's physical distress or pain to be deeply upsetting.[26] In addition to the direct benefit to the child's physical status, therapists who treat pain and physical distress are also indirectly meeting the needs of the family; this may, in turn, reduce the psychological distress of the child-patient and their parents.[27] Parents report pain management as being the aspect of PPC that is most important to them.[28,29] For children, a major source of suffering includes the anticipation of pain or discomfort. Acknowledging, identifying, and working with the family and other providers to aggressively mitigate pain that may be present during rehabilitation, positioning, or functions of daily living, should be part of the ongoing therapy goals to ensure global symptom management and decreased child anxiety, resulting in a higher QoL for the child.[30]

Fatigue and Lethargy

For children and adolescents, functional ability is not only about utility but about coping. Maintaining function, including managing fatigue and lethargy, should be addressed in any symptom management plan.[30] A child's expression of fatigue may be different depending on the developmental age of the child. Research shows that younger children express the physical, rather than emotional, sensations of fatigue, such as only wanting to read or watch television. Adolescents may experience or report not only physical tiredness, but also mental fatigue, and they may be more aware of the meaning that fatigue has for their lives. For instance, adolescents may have more grief and sadness that manifests as fatigue as they can directly associate symptoms with the disease and its treatment (e.g. chemotherapy).[3] This may be further impacted by the realization that it affects their relationships and their engagement in the everyday activities that generally would have been typical for themselves and their peers.[3]

The physical signs of fatigue in children and adolescents, such as weakness, difficulty walking or running, no energy, tiredness, heaviness throughout the body, lethargy, and a desire to rest or lie down, may be most visible to rehabilitation providers who have an ongoing and in-person therapeutic relationship with the child.[3] It is important that providers note differences in energy and function from one therapy session to another, and seek to collaborate with primary care, specialist care, palliative care, and the family to mitigate fatigue symptoms in the child.

Communication and Decision-Making with Parents

Information, education, and support are all facilitated through provider-to-parent communication. Parents value honest, clear, and accessible dialogue,[31] which providers are ethically bound to provide.[12,32] Because children live much longer than adults after initiating palliative care,[6,33,34] communication in care coordination and continuity of care is an integral feature of providing good care to children with life-limiting or life-threatening conditions.

Quality communication is especially important because communication is the mechanism with which parents gather information and learn of options for treatment or maintenance. If this communication is ambiguous or unclear, the parent is unfairly limited in the quality of the decision that they can make. Though communication is exceptionally important at the end of a child's life, adequate information and supportive communication throughout the lifespan of the child gives parents the best foundation from which to make decisions for their child.[35,36] Not surprisingly, decision-making provides ample opportunity for experiencing guilt and decisional regret in parents of seriously ill children. Whether the parent was making a decision to place a gastrostomy tube or not, to place a child in a group home or not, to taper walking interventions or not, or to challenge a child with disabilities to perform better to progress a child's physical therapy regimen, parents voiced that the process of decision-making was inevitably full of guilt and uncertainty.[37–41]

Historically, physicians were the primary decision-makers in pediatric medical care (paternalistic model).[42] However, palliative care philosophy promotes a shared decision-making model as ideal. This model "encourages parents to consider the wishes of their child and to receive the guidance of their child's palliative care team to make the most optimal decision for the care of their child."[9,43,44] According to researcher Bluebond-Langner,[45] practitioners may support parental decision-making by considering these factors when guiding parents: (1) the complex and different roles that clinicians and parents have in the decision-making process; (2) the parent's changing understanding of the child as someone with a future and on whom now-unmet expectations have been placed; (3) that diagnosis of a life-limiting or life-threatening condition is an assault on the life of the family; (4) that for the sake of the family and preserving and maintaining normalcy, parents tend to push against the intrusion of the disease in everyday life; (5) that an individual's and parent's view of illness changes over time; (6) that parents use information in ways that clinicians may not expect; and (7) that parents and clinicians may view the child differently.

Good communication with providers leads to better social and emotional outcomes for the child and family, and inversely, poor communication results in negative social and emotional outcomes for the family.[35,36] When comfort or end-of-life measures become the best options for ill children, communication is integral to allow families to make meaning of the death of a child, *their child*, a death that to many parents seems tragic and "unnatural".[13,46]

Communication with Children and Adolescents

Medical, rehabilitation and psychosocial providers should use communication, interventions, and treatments that are appropriate to the developmental (not chronological) age of the ill child.[13,47] According to the *Textbook of Palliative Care Communication*, "clear and effective communication with children depends on understanding the social, relational, cultural, developmental, and emotional factors that may affect the child's understanding and beliefs about his or her illness."[48] Talking with children and adolescents requires providers to use a framework that focuses on: (1) the information and delivery needs of the child or adolescent; (2) the content of the conversation (what is said); (3) the type of language and delivery (how it is said); and (4) the providers' ability to be reflective in their practice (see Table 2.1).[48]

Summary

Healthcare providers' understanding of the PPC philosophy and developing skills associated with this approach is integral to offering good care to seriously ill children and their families. No longer confined to only the hospital setting or hospice, palliative care philosophy is increasingly being integrated into generalist and rehabilitative practice. A philosophy of palliative care, preventing and relieving suffering, is routinely used in everyday consideration of treatments and QoL for CMC. This lifespan approach to palliative care acknowledges that the needs of the ill child affect the family and that the needs of the family affect the ill child. Researchers and PPC

Table 2.1 Communication with Children and Adolescents

Needs of Child	Content of Conversation	Language and Delivery	Reflective Practice
Take cues from child Use developmental age Pause often to allow for questions or clarifications Encourage the child to echo what you've said to confirm their understanding Reassure the child that they will be cared for by you and others who love the child through the course of their illness	Share literature on the topic you are discussing that is written for children/ adolescents (picture books, comic books, brochures, websites), and is appropriate for their developmental age Only say what you believe to be true	Talk in terms that the child can understand Be concrete Slow down your explanation, be deliberate Avoid euphemisms and overly complex explanations	Listen first Acknowledge and attend to your own beliefs and anxieties Be honest Acknowledge that many children know about death and are aware of its signs even if they don't say or signal their awareness Be willing to say, "I don't know"

Modified from Goldman A, Hain R, Liben S. *Oxford Textbook of Palliative Care for Children*. 2nd ed. New York, NY: Oxford University Press, Inc.; 2012.[48]

healthcare professionals describe that there are key differences between adult and pediatric palliative care. Those differences require providers to acknowledge the unique practice of PPC while offering services not traditionally associated with palliative care, including unique care coordination needs, a focus on continuity of care, whole-family care, communication that acknowledges the surrogate decision-making role of parents, and the need for all providers developing child- and adolescent-informed communication skills. Building skills and increasing understanding of PPC increases the likelihood that rehab providers offer the best care to children and adolescents with life-limiting and life-threatening illness and their families.

References

1 Klick JC. Pediatric palliative care. *Curr Probl Pediatr Adolesc Health Care*. 2010;40(6):120–151.
2 Himelstein B, Hilden J, Boldt A, Weissman D. Medical progress: Pediatric palliative care. *N Engl J Med*. 2004;350(17):1752–1762.
3 Wolfe J, Hinds P, Sourkes B. *Textbook of Interdisciplinary Pediatric Palliative Care: Expert Consult Premium Edition*. London, England: Saunders; 2011.
4 Organization WH. WHO definition of palliative care for children. http://www.who.int/cancer/palliative/definition/en/. Accessed August 21, 2020.
5 Siden H, Davies B. Pediatrics. In: Hanks G, Cherny N, Christakis N, Fallon M, Kaasa S, Portenoy R, eds. *Oxford Textbook of Palliative Medicine*. 4th ed. Oxford, England: Oxford University Press; 2010;1301–1374.
6 Feudtner C, Kang T, Hexem K, et al. Pediatric palliative care patients: A prospective multicenter cohort study. *Pediatrics*. 2011;127(6):1094–1101.

7 Lagman R, Walsh D, Davis M, Young B. All patient refined diagnostic re-
lated group and case mix index in acute care palliative medicine. *J Support Oncol.* 2007;5(3):145–149.

8 National Hospice and Palliative Care Organization. Concurrent Care for
Children Implementation Toolkit. Section 2302 of the Patient Protection and
Affordable Care Act. Alexandria, VA: National Hospice and Palliative Care
Organization; 2012.

9 Jones BL, Koch KD. Neonatal and pediatrics. In: Wittenberg E, Ferrell B,
Goldsmith J, et al., eds. *Oxford Textbook of Palliative Care Communication.* New
York, NY: Oxford University Press; 2016:220–228.

10 Field M, Behrman R. *When Children Die: Improving Palliative and End-of-Life Care
for Children and Their Families.* Washington, DC: Institute of Medicine, Committee on Palliative and End-of-Life Care for Children and Their Families; 2004.

11 Koch K. *Parent decision-making for children with end stage renal disease (ESRD):
Description, interpretation, and implications* [dissertation]. Austin: The University
of Texas at Austin School of Social Work; 2017.

12 Jones BL, Contro N, Koch KD. The duty of the physician to care for the
family in pediatric palliative care: Context, communication, and caring. *Pediatrics.* 2014 February 1;133(Supplement 1):S8–S15.

13 Papadatou D. Training health professionals in caring for dying children and
grieving families. *Death Stud.*1997;21(6):575–600.

14 Simon TD, Berry J, Feudtner C, et al. Children with complex chronic
conditions in inpatient hospital settings in the United States. *Pediatrics.*
2010;126(4):647–655.

15 Cohen E, Kuo D, Agrawal R, et al. Children with medical complexity: An emerging population for clinical research initiatives. *Pediatrics.* 2011;127(3):529–538.

16 Msall M, Tremont M. Measuring functional outcomes after prematurity:
Developmental impact of very low birth weight and extremely low birth
weight status on childhood disability. *Ment Retard Dev Disabil Res Rev.*
2002;8(4):258–272.

17 Tennant P, Pearce M, Bythell M, Rankin J. 20-year survival of children
born with congenital anomalies: A population-based study. *Lancet.* 2010;375:
649–656.

18 Carosella A, Snyder A, Ward E. What parents of children with complex
medical conditions want their child's physicians to understand. *JAMA Pediatr.*
2018;172(4):315–316.

19 Lutenbacher M, Karp S, Ajero G, Howe D, Williams M. Crossing community sectors: Challenges faced by families of children with special health care
needs. *J Fam Nurs.* 2005;11(2):162–182.

20 Adams S, Cohen E, Mahant S, Friedman JN, Macculloch R, Nicholas DB.
Exploring the usefulness of comprehensive care plans for children with
medical complexity (CMC): A qualitative study. *BMC Pediatr.* 2013;13(1):10.

21 Kuo DZ, Robbins JM, Lyle RE, Barrett KW, Burns KH, Casey PH.
Parent-reported outcomes of comprehensive care for children with medical
complexity. *Fam Syst Health.* 2013;31(2):132–141.

22 Bachrach A, Isakson E, Seith D, Brellochs C. *Pediatric Medical Homes: Laying
the Foundation of a Promising Model of Care.* New York, NY: National Center for
Children in Poverty; 2011.

23 Medical Home Initiatives for Children With Special Needs Project Advisory
Committee. American Academy of Pediatrics. The medical home. *Pediatrics.*
2002;110(1):184–186.

24 Knapp C, Baker K, Cunningham C, Downing J, Fowler-Kerry S, McNamara
K. Pediatric palliative care and the medical home. *J Palliat Med.* 2012
June;15(6):643–645. doi:10.1089/jpm.2012.0075.

25 Lafond D. Integrating the Comfort Theory(TM) Into Pediatric Primary Palliative Care to Improve Access to Care. *J Hosp Palliat Nurs.* 2019;21(5):382–389.

26 Muscara F, McCarthy MC, Thompson EJ, et al. Psychosocial, demographic, and illness-related factors associated with acute traumatic stress responses in PARENTS of children with a serious illness or injury. *J Trauma Stress.* 2017;30(3):237–244.

27 Simons LE, Goubert L, Vervoort T, Borsook D. Circles of engagement: Childhood pain and parent brain. *Neurosci Biobehav Rev.* 2016;68(Supplement C):537–546.

28 Pritchard M, Burghen E, Srivastava DK, et al. Cancer-related symptoms most concerning to parents during the last week and last day of their child's life. *Pediatrics.* 2008;121(5):e1301–e1309.

29 Vollenbroich R, Borasio GD, Duroux A, Grasser M, Brandstätter M, Führer M. Listening to parents: The role of symptom perception in pediatric palliative home care. *Palliat Support Care.* 2016;14(1):13–17.

30 Hauer JM, Wolfe J. Supportive and palliative care of children with metabolic and neurological diseases. *Curr Opin Support Palliat Care.* 2014;8(3):296–302.

31 Fiks AG, Jimenez ME. The promise of shared decision-making in paediatrics. *Acta Paediatr.* 2010;99(10):1464–1466.

32 AAP. American Academy of Pediatrics. Pediatric palliative care and hospice care commitments, guidelines, and recommendations. *Pediatrics.* 2013;132(5):966–972.

33 Fromme E, Bascom P, Smith M, et al. Survival, mortality, and location of death for patients seen by a hospital-based palliative care team. *J Palliat Med.* 2006;9(4):903–911.

34 Cheng W, Willey J, Palmer J, Zhang T, Bruera E. Interval between palliative care referral and seen by a hospital-based palliative care team. *J Palliat Med.* 2005;8(5):1025–1032.

35 Contro N, Larson J, Scofield S, Sourkes B, Cohen H. Family perspectives on the quality of pediatric palliative care. *Arch Pediatr Adolesc Med.* 2002;156(1):14–19.

36 Meert K, Thurston C, Sarnaik A. End-of-life decision-making and satisfaction with care: Parental perspectives. *Pediatr Crit Care Med.* 2000;1(2):179–185.

37 Gibson BE, Teachman G, Wright V, Fehlings D, Young NL, McKeever P. Children's and parents' beliefs regarding the value of walking: Rehabilitation implications for children with cerebral palsy. *Child: Care Health Dev.* 2012;38(1):61–69.

38 Carnevale FA, Canoui P, Cremer R, et al. Parental involvement in treatment decisions regarding their critically ill child: A comparative study of France and Quebec. *Pediatr Crit Care Med.* 2007;8(4):337–342.

39 Brotherton A, Abbott J. Mothers' process of decision making for gastrostomy placement. *Qual Health Res.* 2012;22(5):587–594.

40 Jackson JB, Roper SO. Parental adaptation to out-of-home placement of a child with severe or profound developmental disabilities. *Am J Intellect Dev Disabil.* 2014;119(3):203–219.

41 MacDonald H, Callery P. Parenting children requiring complex care: A journey through time. *Child: Care Health Dev.* 2008;34(2):207–213.

42 Raffin T. Withdrawing life support: How is the decision made? *JAMA.* 1995;273(9):738–739.

43 Fiks AG, Jimenez ME. The promise of shared decision-making in paediatrics. *Acta Paediatr.* 2010;99(10):1464–1466.

44 Committee on Hospital Care and Institute for Patient- and Family-Centered Care. Patient- and family-centered care and the pediatrician's role. *Pediatrics.* 2012;129(2):394–404. doi:10.1542/peds.2011-3084.

45 Bluebond-Langner M, Hargrave D, Henderson EM, Langner R. 'I have to live with the decisions I make': Laying a foundation for decision making for children with life-limiting conditions and life-threatening illnesses. *Arch Dis Child.* 2017;102(5):468.

46 Azoulay E, Chevret S, Leleu G, et al. Half the families of intensive care unit patients experience inadequate communication with physicians. *Crit Care Med.* 2000;28(8):3044–3049.

47 Freyer D. Care of the dying adolescent: Special considerations. *Pediatrics.* 2004;113:381–388.

48 Goldman A, Hain R, Liben S. *Oxford Textbook of Palliative Care for Children.* 2nd ed. New York, NY: Oxford University Press, Inc.; 2012.

3   Exercise, Activity in Cancer and Chronic Disease

Jeannette Q. Lee

Introduction

The benefits of exercise and activity in patients with chronic conditions have been reasonably well-described.[1-3] Exercise is safe and valuable before, during, and after cancer treatment, across various cancer types, and serves to mitigate physical and psychological cancer-related impairments across the survivorship spectrum.[4] Evidence also suggests that exercise and other forms of physical activity have a positive impact on the risk, management, and prognosis associated with conditions such as heart failure, chronic kidney disease, Parkinson's disease, and multiple sclerosis, among others (see Chapters 8–16).[5-7]

In general, recommendations regarding the types, frequency, duration, and intensity of exercise and activities for chronic diseases have varied widely. Exercise regimens have been provided in various settings (e.g. home-based, outpatient, hospital-based), as well as with differing levels of supervision. The diversity of disease types, symptom burden, and related treatments have made it challenging to develop specific guidelines for each condition. However, consensus guidelines or general recommendations have been published for cancer survivors[8] and for those with chronic disease and disabilities[9] which have been consistent with the US Department of Health and Human Services (DHHS) activity guidelines for Americans.[10] These guidelines call for at least 150 minutes per week of moderate-intensity aerobic activity or at least 75 minutes per week of vigorous-intensity activity (or a comparable combination). Those who are unable to meet the full recommendations due to their health status or condition are encouraged to be as active as their abilities safely permit, and to "avoid inactivity."[8-10]

Types of Exercise

Aerobic/Cardiovascular Exercise

One of the most common modes of exercise and activity in the chronic disease population is cardiorespiratory, or *aerobic*, exercise. Aerobic exercise improves cardiorespiratory fitness and endurance. Systematic reviews and/or meta-analyses of exercise or physical activity regimens in patients with cancer and other chronic conditions describe several studies that use aerobic exercise, or combined aerobic-mixed activity interventions,[3,4,7,11] (e.g. walking, hydrotherapy, circuit training, self-reported physical activity) including such activities as yoga,[12,13] tai chi,[14,15] or boxing.[16] These studies typically have moderate to vigorous levels of intensity, typically described as a percentage of predicted maximum heart rate or a range in the rate of perceived exertion scale (RPE), though parameters for frequency and/or duration were heterogeneous, ranging in frequency from one to five times per week, from approximately 20 to 60 minutes per session, with durations from a few weeks to over six months. Overall, while there were fewer studies examining lower intensity activities, these exercises and activities still demonstrated improvements in overall functioning over time, particularly if the patient populations were more deconditioned at the start of the exercise regimens or programs.

In individuals with cancer, predominantly aerobic type interventions that were at a moderate to vigorous level of intensity seemed to show more favorable responses in fatigue, health-related quality of life, physical function, and immune responses compared to those who exercised at a lower intensity, or not at all.[17-20] These exercise parameters and resultant findings seem to be consistent in individuals with advanced stage cancer, where Borg's RPE scale ratings ranging from 10 to 15[21-23] were reported, with resulting statistically significant improvements in gait speed, six-minute walk distance, and fatigue severity.[24] For individuals with chronic heart failure, engaging in physical exercise has been theorized to increase systemic arterial compliance, improve stroke volume, counteract muscle atrophy, and inhibit catabolic processes that occur in heart failure.[7,25] Moderate continuous aerobic training is the recommended exercise modality from the Heart Failure Association Guidelines,[26] although interval aerobic training has been posited as a potentially more effective way to build up exercise tolerance in these individuals.[27] For those with Parkinson's disease, where the disease progression can result in quite debilitating sequelae, physical activity may facilitate motor unit recruitment and more efficient energy utilization if used with medication.[28] Several studies have used treadmill training or other aerobic means like a bike or elliptical trainer for individuals with Parkinson's disease as an aerobic modality with significant improvements in walking economy, speed, and distance. Training duration ranged from 3 to 21 weeks.[29,30] Necessary adaptations to the treadmill or elliptical trainer set-up, such as less resistance or shorter initial duration, can be implemented if indicated by the person's health status.[7]

Resistance Exercise

Resistance exercise is another mode of exercise that has been used with success for individuals living with a chronic disease. In people with varying stages and types of cancer, resistance exercise training improves muscular strength and endurance, as well as several psychosocial outcomes like stress, anxiety, body image, and mood.[31] These types of exercises have been used effectively to improve physical outcomes such as muscle wasting and several other quality of life indicators in persons with chronic disease.[7] A preponderance of studies done in these populations usually combine resistance training with some form of aerobic activity/exercise, typically outdoor or treadmill walking or stationary cycling.[3,4,7,31–33] A systematic review of resistance training interventions after cancer treatment noted that only four out of the 24 studies included focused exclusively on resistance training programs.[31] Duration of strength training ranged from 3 to 52 weeks, with many occurring two to three times per week (range 1–5 sessions/week).[4,31,33] Training response was therefore variable, though De Backer et al.[34] has reported that most progression in muscle strength could be attained after the first 12 weeks. Two to three alternating days per week has also been reported as necessary for optimal progression.[35] In general, the total number of exercises performed was variable but ranged from five to nine exercises targeting large muscle groups, performing 8–12 repetitions, and completing one to three sets of each exercise. Common examples were bench press, leg press, seated row, and abdominal crunches. Training intensity was also variable, if described, and was commonly reported as percentages of one repetition maximum (RM) (range: 25–85% of 1 RM). During resistance training of cancer survivors, training intensities typically varied between 60% and 85% of 1 RM for upper and lower body muscles, and 30–60% of 1 RM for abdominal and lower back muscles.[3,31] Training intensities were also reported as ranges on the RPE scale (range 10–16), metabolic equivalents (METs), or included general terms as "moderate," "as tolerated," or "to tolerance."[3,31,32] In individuals with advanced or terminal cancer, resistance exercises were shown to improve fatigue severity and muscle strength, although resistance exercises did not appear to have a strong differential effect when compared to aerobic exercises.[23,36]

A Cochrane review of 37 studies on exercise training for individuals with depression concluded that resistance and mixed-type exercises (aerobic and resistance) were more effective than aerobic exercises alone for mood, and that a greater number of exercise sessions were more beneficial than fewer sessions. It could not, however, make specific recommendations on optimal type, frequency, and/or duration of exercise.[37] Resistance activities have also been used safely for patients with chronic neuromuscular conditions such as Parkinson's disease; individuals with mid-to-severe-stage Parkinson's disease participating in a boxing program showed improved gait velocity and endurance over a traditional exercise group.[16] In individuals with multiple sclerosis, progressive resistance training improved muscle strength and overall positive effects on multiple outcomes like balance and quality of life.[38] Resistance training was previously thought to be contraindicated in individuals with congestive heart failure out of concern that increased vascular resistance from this type of exercise would result in increased cardiac load as compared to aerobic training; however, current evidence shows that combined resistance and aerobic exercise in this population (New York Heart Association class II-III [see Chapter 8]) produces no better or worse results than aerobic exercises, with proper supervision and tailoring of exercises.[7] For individuals with chronic obstructive pulmonary disease (COPD), it has been reported that the addition of resistance training to an aerobic exercise program resulted in greater improvements in strength compared to aerobic exercise alone.[15] Furthermore, with advanced stage COPD, dyspnea during aerobic exercise can limit exercise intensity or progression. Thus, resistance exercises, which may cause less dyspnea, could be an alternative and have the same benefits as endurance training.[39] There are certainly instances where caution must be taken with resistance exercises, such as in rheumatoid arthritis, where high-intensity resistance exercises may lead to more joint damage, particularly if extensive baseline damage was already present prior to the initiation of resistance activities.[7]

Intensity of Strength and Aerobic Exercise

In healthy adults, aerobic and resistance training is more effective when adequate dosages are used. Increased aerobic capacity and endurance are achieved with more efficient myocardial oxygen capacity and cardiac output. Muscle strength improvements are attained when maximal motor units are recruited. The same considerations apply to individuals with chronic disease. Observed training intensities of the evidence presented were mostly in the moderate to high intensity training ranges, with very few adverse events reported. These intensities were safe and well-tolerated in a wide spectrum of chronic diseases and severity, from early to end-stage disease. In fact, compliance was relatively high. However, low-intensity exercise is still beneficial for deconditioned individuals and still positively impacts physical and psychological function. Similarly, positive outcomes were generally observed even with heterogenous frequency and duration, suggesting that exercise recommendations can be flexible and tailored to individuals' preferences and circumstances.

Flexibility

A loss of range of motion may be seen after surgeries or procedures for cancer treatment, or treatment for other chronic diseases like heart, liver, or kidney disease. Exercise recommendations that focus solely on flexibility for these patient populations are relatively scant, though there are reports of improvement of upper and/or lower extremity flexibility with exercise programs where stretching is one component of an overall aerobic and/or resistance exercise regimen in individuals with cancer, including advanced cancer,[4,11,32,40] as well as other chronic conditions like dementia and Parkinson's disease.[7,16] Recent studies have also examined the role of yoga, which may include stretching or flexibility activities, and have reported improved quality of life and reduced severity of fatigue in individuals with varying stages of breast cancer.[12,13] When considering modifiable parameters of flexibility stretching, they include duration, intensity, and frequency.[41] There is little evidence related to chronic conditions with a wide variety of suggestions; recommendations for frail older adults were to stretch to the point of tightness and hold for a few seconds daily.[42] In addition, older adults may require longer hold times (60 seconds versus 15–30 seconds per stretch).[43,44] Key concepts related to intensity of stretch were to avoid aggressive stretching to avoid activating the stretch reflex and minimizing tissue damage and inflammation[41]; this may be accomplished by low intensity, long-duration stretching while avoiding end-range positions of joints when possible.

Timing of Exercise

Exercise interventions for individuals with cancer and other chronic conditions span the survivorship spectrum, from pre-treatment, during treatment, post-treatment, and beyond. It has also spanned early stage, to mid-stage, to advanced or end-stage disease conditions. Typically, the focus of exercise may go from the improvement of functional capacity to maintaining it during treatment, or as the disease progresses. Post-treatment may be a better time point to focus on improving functional capacity once again. If the disease progresses to end-stage, then the focus might shift back to maintaining functional capacity. Exercise and physical activity consistently resulted in physical and psychological benefits, regardless of when it was introduced in the disease trajectory.[4]

Pre-treatment/Early Stage Disease

The concept of pre-treatment exercise or "prehabilitation" is a relatively new one; however, a growing amount of evidence, in particular within oncology rehabilitation, shows that engaging in exercise prior to the initiation of treatment demonstrates improved tolerance to active cancer treatment, reduced hospital length of stays, and aids in return to pre-surgical or pre-treatment functional status.[45,46] For other chronic conditions, the amount of evidence is scant though gains have also been shown when exercise training is initiated in the early stages of the disease, or when deficits are still light. In the case of multiple sclerosis or Parkinson's disease, for example, it has been hypothesized that exercise interventions during the early stages of disease may impact the disease pathology, exert a neuroprotective effect, and slow down progression; a mix of fitness and muscle training produced gains in strength and quality of life.[7,38,47]

During Treatment/Advancing Disease/Disease Exacerbations

Functional declines are typically seen with active treatment, or with disease progression, and may be attributed to factors including: reduced levels of usual activity; abnormalities in blood counts; increased oxygenation needs;

anxiety; and isolation. Current evidence suggests that when performed during active treatment, exercise helps to maintain or even improve physical capacity and treatment-related symptoms and impairments, as opposed to a decline in function or exacerbation of symptoms in those not receiving or participating in exercise.

In individuals with various types of cancer, the benefits of exercising during active treatment have included a decrease in cancer-related fatigue, improvements in quality of life, as well as various indicators of physical function.[13,31,40,48,49] A better tolerance of adjuvant cancer treatment (i.e. chemotherapy, radiation therapy, or both), better treatment completion rates, and restoration or prevention of specific body structure impairments or complications were also noted.[11,40,50–52] No significant adverse events have been associated with exercise during cancer treatment, though several reviews point out that the phase of treatment should be considered, as well as exercise intensity and/or duration, in order to maintain safe blood counts.[11,13,48]

In other chronic conditions where disease exacerbations/flare-ups, or later stage symptoms, might result in heavier disease burden, alternatives to more traditional training formats may be needed to account for symptom control. In individuals with advanced COPD, non-linear exercise training, where the volume, duration, and intensity of exercise is altered frequently, was used with more success as compared to traditional exercise training; altering exercise parameters helped to take into account the various causes of exercise intolerance in advanced COPD (e.g. dyspnea, oxygen desaturation, fatigue).[53] In individuals with heart failure where ejection fraction was <40%, engaging in exercise resulted in clinically significant improvements in health-related quality of life and lower heart failure-related hospitalizations.[7] An exercise program consisting of flexibility, balance, and functional exercises resulted in improved adherence and overall physical function in individuals with mid-stage Parkinson's disease.[30]

Terminal Disease

Improving and/or maintaining function and independence have been identified as important goals of patients toward the end of life.[54] In fact, individuals who have terminal or advanced disease arguably would benefit the most from interventions that can improve quality of life. However, the evidence regarding exercise for individuals at end of life is relatively sparse. Heywood, McCarthy, and Skinner[32] reviewed the safety of exercise in individuals with advanced cancer and found it to be safe. Less than 1% out of almost 1,100 participants included in the review reported an exercise-related adverse event, all of which were minor in nature.[32]

In individuals with terminal cancer, variably defined in studies as "palliative," "advanced cancer," "stage IIIB-IV," or "life expectancy <2 years," multiple modes of exercise (aerobic, resistance, mixed, or alternatives like Qigong or yoga) resulted in improvements in self-reported health-related quality of life, fatigue severity, sleep quality, physical function, and psycho-social outcomes, as well as objective outcomes such as the six-minute walk test, short physical performance battery (SPPB), peak VO_2 max, and 1 RM tests.[55,56] Cancer diagnoses spanned many different types, but many of the studies examined individuals with lung, hematological, breast, and prostate cancers.[32,55,56] Safety, slower or more conservative exercise progressions, and supervision by a trained or qualified practitioner were common elements in many studies. The heterogeneity of exercise duration and frequencies, and usually smaller sample sizes, suggest that challenges remain around optimal dosing, though there is evidence that patients near end of life or with terminal disease can safely participate in, and benefit from, moderate intensities of exercise.[55]

For individuals with advanced, progressive, or chronic illnesses such as end-stage heart failure or COPD, the disease trajectory often results in intractable symptoms and decline. While the provision of quality end-of-life care is a priority, the role of exercise may be more equivocal depending on the disease or symptom burden. Exercise, with supplemental measures in place, may help to alleviate the most debilitating symptoms, resulting in enhanced quality of life or preservation of function. In individuals with advanced/end-stage COPD, exercise, including pulmonary rehabilitation and ventilatory muscle training, is one of the more effective non-pharmacological approaches for re-conditioning and for managing dyspnea.[57,58] While exercise parameters were variable, a recommendation of at least four weeks duration was reported.[58] For end of life, the most common strategies used to support exercise tolerance were a fan, energy conservation techniques, and breathing and relaxation techniques.[57] A home-based circuit training exercise regimen with a focus on functional exercises and dual-tasking was shown to be effective in reducing the incidence of falls in individuals with advanced Alzheimer's disease.[59] In individuals with advanced chronic heart failure (NYHA IIIb or higher), exercises performed over 12 weeks, including walking, cycle ergometry, and calisthenics led to an improvement in left ventricular function and ejection fraction, as well as an improvement by as much as 16% VO_2max.[60] Over-all, individuals with progressive disease with potential for significant disease burden may derive the most benefit if exercises are taught early, preferably before, the end-of-life phase.

Setting

Exercise regimens for individuals with chronic, progressive conditions were performed in an assortment of settings, mostly ambulatory, including gyms, re-habilitation clinics, and community centers.[4,7] With disease progression, there were more exercise regimens that were implemented in hospital-based settings or home-based settings.[55,56] An environment that was compatible with exercise and physical activity, but also accepting of illness and varying performance levels, was seen as positive.[56] Exercising at home also had the added benefit of involving the caregiver and/or tailoring exercises to address the individual's goals. For individuals with dementia, who may be confined to nursing institutions, the use of music, having a home-like atmosphere, and functional modifications to account for differing levels of functional status were associated with positive results on levels of activity.[61] In general, across all settings, exercise programs were generally safe and few adverse events were reported.[4,7,32]

Supervision during Physical Activity

Overall, supervised exercise programs resulted in better exercise adherence, health-related quality of life, and various indicators of physical and psychosocial indicators compared to non-supervised exercise programs.[7,17,49] Structured programs, (i.e. followed a set of exercises or movement-based classes), also had better outcomes compared to controls, (i.e. "usual care", "no intervention"), or general education.[7,13] It might be posited that individuals may feel more supported, or have a better personalized experience, when exercise activity is being supervised by a qualified practitioner. There is a consensus that for individuals who are new to exercise or are in the initial training period, supervision and monitoring are ideal.[7] In instances where disease progression has resulted in functional decline or increased symptom severity, supervision might be prudent and necessary.

Safety and Other Considerations

For the sake of safety and caution, assessment by a qualified healthcare practitioner may be warranted prior to the initiation of exercise, particularly as disease burden gets heavier. Exercise tolerance may be decreased on specific days or periods, such as during the day of treatment or immediately following or during a disease flare-up or exacerbation. There may be disease-specific limiting issues as well. For example, individuals with multiple sclerosis have temperature sensitivities, so care must be taken so the individual does not overheat or become chilled during exercise. Individuals who are osteoporotic should perform exercises that have minimal to no fall risk. For individuals at end of life, a home-based setting for performing exercises may be preferred over other settings and is easier to tailor to the individual's specific needs or goals. Other measures such as starting with shorter sessions and lower exercise intensities, slower exercise progressions, supervision by a qualified practitioner during exercise, or exercising with supplemental oxygenation for those with dyspnea at rest or low oxygen saturation may be considered,[7,8] with the goal of continuing with exercise and physical activity in a safe and meaningful manner.

Summary

Physical activity and exercise within the context of advanced chronic disease and cancer have a substantial body of literature that establishes its safety and clinical efficacy. Exercise may be introduced at any phase of the disease journey, but it is anticipated that the earlier that exercise is introduced, the more physical, mental, and emotional benefits will be appreciated. Once intro-duced, exercise is deemed safe, effective and can improve a variety of physical factors, including pain, fatigue, strength, and overall quality of life. Due to the medical complexity of advanced disease processes, close supervision and sup-port are increasingly necessary during exercise prescription and performance near the end of life.

References

1   Campbell KL, Winters-Stone KM, Wiskemann J, et al. Exercise guidelines for cancer survivors: Consensus statement from international multidisciplinary roundtable. *Med Sci Sports Exerc.* 2019;51:2375–2390.
2   Hayes SC, Spence RR, Galvao DA, Newton RU. Australian Association for Exercise and Sport Science position stand: Optimising cancer outcomes through exercise. *J Sci Med Sport.* 2009;12:428–434.
3   Kujala UM. Evidence on the effects of exercise therapy in the treatment of chronic disease. *Br J Sports Med.* 2009;43:550–555.
4   Stout NL, Baima J, Swisher AK, Winters-Stone KM, Welsh J. A systematic review of exercise systematic reviews in the cancer literature (2005–2017). *PM&R.* 2017;9:S347–S384.
5   Cattadori G, Segurini C, Picozzi A, Padeletti L, Anza C. Exercise and heart failure: An update. *Esc Heart Fail.* 2018;5:222–232.
6   Wilkinson TJ, Shur NF, Smith AC. "Exercise as medicine" in chronic kidney disease. *Scand J Med Sci Spor.* 2016;26:985–988.
7   Pedersen BK, Saltin B. Exercise as medicine - evidence for prescribing exercise as therapy in 26 different chronic diseases. *Scand J Med Sci Sports.* 2015;25(Supplement 3):1–72.
8   Schmitz KH, Courneya KS, Matthews C, et al. American College of Sports Medicine roundtable on exercise guidelines for cancer survivors. *Med Sci Sports Exerc.* 2010;42:1409–1426.
9   Gordon BT DJ, Painter PL, Moore GE. Basic physical activity and exercise Recommendations for persons with chronic conditions. In: Moore GE DJ, Painter PL, eds. *ACSM's Exercise Management for Persons with Chronic Disease and Disabilities*, 4th ed. Champagne, IL: Human Kinetics; 2016.
10 Committee PAGA. 2018 Physical Activity Guidelines Advisory Committee Scientific Report. Washington, DC: U.S. Department of Health and Human Services; 2018.
11 Speck RM, Courneya KS, Masse LC, Duval S, Schmitz KH. An update of controlled physical activity trials in cancer survivors: A systematic review and meta-analysis. *J Cancer Surviv.* 2010;4:87–100.
12 Cramer H, Lange S, Klose P, Paul A, Dobos G. Yoga for breast cancer patients and survivors: A systematic review and meta-analysis. *BMC Cancer.* 2012;12:412.
13 Mishra SI, Scherer RW, Snyder C, Geigle PM, Berlanstein DR, Topaloglu O. Exercise interventions on health-related quality of life for people with cancer during active treatment. *Cochrane Database Syst Rev.* 2012;8:CD008465.
14 Song R, Grabowska W, Park M, et al. The impact of Tai Chi and Qigong mind-body exercises on motor and non-motor function and quality of life in Parkinson's disease: A systematic review and meta-analysis. *Parkinsonism Relat Disord.* 2017;41:3–13.
15 Nolan CM, Rochester CL. Exercise training modalities for people with chronic obstructive pulmonary disease. *COPD.* 2019;16:378–389.

16 Combs SA, Diehl MD, Chrzastowski C, et al. Community-based group exercise for persons with Parkinson disease: A randomized controlled trial. *NeuroRehabilitation.* 2013;32:117–124.

17 Buffart LM, Kalter J, Sweegers MG, et al. Effects and moderators of exercise on quality of life and physical function in patients with cancer: An individual patient data meta-analysis of 34 RCTs. *Cancer Treat Rev.* 2017;52:91–104.

18 Granger CL, McDonald CF, Berney S, Chao C, Denehy L. Exercise intervention to improve exercise capacity and health related quality of life for patients with non-small cell lung cancer: A systematic review. *Lung Cancer.* 2011;72:139–153.

19 Fong DY, Ho JW, Hui BP, et al. Physical activity for cancer survivors: Meta-analysis of randomised controlled trials. *BMJ.* 2012;344:e70.

20 Smits A, Lopes A, Das N, Bekkers R, Massuger L, Galaal K. Exercise Programme in Endometrial Cancer; Protocol of the Feasibility and Acceptability Survivorship Trial (EPEC-FAST). *BMJ Open.* 2015;5:e009291.

21 Coleman EA, Coon S, Hall-Barrow J, Richards K, Gaylor D, Stewart B. Feasibility of exercise during treatment for multiple myeloma. *Cancer Nurs.* 2003;26:410–419.

22 Kuehr L, Wiskemann J, Abel U, Ulrich CM, Hummler S, Thomas M. Exercise in patients with non-small cell lung cancer. *Med Sci Sports Exerc.* 2014;46:656–663.

23 Litterini AJ, Fieler VK, Cavanaugh JT, Lee JQ. Differential effects of cardiovascular and resistance exercise on functional mobility in individuals with advanced cancer: A randomized trial. *Arch Phys Med Rehabil.* 2013;94:2329–2335.

24 Kemoun G, Thibaud M, Roumagne N, et al. Effects of a physical training programme on cognitive function and walking efficiency in elderly persons with dementia. *Dement Geriatr Cogn Disord.* 2010;29:109–114.

25 Hambrecht R, Gielen S, Linke A, et al. Effects of exercise training on left ventricular function and peripheral resistance in patients with chronic heart failure: A randomized trial. *JAMA.* 2000;283:3095–3101.

26 Ponikowski P, Voors AA, Anker SD, et al. 2016 ESC Guidelines for the diagnosis and treatment of acute and chronic heart failure: The Task Force for the diagnosis and treatment of acute and chronic heart failure of the European Society of Cardiology (ESC). Developed with the special contribution of the Heart Failure Association (HFA) of the ESC. *Eur J Heart Fail.* 2016;18:891–975.

27 Wisloff U, Stoylen A, Loennechen JP, et al. Superior cardiovascular effect of aerobic interval training versus moderate continuous training in heart failure patients: A randomized study. *Circulation.* 2007;115:3086–3094.

28 LeWitt PA, Bharucha A, Chitrit I, et al. Perceived exertion and muscle efficiency in Parkinson's disease: L-DOPA effects. *Clin Neuropharmacol.* 1994;17:454–459.

29 Goodwin VA, Richards SH, Taylor RS, Taylor AH, Campbell JL. The effectiveness of exercise interventions for people with Parkinson's disease: A systematic review and meta-analysis. *Mov Disord.* 2008;23:631–640.

30 Schenkman M, Hall DA, Baron AE, Schwartz RS, Mettler P, Kohrt WM. Exercise for people in early- or mid-stage Parkinson disease: A 16-month randomized controlled trial. *Phys Ther.* 2012;92:1395–1410.

31 De Backer IC, Schep G, Backx FJ, Vreugdenhil G, Kuipers H. Resistance training in cancer survivors: A systematic review. *Int J Sports Med.* 2009;30:703–712.

32 Heywood R, McCarthy AL, Skinner TL. Safety and feasibility of exercise interventions in patients with advanced cancer: A systematic review. *Support Care Cancer.* 2017;25:3031–3050.

33 Hashida R, Kawaguchi T, Bekki M, et al. Aerobic vs. resistance exercise in non-alcoholic fatty liver disease: A systematic review. *J Hepatol.* 2017;66:142–152.

34 De Backer IC, Van Breda E, Vreugdenhil A, Nijziel MR, Kester AD, Schep G. High-intensity strength training improves quality of life in cancer survivors. *Acta Oncol.* 2007;46:1143–1151.

35 Kraemer WJ, Ratamess NA. Fundamentals of resistance training: Progression and exercise prescription. *Med Sci Sports Exerc.* 2004;36:674–688.

36 Jensen W, Baumann FT, Stein A, et al. Exercise training in patients with advanced gastrointestinal cancer undergoing palliative chemotherapy: A pilot study. *Support Care Cancer.* 2014;22:1797–1806.

37 Cooney GM, Dwan K, Greig CA, et al. Exercise for depression. *Cochrane Database Syst Rev.* 2013;9:CD004366.

38 Kjolhede T, Vissing K, Dalgas U. Multiple sclerosis and progressive resistance training: A systematic review. *Mult Scler.* 2012;18:1215–1228.

39 Iepsen UW, Jorgensen KJ, Ringbaek T, Hansen H, Skrubbeltrang C, Lange P. A systematic review of resistance training versus endurance training in COPD. *J Cardiopulm Rehabil Prev.* 2015;35:163–172.

40 Cheema B, Gaul CA, Lane K, Fiatarone Singh MA. Progressive resistance training in breast cancer: A systematic review of clinical trials. *Breast Cancer Res Treat.* 2008;109:9–26.

41 Apostolopoulos N, Metsios GS, Flouris AD, Koutedakis Y, Wyon MA. The relevance of stretch intensity and position-a systematic review. *Front Psychol.* 2015;6:1128.

42. Aguirre LE, Villareal DT. Physical exercise as therapy for frailty. *Nestle Nutr Inst Workshop Ser.* 2015;83:83–92. doi:10.1159/000382065

43 Page P. Current concepts in muscle stretching for exercise and rehabilitation. *Int J Sports Phys Ther.* 2012;7(1):109–119.

44 Feland JB, Myrer JW, Schulthies SS, Fellingham GW, Measom GW. The effect of duration of stretching of the hamstring muscle group for increasing range of motion in people aged 65 years or older. *Phys Ther.* 2001 May;81(5):1110–1117.

45 Sebio Garcia R, Yanez Brage MI, Gimenez Moolhuyzen E, Granger CL, Denehy L. Functional and postoperative outcomes after preoperative exercise training in patients with lung cancer: A systematic review and meta-analysis. *Interact Cardiovasc Thorac Surg.* 2016;23:486–497.

46 Singh F, Newton RU, Galvao DA, Spry N, Baker MK. A systematic review of pre-surgical exercise intervention studies with cancer patients. *Surg Oncol.* 2013;22:92–104.

47 Alonso-Frech F, Sanahuja JJ, Rodriguez AM. Exercise and physical therapy in early management of Parkinson disease. *Neurologist.* 2011;17:S47–S53.

48 Bergenthal N, Will A, Streckmann F, et al. Aerobic physical exercise for adult patients with haematological malignancies. *Cochrane Database Syst Rev.* 2014;11:CD009075.

49 Meneses-Echavez JF, Gonzalez-Jimenez E, Ramirez-Velez R. Effects of supervised multimodal exercise interventions on cancer-related fatigue: Systematic review and meta-analysis of randomized controlled trials. *Biomed Res Int.* 2015;2015:328636.

50 Carvalho AP, Vital FM, Soares BG. Exercise interventions for shoulder dysfunction in patients treated for head and neck cancer. *Cochrane Database Syst Rev.* 2012;4:CD008693.

51 Cheifetz O, Haley L, Breast Cancer A. Management of secondary lymphedema related to breast cancer. *Can Fam Physician.* 2010;56:1277–1284.

52 Courneya KS, Segal RJ, Mackey JR, et al. Effects of aerobic and resistance exercise in breast cancer patients receiving adjuvant chemotherapy: A multi-center randomized controlled trial. *J Clin Oncol.* 2007;25:4396–4404.

53 Klijn P, van Keimpema A, Legemaat M, Gosselink R, van Stel H. Nonlinear exercise training in advanced chronic obstructive pulmonary disease is superior to traditional exercise training. A randomized trial. *Am J Respir Crit Care Med.* 2013;188:193–200.

54 Kaldjian LC, Curtis AE, Shinkunas LA, Cannon KT. Goals of care toward the end of life: A structured literature review. *Am J Hosp Palliat Med.* 2008;25:501–511.

55 Heywood R, McCarthy AL, Skinner TL. Efficacy of exercise interventions in patients with advanced cancer: A systematic review. *Arch Phys Med Rehabil.* 2018;99:2595–2620.

56 Albrecht TA, Taylor AG. Physical activity in patients with advanced-stage cancer: A systematic review of the literature. *Clin J Oncol Nurs.* 2012;16:293–300.

57 Spathis A, Booth S. End of life care in chronic obstructive pulmonary disease: In search of a good death. *Int J Chron Obstruct Pulmon Dis.* 2008;3:11–29.

58 McCarthy B, Casey D, Devane D, Murphy K, Murphy E, Lacasse Y. Pulmonary rehabilitation for chronic obstructive pulmonary disease. *Cochrane Database Syst Rev.* 2015;2:CD003793.

59 Ohman H, Savikko N, Strandberg T, et al. Effects of exercise on functional performance and fall rate in subjects with mild or advanced Alzheimer's disease: Secondary analyses of a randomized controlled study. *Dement Geriatr Cogn Disord.* 2016;41:233–241.

60 Erbs S, Hollriegel R, Linke A, et al. Exercise training in patients with advanced chronic heart failure (NYHA IIIb) promotes restoration of peripheral vasomotor function, induction of endogenous regeneration, and improvement of left ventricular function. *Circ Heart Fail.* 2010;3:486–494.

61 Anderiesen H, Scherder EJ, Goossens RH, Sonneveld MH. A systematic review--physical activity in dementia: The influence of the nursing home environment. *Appl Ergon.* 2014;45:1678–1686.

4 Role of Therapists and Palliative Care Models

Christopher M. Wilson and Amy J. Litterini

Introduction

Rehabilitation professionals and physical activity providers have been providing care to those with a terminal or life-threatening illness since the inception of their respective professions; however, there is little focus and training for the unique care needs of those with advanced or terminal illness. As a disease progresses or symptoms worsen, the care philosophy of the medical team and therapists must also change and adapt to the new events and findings. Even in the event that a person's physical status may remain stable, there may be extreme variability to a person's emotions, mood, psychological, or psychosocial status that will require unique, individualized, and patient-centered approaches to provide optimal care.

Palliative Rehabilitation

In 1981, Dietz[1] described four general approaches to cancer rehabilitation – Preventative, Restorative, Supportive, and Palliative. This was one of the first examples of the consideration of the role of a therapist in participating in the care of a terminally ill individual. In 1984, Jane Toot[2] published a perspective on the therapist's role within the context of hospice care. She described that therapists often already had many of the tools and techniques available to provide direct care; she contended that an understanding of the terminally ill individual's circumstances and the care being received was the gap in knowledge that many therapists have when working with individuals near the end of life (EoL). In this seminal article, she advocated several domains for therapists to best learn about end-of-life care: (1) attitudes of death and dying; (2) appreciation of patients' needs (for adults and children); (3) alternatives of care; and (4) interactions with other healthcare professionals.

Therapists' Role in Chronic Disease and Palliative Care

Although therapists receive extensive entry-level training in restoring and mitigating impairments, functional limitations, and participation restrictions for a variety of degenerative or chronic conditions, therapists have reported receiving little to no education or training in advanced diseases, palliative care (PC), or hospice.[3] In order for therapists to best approach designing a cohesive and effective plan of care, it is useful to understand the interaction between cellular and physiologic changes and its impact on function and participation. The World Health Organization (WHO) developed the International Classification of Functioning, Disability, and Health (ICF) in 2002 and it has been widely adopted for use by professional associations and organizations (Figure 4.1).[4]

Although therapists with experience caring for individuals with chronic, degenerative, or terminal disorders may already utilize the concepts of the ICF, one of the key roles for therapists is to be able to concisely communicate the positive impact and unique clinical skills that can be provided once they are consulted. In order to best convey this impact, the format and language of the ICF model can assist other providers to understand the role of physical activity and rehabilitation in palliative and end-of-life care.

Within the ICF model, there are interacting domains to describe the different influences on an individual's ability to interact with their world and society. In order to illustrate the interacting factors of the ICF model, we will examine the case of a 63-year-old female with stage IV breast cancer.

Health Condition

The underlying cause is a disease pathology or disorder known in the ICF model as the *Health Condition*. At the disease/pathology level in the case example, the initial cellular change is the breast neoplasm itself. Unless a neoplasm is exceptionally large, inflamed, or compressing sensitive or critical structures

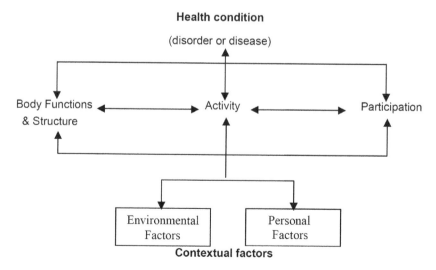

Figure 4.1 Conceptual Model of the International Classification of Functioning Disability and Health. Reprinted with permission.

(e.g. nerves, blood vessels), it may not cause substantial physical impairments or pain. Concurrently, additional Health Conditions may arise as side effects of treatments. For example, a mastectomy and lymph node excision will result in disruption to soft tissues, muscles, nerves, blood vessels, lymphatic tracts, and other structures in the surgical area. This may worsen as the tissues are healing and may involve scarring or adhesions around the surgical sites. If this individual also receives external beam radiation for her breast cancer, there may be Health Condition changes such as desquamation of the skin and radiation-induced fibrosis in this area. These are a result of damage to the DNA and impaired collagen and myofascial tissue reactions. Finally, at the Health Condition level, chemotherapy will have a multisystem impact on a variety of tissues throughout the body. Depending on the type of chemotherapy, this may include cardiotoxicity, neurotoxicity, or cancer-related fatigue.

The next three components are *Impairments of Body Structures and Functions*, *Activity Limitations*, and *Participation Restrictions*. Within the ICF model, there are interacting influences between these three domains.

Impairments of Body Structures and Functions

"*Body Functions* are physiological functions of body systems (including psychological functions). *Body Structures* are anatomical parts of the body such as organs, limbs and their components."[4] More than one health condition can impact a body structure/functional impairment. After the breast cancer surgery and treatments, the tissue-level changes have caused regional impact on the patient's shoulder arthrokinematics and ability to generate muscle forces. This will result in a limitation to the individual's ability to use her arm as her range of motion and strength have become impaired, and it may be painful for her to move as well. In addition, systemic treatments like chemotherapy may result in impaired proprioception and cardiovascular functioning.

Activity Limitations

With these new impairments to body structures/functions arises *Activity Limitations*. The ICF defines *activity* as "the execution of a task or action by an individual" while *activity limitations* are "difficulties an individual may have in executing activities."[4] In the case of breast cancer, its treatments, and resulting impairments, this individual will have a limitation in performing her activities of daily living (ADL). As the breast cancer diagnosis and its treatments have affected her dominant arm, she will have difficulty with tasks like bathing, grooming, dressing, driving, and meal preparation. As chemotherapy has resulted in impaired sensation, proprioception, and cardiovascular function, this individual will have decreased ability to walk extended distances and she may demonstrate gait deviations resulting in an increased risk of falling. Conversely, activity limitations may also result in new impairments to body structures and functions. For example, if this individual's shoulder dysfunction is not addressed and she attempts to continue to use her right shoulder while it is stiff, weak, and painful, it may result in poor bio-mechanical movement patterns which could result in a rotator cuff impingement. This may result in pain and tissue damage, such as fraying or rupture of the supraspinatus tendon.

Participation Restrictions

At the participation level, because of the patient's activity limitations and cancer-related fatigue, her ability to participate in life activities in her immediate community, according to her individual societal roles, will be affected. The WHO defines *Participation Restrictions* as "problems an individual may experience in involvement in life situations."[4] With the onset of these interacting factors, she may not be able to walk long enough distances to get to the grocery store, she may be too fatigued to work, and she may not be able to perform her normal societal roles, such as caring for her grandchildren or playing recreational golf with her social group. Participation Restrictions can lead to Activity Limitations and Impairments to Body Structures and Functions. In the case example, if the person was not able to participate in her recreational golf activities, which was her main form of cardiovascular exercise, she may become progressively deconditioned. Her cardiac function may become further impaired which would lead to an increasingly sedentary lifestyle, further affecting her cardiovascular status and capacity to perform her ADLs.

Personal and Environmental Factors

Finally, the ICF model describes the *Personal Factors* and *Environmental Factors* that also impact a person's ability to function. "*Environmental Factors* make up the physical, social, and attitudinal environment in which people live and conduct their lives."[4] Internal *Personal Factors* include "gender, age, coping styles, social background, education, profession, past and current experience, overall behaviour pattern, character and other factors that influence how disability is experienced by the individual."[4] Personal and Environmental Factors can be facilitators or barriers. For example, if our individual with breast cancer has a strong social support network to help her through her treatments and to coach her during the challenging times in her disease treatment process, she is more likely to be able to achieve her ongoing goals and stay consistent with her treatment regimen. Conversely, if this patient is in a home with a substantial number of stairs and she is not able to safely navigate those stairs, there is an increased likelihood of not being able to safely function in her own home, which can result in a fall. As can be imagined, contextual factors are highly individualized and a similar factor may have a greater or lesser impact on each person's health outcomes and quality of life (QoL). This knowledge of the likely and potential impact of these ICF domains on a person's life activities often requires the skill of a trained, educated therapist to recognize what domains are most affected and which are the most effective means to address them.

Patterns of Disease Trajectories

An important component of the participation of therapists in planning the care of individuals with a life-threatening illness is an understanding of the patterns of disease trajectories. This will assist the therapist in setting goals and understanding when an individual may experience a physical decline. In 2003, Lynn and Adamson[5] published a white paper entitled *Living Well at the End of Life*. Within that publication, they proposed three disease trajectories to assist healthcare providers in understanding the functional trajectory of individuals with similar diagnoses. In this chapter, the authors of this text propose some minor refinements to Lynn and Adamson's disease trajectories and describe additional disease trajectories that may further assist the therapist in anticipating or understanding a person's disease journey (Figure 4.2).

The first diagnosis category that was described was a short period of evident decline (Figure 4.2A). This disease trajectory is typical of cancer (see Chapter 9). This disease process is characterized by retention of fairly high functional

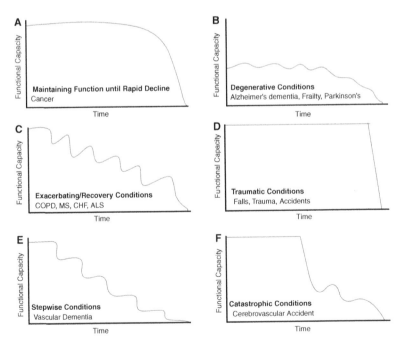

Figure 4.2 Functional Trajectories for Disease Categories. Adapted with Permission of the Rand Corporation.

capacity until the disease process or its treatments overwhelm the person's body systems physiologically. At that time, there is a steady and rapid decline. This decline may occur at variable rates depending on individual circumstances of the person and the disease.

The second of Lynn and Adamson's disease trajectories is prolonged dwindling (Figure 4.2B). This is typical of neurological disorders, such as Alzheimer's dementia, Parkinson's disease, amyotrophic lateral sclerosis (ALS), and frailty (see Chapter 13). This disease trajectory pattern is characterized by a longer duration of slow, progressive loss of physical or cognitive functions. This cognitive decline may or may not immediately result in activity limitations in conditions such as Alzheimer's dementia, but as the disease process advances, activity limitations and participation restrictions frequently emerge.[6]

The third disease trajectory described by Lynn and Adamson includes a series of exacerbations with subsequent recovery (Figure 4.2C). This recovery is generally not a full return to baseline but at some diminished capacity. This may be typical of conditions such as chronic obstructive pulmonary disorder (COPD, see Chapter 11), congestive heart failure (CHF, see Chapter 8), and multiple sclerosis. With each exacerbation, the person's functional status does not fully recover, which continues through the life cycle until the person is hospitalized or an exacerbation is too overwhelming for the body systems, resulting in death. On some occasions this may also occur after a peripherally related medical issue, like a deep vein thrombosis or myocardial infarction.

In a further refinement of Lynn and Adamson's theoretical patterns of disease trajectory, Lunney et al.[7] described functional decline in the context of trauma or severe injury (Figure 4.2D). Lunney et al. depicted an initially very high functional status without significant limitations; once the trauma occurred, a near vertical decline in functional status was depicted. While this may be applicable for individuals who experience a traumatic event that results in sudden death (e.g. severe motor vehicle accident), if the condition does not result in immediate or near-term mortality, there is generally a period of progressively worsening functional status until death (see Chapter 10). A characteristic case for this includes traumatic motor vehicle accidents or falling down the stairs. If the injury did not immediately take the patient's life, there will be efforts to stabilize the person and attempt to provide acute, subacute, or inpatient rehabilitation. If these are unsuccessful, progressive loss of function and an overwhelming medical status may occur, resulting in death.

In addition to the aforementioned disease trajectories, the authors propose two additional patterns of functional decline to further refine therapists' understanding of possible disease trajectories nearing death. The first one is a stepwise decline in function that is most characteristic of non-progressive but subsequent medical events (Figure 4.2E).[8-10] This may occur in conditions such as vascular dementia, where an individual experiences multiple episodes of vascular ischemia, with periods of stability to their cognitive and physical function or repeated episodes of kidney failure (see Chapter 15). Another example is if an individual experiences repeated small pulmonary emboli from a hypercoagulable state, that causes a stepwise decrease in pulmonary function. This pattern may hold some similarities to the exacerbating/recovery trajectory (Figure 4.2C) and the prolonged dwindling trajectory (Figure 4.2B), however, is unique from both of them because of the stepwise fashion of decline with little to no clear recovery between steps.

Finally, the last newly proposed disease trajectory pattern is entitled catastrophic conditions (Figure 4.2F). Diagnoses in this trajectory include a cerebrovascular accident (see Chapter 12), spinal cord injury, or traumatic brain injury. It should be noted that many of these conditions are not consistently terminal and therefore would not likely take a person's life immediately. The individual may have years of long-term stability or a slow, age-related decline in function. As these individuals often benefit from PC services and skilled maintenance, they are important for therapists to understand and establish long-term therapeutic relationships. Some individuals may experience repeated health issues or functional decline resulting in a more rapid physical decline and death. As can be seen in Figure 4.2F, this catastrophic condition is preceded by high-level baseline functioning with a precipitous drop off (similar to trauma); however, after this change in functional status, there is an indeterminate duration of significantly impaired functional status for the remainder of the person's life.

Role of Physical Therapy in Palliative Care

As described by Toot[2] in 1984, as a person's disease worsens it generally results in further deviations from normal physical activity and conventional rehabilitative care activities. This is attributed to the fact that the care needs, contextual factors, and medical issues become more variable and complex in the progressive disease process.

In 2017, Wilson et al.[3] completed a qualitative study of 20 physical therapists (10 from the United States and 10 from Canada) who provided hospice and palliative care (HPC). From this study, a conceptual model was developed to describe the role of therapists within HPC across the disease spectrum. This conceptual framework was further refined in 2020 while interviewing 14 other physical therapists from eight additional nations with advanced integration of PC into their respective medical systems (Figure 4.3).[11] Within the large oval is the therapists' role as it relates to HPC across the entire continuum of a disease process, regardless of an individual patient's specific disease status. This includes provision of patient and family care, being an interdisciplinary team member, and fulfilling professional responsibilities related to the therapists' role in assisting those near the EoL.

The large bi-directional arrow represents the shifting patient care priorities across the continuum as individuals advance through their disease trajectory from initial diagnosis through the EoL. These shifting priorities include

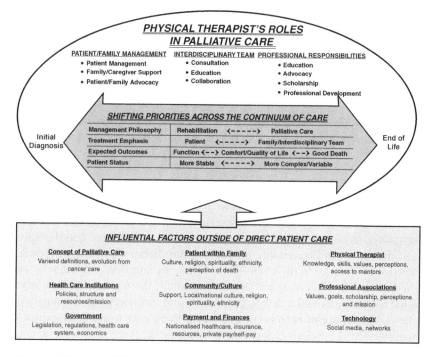

Figure 4.3 Roles of Physical Therapists in Palliative Care. Republished with permission from BMJ Supportive and Palliative Care.

therapists' management philosophy moving from rehabilitation to PC. With disease progression, treatment emphasis shifts from the patient to the family and interdisciplinary team. In addition, expected outcomes shift from optimizing function to focusing on QoL and comfort, and finally shifting focus toward achieving a good death.

Below the large oval that outlined the therapists' role in HPC is a large rectangle with an arrow at the top that reflects influential factors outside of direct therapist care. These factors include influences inherent to an individual therapist's scope and comfort level, knowledge, and skills. In addition, influences include the community, government, and related professional associations. Furthermore, payment and finances, healthcare institutions' policies and missions, and the personal/family circumstances and preferences were influential factors on provision of therapy outside of direct care. Due to these external influences, therapists should work to shift the perceptions of those individuals involved in these outside influences. This will assist in facilitating the development of a positive perception of therapist services within provision of care for those with a life-threatening illness.

Decision-Making for Therapists in End-of-Life Care

Briggs[12] published five theoretical practice models for therapists to be able to modify their clinical approach based on the person's individualized needs. In this portrayal, Briggs noted that the patient may benefit from more than one of these models at any point in time and may shift from one model to another depending on the individual's personal and medical circumstances. In the authors' experience, many seasoned therapists have applied some of these models (if not all of them) during their clinical practice; however, they may not have realized that they were providing these unique models of care.

Rehab Light

One of the common concerns about involving activity professionals and therapists in the PC plan is the concern of therapist interventions increasing pain, fatigue, or causing stress or disruption in care.[3] Some non-therapist providers may not consistently understand the therapist's ability to remain effective by decreasing the intensity, frequency, or duration of therapeutic or physical activity interventions.[13] In Rehab Light, the therapist is cognizant of the patient's motivation levels, pain levels, and functional reserve capacity, where a high dose of exercise or physical activity may worsen the patient's condition. In the Rehab Light treatment approach, there is an expectation of improvement to physical capabilities, functioning of body structures, and participation; however, aggressive interventions may hinder this improvement, as opposed to helping it further.[14] A slow, well-paced intervention plan will set the patient up for success.

In these cases, an astute therapist will utilize clinical judgment to moderate the frequency or intensity of services or focus interventions more on education and pacing. Clinically, this may involve decreasing frequency of visits to fewer times per week or decreasing duration of visits (e.g. from 45 to 30 minutes). This may also include using decreased resistance to exercise, decreased rating of perceived exertion (RPE) during activity, or providing more frequent and meaningful rest breaks for the patient.

Case example: A 97-year-old female, IG, has been living with end-stage congestive heart failure. Upon the therapist's initial interaction in the home health setting, she was ambulating with a four-wheeled walker approximately 20 feet with fair balance. She required a three-minute rest between ambulation sessions before recovering enough to ambulate again. Her personal goal was to get back to church every Sunday. Despite her activity limitations, IG was motivated to continue home care physical therapy. Per her physician, she was borderline to transition to hospice care, but she was not open to it as she "has a lot of living to do!". Clinically, her cardiac ejection fraction was 20% (normal is 55–60%) and her RPE on the Borg scale was 14/20 during ambulation. She wanted to do as much therapy as she could but became fatigued on being pushed too hard. In this case, there was an expectation of improvement clinically via a well-dosed physical activity regimen; however, if IG's cardio-vascular system was taxed excessively, it may have slowed her recovery or re-duced her quality of life. In this case, the therapist employed the Rehab Light philosophy which focused on smaller bouts of activity, decreased frequency of therapy sessions throughout the week, and maintained lighter activity resis-tance and duration to position IG for clinical improvements to optimize her quality of life.

Rehabilitation in Reverse

A critical step for the therapist is to consider the patient's disease trajectory during treatment planning. This will help to address the impairments, activity limitations, and participation restrictions that the patient is currently experi-encing, but also address issues that *will be encountered in the future*. This therapist will then deliver proactive, preventative interventions to prepare the individ-ual for these issues before they occur. One example of this would be a person with a progressive, degenerative neurological disorder (e.g. ALS). In the early stages of disease, the person may be fully independent and participating in recreational activities at a high level, such as running or jogging. During this timeframe, the therapist would facilitate performance of a running program while also preparing for a successful transition to a future walking or biking program, in anticipation of future symptoms and impairments. As the ALS progresses, the therapist is able to teach pacing techniques, adapted ADL techniques, and using a cane to ambulate. In addition, this patient is expected to experience future muscular weakness and activity limitations; therefore, teaching seated dressing and bathing techniques would be appropriate in light of the advancing disease process. Although using the cane currently is appro-priate and may be functionally safe, in anticipation of this future functional decline, the therapist would begin to teach the patient how to use another safer assistive device, such as a walker or wheelchair.[14] Finally, as the patient approaches death at the end stage of disease, the therapist can teach family members how to safely assist with ADLs or utilize a mechanical lift for getting in and out of bed.

Conveying the appropriate message to the patient during Rehab in Reverse is extremely important. If the therapist abruptly teaches the patient how to use a walker or wheelchair without the proper context when they are still functioning adequately with a cane, it could create emotional distress and result in the patient losing hope and confidence in their therapist. A beneficial portrayal of this scenario may be employing verbiage such as, "We all have good days and bad days and it is prudent life practice to prepare for a rainy day." Another useful communication example applicable in this scenario may include, "Most of the time you will not need the walker or wheelchair, but you can feel better knowing that it is close and available to you in case you ever need it. If you don't need it, you can leave it in your closet and be confident that it is there as a backup plan."

Finally, other useful analogies to assist the individual's acceptance of these skills or devices include comparing them to a fire extinguisher or an automobile seat belt – "Most of the time you don't need it but that one time you do need it, you are very glad it is there!"

Other examples of Rehabilitation in Reverse include educating an individual on fall prevention and fall recovery before a fall occurs. If the patient is anticipating balance or strength impairments, the patient may have an increased risk of falls and if they do fall, training on procedures to take after this fall may be helpful.[15] This may include how to fall without injuring themselves or how to get up from a fall, inspect their body for any injuries, and notify family or other medical personnel if needed. A study by Cox and Williams[16] identified trends in reducing fear of falling in older adults after training in fall recovery; however, the trend did not achieve statistical significance.

Case example: WW was a 51-year-old male diagnosed with a spinal metastatic lesion and T12 cord compression from lung cancer. Approximately three weeks ago he was able to walk without an assistive device. Upon the occupational therapist's (OT's) evaluation, he was using a cane and getting more unsteady with his legs buckling more. He required moderate assistance from two people during walking for safety due to the unexpected leg buckling. His doctor had prescribed a thoraco-lumbar-sacral orthosis to protect this area. His spinal lesion was not responsive to radiation and palliative chemotherapy, as it continued to grow in size upon repeat imaging. WW's goal was to stay home and be mobile around the house without injuring his family or falling and injuring himself. In anticipation of progressive loss of lower extremity function, the OT began to proactively train WW in the use of a wheeled walker, a wheelchair, transfers, and proper use of a bedside commode. Although WW did not need these devices yet, they were procured in anticipation of the advancing disease process.

Case Management

In this practice model, the therapist may not be seeing the patient or providing interventions on a regular basis. The therapist may only see the individual once every several weeks (or even less often) to provide periodic screenings or to prescribe or update physical activity regimens. This case management model also allows for early identification of emerging health issues that may not have been otherwise detected, or for which the patient may not have pursued medical attention. An example of this may be an early stage identification of a lymphedema exacerbation. During this routine screening, assessment, and updating of an exercise regimen, the therapist may discover these issues and elect to initiate treatment or refer to another medical professional as indicated by the individual patient's situation and preferences. After completion of a regular series of interventions, instead of abrupt cessation of therapist services, the therapist would schedule a monthly periodic follow-up visit to update the individual's exercise regimen or restart therapy services if needed.

Case example: EB was a 56-year-old female with stage 2 (moderately severe) chronic obstructive pulmonary disorder (COPD). At the time of her evaluation, her COPD was not significantly affecting her quality of life. Her physician provided a prescription for two long-acting inhalers. Within the past two months, her airflow restriction began to worsen and was now easily detectable on a spirometry test. She was beginning to experience increased coughing and sputum production. Clinically, she demonstrated good balance and coordination and was able to ambulate 380 meters in the six-minute walk test without an assistive device. She wanted to have a therapist prescribe an exercise program and have periodic advancements or updates. In this case, the therapist would prescribe a moderate-intensity exercise program of 150 minutes of aerobic activity weekly as well as a muscle-strengthening regimen. EB was instructed to contact the therapist if any questions or issues arose with this regimen; otherwise, a follow-up visit was scheduled in one month to further evaluate and advance her exercise regimen.

Skilled Maintenance

In the skilled maintenance practice paradigm (see Chapter 1), there may be clinical situations where therapy services are indicated to be delivered by a skilled professional and without these services, an individual's condition would worsen at a faster rate or certain physical tasks would not be able to be accomplished. Depending on the jurisdiction of the practicing therapist and patient insurance payer regulations, skilled maintenance therapy may not be an available practice model.[17]

In 2014, the United States federal government entered into a settlement agreement entitled Jimmo versus Sebelius. The Center for Medicare and Medicaid Services (CMS) policies were contested in court because of the misperception among providers and patients that an individual required the capacity for physical or functional improvement to continue to receive skilled services, including rehabilitation (i.e. physical therapy, occupational therapy or speech-language pathology).[18] This settlement agreement clearly outlined that if the patient required skilled professionals to maintain or slow the decline of a condition that the services are eligible for payment from CMS. In this scenario, the payment for services rendered hinges heavily on the therapist's clinical documentation.[19] If the clinical documentation does not clearly establish what impairments, activity limitations, or participation restrictions may manifest or worsen if the services are not rendered, CMS may deem them not medically necessary. In addition, the clinical documentation must demonstrate why rendering the services requires the skill and training of the specified healthcare provider (e.g. physical therapist), as opposed to a layperson or a lesser-qualified individual (e.g. carer, nursing aide). In addition, the therapist who is providing this clinical documentation should clearly document the potential long-term consequences if these services are not rendered. For example, if the patient does not get therapy services, they might be more likely to have a fall, be hospitalized, require higher dosages of pain medications, or have a heightened need for emergency medical services.

Case example: LG was a 77-year-old male who was diagnosed with metastatic prostate cancer with a large bone metastasis to the right tibia. The lesion encompassed approximately 80% of the cross-sectional diameter of the tibial cortex. The orthopedic oncologist recommended a partial weight bearing status of less than 5% weight bearing of the right leg to avoid pathologic fracture and noted that the patient was not a candidate for prophylactic internal fixation surgery. LG's personal goal was to not use a bedside commode or bedpan.

Upon observation, the OT noted that the person demonstrated unsafe movement patterns when ambulating with an assistive device but knew the basic concepts of standard walker use. Based on the amount of guarding and feedback the patient needed, the patient should not ambulate without a therapist to ensure safety. There was no anticipation of improvement in gait or function due to the person's medical status. In order to achieve this patient-centered goal, focus on training in proper walker use to protect the tibial metastasis required the skill of a licensed OT. As a component of his OT treatment plan, maintaining ambulatory status to the bathroom was emphasized, in addition to modifying ADLs to avoid violating his weight bearing status. The OT was deliberate in the clinical documentation in order to clearly detail the anticipated disease progression without OT, why the services required a licensed OT, and what medical consequences may occur if the weight bearing status was violated. Once LG and his family were independent in walker use, wheelchair propulsion, and lateral transfers to the toilet, regular OT services were held until needed again in the future.

Supportive Care

Near the EoL and in advanced disease processes, there are a number of skills, direct interventions, and educational interventions that would assist in providing care for the person at the EoL. As some of these skills may not directly require the therapist to administer them, it may be beneficial for a therapist to educate caregivers, families, and healthcare team members in the provision of these activities. Near the EoL, patients are more sedentary, weaker, and have immediate and predictable associated physical, psychological, and emotional issues. Within the therapist's skill set is a series of interventions to assist patients to maintain their dignity, safety, and optimize comfort at a time when they are very physically and emotionally challenged.

Case example: GF was a 67-year-old male with end-stage renal disease and advanced metabolic encephalopathy. Clinically, he required maximum assistance of two people for bed mobility and turning and was not able to assist with any upright or out-of-bed activity. He was confused and disoriented most of the day. He was at a very high risk of developing sacral pressure ulcers and had poor nutritional intake. He reported pain and stiffness in his thighs and legs that was alleviated with passive range of motion. His family needed education on a turning schedule and proper positioning for skin protection. His family was not open to hospice at the time due to their beliefs, but he would be a candidate for hospice/end-of-life care. The therapist provided extensive family and caregiver education in safe patient handling techniques to assist with using a bedpan, proper technique in lower extremity range of motion, how to provide massage to GF to comfort him at the EoL, and the proper technique of turning schedules and positioning for prevention of decubitus ulcers to his bony prominences. This was completed in two visits with the therapist; however, the family and therapist remained in contact to reinforce compliance, assure proper performance, and troubleshoot any emerging issues.

Value of Briggs' Models

One of the primary values of Briggs' models is the ability to communicate among practitioners the specific circumstances, thought processes, and overall considerations for prognosis by stating which practice model a therapist is working on at any specified point in time. For example, if a therapist is handing off care to another provider, the evaluating therapist could report that they were working on *Skilled Maintenance* or *Rehabilitation in Reverse* care model. If both providers are knowledgeable about these care models, it helps to concisely and accurately convey the specific focus based on the individual's disease trajectory and circumstances.

Summary

Across the disease spectrum of chronic and life-threatening illnesses, the roles of therapists change and adapt frequently. In order to facilitate treatment planning and goal setting, an understanding of the varying disease trajectories and associated functional changes are warranted. Based on the person's disease process and capacity for physical gains, a number of practice models can be applied by the therapist. These include *Rehab Light, Rehabilitation in Reverse, Skilled Maintenance, Case Management,* and *Supportive Care.* Although experienced therapists may frequently apply some aspects of these models, some of their value is conveying the varying roles of therapists in life-threatening illness to interdisciplinary team members, patients, and families. This clear understanding will facilitate access and referrals to therapists. Without facilitation of these referrals, individuals facing life-threatening illnesses may not have consistent access to therapist services and reduced QoL may ensue.

References

1 Dietz JH. *Rehabilitation Oncology*. New York, NY: John Wiley & Sons; 1981.
2 Toot J. Physical therapy and hospice: Concept and practice. *Phys Ther.* 1984;64(5):665–671.
3 Wilson CM, Stiller CH, Doherty DJ, Thompson KA. The role of physical therapists within hospice and palliative care in the United States and Canada. *Am J Hosp Palliat Med.* 2017;34(1):34–41. doi:10.1177/1049909115604668.
4 World Health Organization. *Towards a Common Language for Functioning, Disability, and Health ICF.* Geneva, Switzerland: World Health Organization; 2002.
5 Lynn J, Adamson DM. Living well at the end of life: Adapting health care to serious chronic illness in old age. Rand Corporation. https://www.rand.org/content/dam/rand/pubs/white_papers/2005/WP137.pdf. Published 2003. Accessed June 1, 2020.
6 Liu-Seifert H, Siemers E, Sundell K, et al. Cognitive and functional decline and their relationship in patients with mild Alzheimer's dementia. *J Alzheimer's Dis.* 2015;43(3):949–955.
7 Lunney JR, Lynn J, Foley DJ, Lipson S, Guralnik JM. Patterns of functional decline at the end of life. *JAMA.* 2003;289(18):2387–2392.
8 Rockwood K. Vascular cognitive impairment and vascular dementia. *J Neurol Sci.* 2002;203:23–27.
9 Gustaw-Rothenberg K, Kowalczuk K, Stryjecka-Zimmer M. Lipids' peroxidation markers in Alzheimer's disease and vascular dementia. *Geriatr Gerontol Int.* 2010;10(2):161–166.
10 Roh JH, Lee J. Recent updates on subcortical ischemic vascular dementia. *J Stroke.* 2014;16(1):18–26.
11 Wilson CM, Stiller CH, Doherty DJ, Thompson KA, Smith AB, Turczynski KL. Physical therapists in integrated palliative care: A qualitative study. *BMJ Support Palliat Care.* doi:10.1136/bmjspcare-2019-002161.
12 Briggs RW. Clinical decision making for physical therapists in patient-centered end-of-life care. *Top Geriatr Rehabil.* 2011;27(1):10–17.
13 Spill GR, Hlubocky FJ, Daugherty CK. Oncologists' and physiatrists' attitudes regarding rehabilitation for patients with advanced cancer. *PM&R.* 2012;4(2):96–108.
14 Wilson CM, Mueller K, Briggs R. Physical therapists' contribution to the hospice and palliative care interdisciplinary team: A clinical summary. *J Hosp Palliat Nurs.* 2017;19(6):588–596. doi:10.1097/NJH.0000000000000394.
15 Hofmeyer MR, Alexander NB, Nyquist LV, Medell JL, Koreishi A. Floor-rise strategy training in older adults. *J Am Geriatr Soc.* 2002;50(10):1702–1706.
16 Cox TB, Williams K. Fall recovery intervention and its effect on fear of falling in older adults. *Act Adapt Aging.* 2016;40(2):93–106.
17 Tovino S. Disparities in private health insurance coverage of skilled care. *Laws.* 2017;6(4):21.
18 Gladieux JE, Basile M. Jimmo and the improvement standard: Implementing Medicare coverage through regulations, policy manuals and other guidance. *Am J Law Med.* 2014;40(1):7–25. doi:10.1177/009885881404000101.
19 Wilson CM, Boright L. Documenting medical necessity for palliative care and degenerative or chronic conditions. *Rehabil Oncol.* 2017;35(3):153–156. doi:10.1097/01.REO.0000000000000066.

5   Caregivers in Patient- and Family-Centered Care

Amy J. Litterini and Christopher M. Wilson

Introduction

At the center of healthcare, especially the care of the patient with a life-threatening or terminal illness, is the concept of patient- and family-centered care. This aligns closely with the concept of a "good death" and "death with dignity". As much of the care burden rests on the family, in order for the terminally ill individual to receive high-quality care, the caregiver must obtain key skills and knowledge from the care team. These include activities such as body mechanics training, safe equipment use, and other therapeutic skills. Equally important is the psychosocial and emotional state of the caregiver because if the caregiver becomes burnt-out or becomes ill, they will not be able to provide the key care activities. Frequently the patient's and the family's interests, values, and care goals align; however, there are situations where there are discrepancies between the patient's and the family's goals of care or objectives, and the therapist is often integrally involved with this dilemma. This chapter will outline best practices relevant to caregiver training, skills, coping, stress management, and conflict resolution to accomplish the goal of patient-centered care.

The Critical Role of the Caregiver

Some of the most significant unsung heroes of palliative care (PC) and hospice care are the caregivers. Playing a critical role for individuals with life-threatening illnesses on many levels, and in several different capacities, caregivers are at the forefront of the day-to-day care of individuals with life-threatening illnesses. The concept of the caregiver role extends from paid individuals such as skilled clinicians or support personnel to unpaid volunteers, family members, and friends, with the majority of care for individuals in the home provided by unpaid caregivers.[1] In the case of older adults at the end of life (EoL), unpaid caregivers often live with the individual and frequently face their own health challenges, such as advanced age.

According to Ornstein et al.[1] nearly nine in ten caregivers for patients at the EoL are unpaid. The prospective data collected by these authors represented 900,000 community-dwelling Medicare beneficiaries receiving care in the

United States who died within one year. They found the physical demands to be greatest for EoL caregivers of patients with dementia, while financial and emotional difficulties were greatest among caregivers of patients with cancer.[1] Additionally, the prevalence of caregiving-related physical difficulties associated with patient care and the time spent providing it, are greater for EoL caregivers when compared to caregivers of individuals not facing EoL.[1] Not surprisingly, the costs for paid caregiving increase substantially when individuals require admission to facilities and are no longer able to remain in their home setting. Based on these heavy personal and financial demands on society, if adequate attention is not paid within healthcare systems to supporting the caregiver, the entire system performs inefficiently and is at risk for failure.

In ideal circumstances, patient care extends directly from the interprofessional team to both the patient and family unit. In this framework, family members and loved ones are included as an important extension of the support structure provided during patient/family-centered care. Specific attention should be paid not only to the needs of the patient but to the needs of the entire patient/family unit in order to support the appropriate environment for patient care. An interprofessional or multidisciplinary approach to patient/family-centered care includes an emphasis on the needs of the entire family, with services provided when and as needed by the appropriate disciplines. This approach extends in a trans-disciplinary fashion from the dietitian counseling on proper nutrition and appropriate intake to the social worker providing emotional support, to the rehab therapists prescribing physical activity and working on body mechanics training and equipment needs for safety.

Care Provision Models to Facilitate Quality Care

With the challenges of caring for an individual at EoL, there are numerous innovative care models to attempt to improve these activities. The concept of a Patient-Centered Medical Home (PCMH) is a care model that was originally developed to strengthen primary care medicine in the setting of care for children with special needs.[2] With the goal of improving access to comprehensive care geared toward patient safety and improved quality, PCMH has gained traction in other care settings as well, including geriatrics, oncology, and community-based palliative care (CBPC). With the fundamental goals to (1) provide structure for CBPC by enhancing patient-family-provider communication while addressing gaps that can fragment care, and (2) extend the reach of specialized medical care into the home through the PCMH, the potential outcomes provided can be numerous. Proponents suggest it can improve care quality and enhance care coordination while simultaneously supporting improved self-management and adherence to treatment plans. The PCMH model has been operationalized into routine clinical practice in the United States with the goal of improved patient-provider communication, thus reducing emergency room visits and hospital admissions. As patients with complex medical needs associated with life-threatening illnesses require more comprehensive, coordinated care, hospice care and PC as an extension of PCMH appears to be a logical framework and has been the philosophy of practice since hospice's inception. Any viable medical model that stands to permit a patient to remain safely in their home for the longest duration of time possible and reduce the fragmentation of care frequently experienced by patients, families, and clinicians, should be considered where accessible and advocated for when unavailable. When matching the right discipline with the right patient, at the right time, with the appropriate level of intensity of care when necessary, the healthcare system stands to streamline what is otherwise an extremely costly subset of patient care activities. It is always important as part of the care team to discern if the decisions being made are truly patient-centered and directed and not for the convenience of the provider organization.

Learning Caregiving Skills

Body Mechanics for Reduced Risk of Injury

As chronic illnesses progress, an individual gradually loses functional mobility and the capacity to be independent with activities of daily living (ADL). Subsequently, the overall demands on caregivers often increase exponentially. Specifically, the physical demands of ADLs such as bed mobility, positioning, transfers, toileting, bathing and dressing, and eating require significant effort from the caregiver for routine completion on a day-to-day basis. The efficiency with which these activities are performed matters greatly in reducing the risk of acute and/or chronic use injuries for caregivers, and overall safety for patients. Generally speaking, most individuals don't routinely consider concepts such as proper form and/or technique in their daily movement until the repetition and chronicity of an activity draws their attention, possibly secondary to the onset of pain. Caregiver training, the acquisition of appropriate durable medical equipment, and specialized safe patient handling and mobility programs geared toward this focus, are essential for promoting proper body mechanics and safety during patient care.

According to the National Institute for Occupational Safety and Health (NIOSH), injuries to the musculoskeletal system are among the highest in the US healthcare industry.[3] It is estimated that hospital employees experience twice the national average for work-related injuries across all industries, while nursing home employees suffer three times the national average.[3] Due to this high rate of injury resulting in a significant expense to the healthcare industry, a lifting equation developed by NIOSH calculated 35 pounds (16 kg) as the maximum acceptable weight for the reduction of risk of injury in the most ideal, low-risk situation.[4] However, it should be noted that some authors caution against using this threshold as a strict policy, and that, in fact, no safe lifting of weight can actually be advised as patients, caregivers, and conditions vary widely across healthcare settings.[5] These realizations assisted in the initiation of the "no lift" facility movement, although most individuals working in facilities will admit that this is an unrealized and unrealistic initiative. Momentum for safety awareness and reduced disability in the workforce has, however, served to create a paradigm shift towards safe patient handling and mobility program development across the United States and worldwide. Examples of mechanical lifts and further information on alternatives to lifting procedures can be found in Chapter 20.

Caregiver Training

As many individuals with life-threatening illnesses are elderly, likewise, their unpaid caregivers are often elderly spouses or family members at risk of their own personal injury. However, both paid and unpaid caregivers of any age or physical stature are at risk of injury secondary to caregiving. Training and education on things such as lowering one's center of gravity and widening one's base of support during patient repositioning and/or transfers, using short lever arms, and keeping loads close to one's center of mass, all can be helpful for injury risk reduction. Additionally, caregiver training in proper bed mobility and transfer techniques with appropriate devices can, in turn, reduce the risk of injury for the patient themselves. Particularly for those patients who cannot actively assist in functional mobility, or who are cognitively unable to follow basic sequencing commands for mobility, technique on the part of the caregiver is critical for protection of joints and the skin integrity of the patient. Finally, caregivers should be able to recognize when a technique or procedure excessively exposes himself or herself to increased risk of injury and perform the needed technique in a different manner.

Educational programs that incorporate caregiver training deliberately into the patient's plan of care have proven to be a novel approach for patients with life-threatening illnesses. Particularly when the goal is to return home, the emphasis on caregiver training needs to be prominent in the care planning. Some innovative programs often referred to as "Caregiver Boot Camps" have successfully demonstrated the concept of caregiver training emphasis in very deliberate ways. One such example, the Beaumont Short Stay Family Training program (see next), is a revolutionary inpatient rehabilitation program with the primary focus of allowing patients to be discharged to home with the best care possible from their caregivers. Other facilities, such as The Memory Care Center in Greensboro, North Carolina, USA, provide hands-on skills training for loved ones caring for a person with dementia or other chronic illness.[6] A third example is the University of California-Los Angeles' Alzheimer's and Dementia Care Program, which provides skills training courses for both English- and Spanish-speaking caregivers of persons with dementia.[7] One of the important concepts of each of these programs is individualizing the caregiver skills based on the patient's current and anticipated care needs as symptoms and disease burden evolve. For example, teaching how to assist with a pivot transfer may be counterintuitive for the family of a currently ambulatory person, though as the patient becomes weaker, the caregiver will have the skills for these potential circumstances.

Beaumont's Short Stay Inpatient Rehabilitation Program: Family Training in Patient Care Procedures

In addition to three hours of intensive rehabilitation services, a standard requirement for admission to inpatient rehabilitation (IPR) is generally being able to demonstrate substantial gains in functional mobility, activities, and participation in life activities. In cases where an individual with a life-threatening or degenerative illness is considering IPR, this threshold or expectation may be too great. This often leaves those with significant physical disability two main options after hospitalization: (1) to return home, or (2) to discharge to an extended care facility (ECF). As has been highlighted several times throughout this text, very few individuals wish to spend their last months of care in a setting other than their home, and the authors have heard many individuals express fears that if they are admitted to a nursing facility or ECF, they may not be able to accomplish their goal of getting home. This creates an opportunity and a paradigm shift for traditional IPR to instead focus on the training of the family (see Chapter 19). IPR is optimally situated to provide intensive physical training and educational opportunities for patients and caregivers. Historically, IPR has focused on the provision of care for patients while also occasionally teaching family caregivers to assist with some tasks. A new model of IPR care for patients in PC is via a short stay family training (SSFT) visit. During the SSFT admission, there is no expectation of improvement in the patient's functional capacity, strength, or impairments; however, there is a clear expectation that after specialized patient/family training, the patient/ family unit can be independent in performing complex daily tasks to achieve the goal of returning home. There remains the requirement for three hours of rehabilitation, but instead of physical performance of tasks consistently by the patient, the emphasis is on training the patient's *family* (and by proxy, the patient themselves) in performing the required physical mobility-related tasks. Examples may include positioning in bed, lower body dressing, car transfers, wheelchair use, and toilet or bathing transfers.

In order to identify if a patient is appropriate for the SSFT approach in IPR, several key steps must be identified. First, the patient must be medically stable or approaching medical stability to be discharged from the hospital. Second, it must be determined if the patient and family will be able to safely learn how to perform targeted daily activities at home. All aspects of home life must be considered, including the ability to perform the most basic of tasks such as toileting, bathing, dressing, and grooming, as well as meal preparation. If these basic tasks cannot be completed in the home, it would be appropriate to consider an alternative care plan, such as privately hired help for these activities or discharge to an ECF. Finally, if the patient's long-term goal is to go home and not to an ECF, then this person may be appropriate for SSFT in

IPR. Another key discussion point is if the family or caregiver has the physical and mental capacity, as well as the motivation and resources, to assist with the care of the individual with a life-threatening illness. There may be certain scenarios where the person may be physically able, but not mentally or emotionally able, to carry out these care tasks. In cases such as these, admission to IPR for SSFT may not be the best choice. In these cases, alternative arrangements including further discussion of placement in an ECF, or a residential hospice facility, may be appropriate. It is also an important consideration if the caregiver who is willing to participate in the three hours of daily training in IPR is going to be the person who is primarily caring for the terminally ill individual at home. If all of these criteria are met, then various admission approvals may be pursued.

Although when published by Smith et al.[8] the SSFT was described in IPR, there may be other opportunities to perform this program in other settings. If the patient only needs training in one or two tasks with their caregivers, a worthwhile discussion is *'can the patient's hospital stay be extended to perform this training during the acute care hospitalization?'* For example, if a patient is not able to leave the bed and the family is interested in procuring and using a mechanical lift system, then a dedicated training session lasting several hours may be a beneficial use of acute care therapist resources as opposed to an extended stay at greater expense in the IPR setting.

Clinical Pearl from Rich Briggs, PT:

The potential for a mechanical lift...is often a desired and offered option. In practice with home hospice, I have found that most often it takes two able caregivers to successfully use. Complications at home include carpeted surfaces (shag is the worst) and narrow spaces. It is often worth a conversation with the family, perhaps when at home and they experience the difficulty of operation. It may become clear there (or in the hospital) that just doing bed care is the likely, if undesired alternative. All part of the process, to be expected, and not a failure.

A key role in palliative IPR via the SSFT approach is nursing, enabling the patient and family caregiver to complete more ADL tasks on their own in anticipation of discharge from the IPR setting. Upon initial admission, the nursing staff may be assisting with almost all daily tasks including dressing, bathing, toileting, and physical mobility. Through coaching and encouragement, the patient and family are progressively able to use more of the skills that are learned in physical therapy and occupational therapy to achieve more independence and confidence in anticipation of discharge home. In addition to learning these critical ADL tasks, the caregiver and patient are trained in using adaptive medical equipment, such as wheelchairs, mechanical lifts, and transfer boards, and are also taught safe patient-handling and mobility techniques to prevent caregiver injury. In addition, the social worker can focus on not just coping strategies for the patient with an advanced illness, but self-care strategies for the caregiver. If a caregiver gets burnt out or injured, and is no longer able to perform their tasks to care for their loved one, then further physical and functional failure may ensue for the patient. This may result in subsequent hospitalization, need for further medical or diagnostic services and interventions, or admission for a higher level of daily skilled care.

Durable Medical Equipment

Having the proper durable medical equipment available at the right time, for the right application, for the right patient, can make caregiving not only easier but actually physically and logistically possible. For the caregiver at a mechanical disadvantage in strength or size compared to the patient, proper equipment allows for safe mobility in circumstances where it would be otherwise physically unsafe and inappropriate to attempt. Examples of equipment that improves mechanical advantage include mechanical lifts, stand-assist devices, transfer boards, and transfer discs. Equipment necessary for the protection and maintenance of skin integrity and comfort in positioning includes specific seating systems made from air, foam, or gel, wedge cushions for angled positioning and mattresses for reduced and/or alternating pressure.

Prior to the need for progression to wheelchair use, technological advances have provided adaptations in options for standard four-legged chairs. Considering the difficult task of moving individuals forward/backward, and to/from tables and counters for dining, recreational activities, or while performing other ADL tasks, equipment that reduces the strain on caregivers and effort by patients can be a game changer. Companies such as Canadian ComforTek (ComforTek Seating, Inc, Alberta, Canada) are designing furniture and locking, wheeled-base frames for existing furniture, in order to reduce the effort associated with manipulating existing chairs (see Figure 5.1). Some models also allow the seating surface to swivel, at the control of either the patient or the caregiver, in order to alter orientation in the room for ease in transfers.

As the ability to safely and independently ambulate declines, the progression to at least intermittent use of a wheelchair should receive serious consideration. The plan of care should include both an appropriate fit of the patient to the specific chair indicated and proper training in wheelchair mobility as a means of continued independence. Additionally, wheelchairs with specific capabilities for tilted and reclined positions, and pressure reduction, can also be beneficial for promoting sitting tolerance and time out of bed in later stages of disease. For patients unable to safely self-propel, a basic transport chair is indicated for use by the caregiver as these are generally lighter and narrower in width overall.

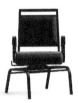

Figure 5.1 ComforTek Seating Options.
Source: Reprinted with permission, ComforTek Seating, Alberta, Canada.

Cost is often a concern and a potential barrier in the acquisition of durable medical equipment, as insurance coverage can be limited or equipment access and availability in one's region can be problematic. Routine equipment needs may be covered by private insurance and/or through one's hospice benefit, but the type of item selected and actual costs covered are often determined by the agency providing services (e.g. custom, high-end items are generally not covered). The price and accessibility of a device ranges substantially based on the capabilities provided and the materials and procedures necessary in the construction. Furthermore, the expense also fluctuates based on items purchased over the counter versus those which are custom fit and ordered specifically for the patient. Additionally, constraints in one's living space such as small sleeping quarters, narrow hallways and door frames, and inadequate or narrow kitchen and bathroom setup can also pose challenges. Particular attention should be paid to the correct installation of mobility equipment, such as grab bars, to ensure that they are, in fact, compliant with any legislative or regulatory standards (e.g. Americans with Disabilities Act) and installed into the wall studs for safe use.

Creativity and ingenuity can allow for effective movement in a safe environment. Ideally, in-home care consultation and treatment from a physical therapist (PT) or an occupational therapist (OT) would be provided in order to maximize the options for the patient and family in their existing circumstances. Likewise, borrowed equipment can be an appropriate alternative to purchasing new items when possible. In nearly all jurisdictions, many lending closets and local philanthropic organizations repurpose and redistribute items donated for use within their local communities such as walkers, wheelchairs, bedside commodes, canes, and crutches. Such organizations include local religious institutions, Lions Clubs, Kiwanis Clubs, and lending closets set up directly within a city, town, or municipality. A state-wide example across California, USA, is Ability Tools, which runs Device Lending and Demonstration Centers and Reuse Centers with support from the California Foundation for Independent Living Centers.[9]

Clinical Pearl from Rich Briggs, PT

Experience has shown that most often when the equipment has been ordered by the discharge planner or nurse without consultation or evaluation by a PT/OT, the equipment is likely not the most efficient for use or effective in the environment. Case example: I had a patient who had three different wheelchairs delivered in succession until PT referral to determine the optimal fit and type for use. Frustrating and inefficient.

LGBTQ and Terminal Illness

Although each individual person's life context and personal situation is unique and highly variable, there may be unique care needs for individuals who identify as lesbian, bisexual, gay, transgender, or queer (LGBTQ) of which the therapist should be aware. As with any individual, care should be taken to avoid stereotyping or assuming the trends of a group apply to an individual, but it is hoped that some noted trends may assist a therapist to inquire about an individual's life circumstances. This will help the therapist to best tailor the care to the individual's care needs within the context of their life situation. In addition to existing national, religious, or cultural stigmas that may suppress an individual's desire to speak about their sexuality or sexual identity, some individuals' family members may not be aware of their status, or the individual themselves does not wish for them to know. These influences may hinder a person's comfort with discussing topics related to their personal history; a therapist's declaration that any information will be handled confidentially and nonjudgmentally may be helpful. The therapist should also be aware that the topic of a person's sexuality or sexual identity has the potential to cause stress and family discord at an already stressful time, so careful navigation is warranted. It is good clinical practice in providing care for those with life-threatening illnesses to not assume that the person in the room is an immediate family member and even if they are, they may not wish sensitive information disclosed.

In some terminal illness situations, it is often assumed that the spouse/partner, parents, or children will provide end-of-life care tasks but family dynamics are often complex and wrought with emotion and history. For example, an individual who is gay may be estranged from disapproving parents and thereby this option for providing caregiver support may not be a feasible option. In some jurisdictions, gay marriage or other civil unions may not be legally recognized or available, which may limit who can assist in EoL decision-making and sometimes who can even be in the room during certain procedures or discussions. Finally, the statistical likelihood of LGBTQ older adults who have children is lower, which also limits the options of having a network of children to provide care for them in advanced illness. Alternate means of engaging their personal network or seeking alternate means to provide supportive care is warranted and necessary to assure care with comfort and dignity. Finally, as with any challenging family dynamics and history, terminal illness and end-of-life care bring forth a new opportunity for making amends, healing, and reconciliation. One of the rich benefits of being a therapist practicing in PC is to participate in these healing events, but the therapist should anticipate these events and be flexible in the administration of therapeutic interventions. One practice that may help guide the therapist in this process is attendance at IDT meetings where new patients are introduced. The nurse and social worker will likely have explored family relationships for the care planning process and share their insight with other team members. Review of their documentation, or direct personal contact prior to a therapist visit, will assist in understanding the person's social and care circles.

Distress, Emotional Health, and Caregiver Sustainability

As the toll of a chronic illness persists over time, family members can, directly and indirectly, feel the effects of the diagnosis on their loved ones. The burden of having to witness the deterioration of those in their care, often slowly suffering in multiple ways, can be cumulative and cause substantial emotional distress. This distress, in turn, can result in physical, mental, and emotional issues which potentially limit one's ability to provide caregiving. Therefore, it is incumbent on the healthcare system to maximize the overall health of the caregiver in order to strengthen the entire patient/family unit. Ideally, this would occur through training to perform the physical aspects of care, as discussed earlier, and for mental and emotional health through routine screening and referral for intervention by a licensed mental health professional. Interventions such as couples counseling, individual counseling, and/or family counseling should be available, offered routinely and proactively, and utilized. Participation in regular family meetings is recommended to allow for the transfer of information, open communication, and dialogue about status and prognosis. Training in self-care and relaxation techniques for caregiver wellness should also be incorporated.

Particular attention should be paid to the children of individuals with life-threatening conditions in order to best prepare them for further decline, and the ultimate loss, of their parent. As anticipatory grief is likely to occur following a life-threatening diagnosis, early intervention from a social worker and/or licensed counselor for grief counseling is indicated. For families receiving hospice care, grief counseling following the loss of a loved one is recommended to continue for a minimum of one year during the initial bereavement period. All significant dates within that time period, such as birthdays, anniversaries, and holidays, should be noted with special attention and support. Specific bereavement groups pertaining to the circumstances of a particular loss, such as motherless daughter groups, loss of a spouse, and groups designed for children following the loss of a parent, are recommended for professional and peer support. Many hospice agencies have grief support groups that are open to survivors within their community, even if the person/their loved one was not on hospice care. Spiritual counseling from a chaplain, and/or the individual's clergy of their religion of choice, is also considered standard of care during and after a life-threatening illness in the family. Having a medical chaplain as part of the interdisciplinary team is critical for comprehensive care for all involved with patients at the EoL.

A notable issue that may cause substantial emotional stress is when the care goals of the patient do not match those of the family. This may occur when a patient wishes to pursue comfort measures and simply engage in remaining life events and the family caregivers want the patient to "keep fighting" and pursue aggressive medical care measures. As therapists, our physical activity interventions may be perceived to be aggressive and therefore helpful by family, while perhaps simultaneously difficult and/or uncomfortable for the patient (if not properly dosed). Families may provide pressure on or influence the patient or the therapists to participate in, or continue, unwarranted physical activity due to this disconnect in perspective. Effectively and delicately navigating this narrow space is a vital role for the therapist. In a study of 13 PC physiotherapists from different nations discussing the roles of PTs, a key role was to advocate for the patient; oftentimes this means to advocate for the patient and the family as a cohesive unit.[10] In this case, the therapist's role is to advocate for the patient within their family.[10] The therapist should employ communication skills to educate the family as to the patient's voiced wishes. In addition, it should be communicated that the requested intensity of physical activity may not be conducive to the overall goals of care and comfort of the patient. Engaging the support of IDT members such as the social worker and nurse can help negotiate this potential family conflict.

Public Advocacy

Advocacy often becomes a passion for family members and loved ones of an individual with a life-threatening illness, and often the patient themselves. Whether campaigning or personally fundraising for research allocations related to a specific disease, or increasing awareness both within their community or nationally, the desire is often to become part of the solution. This drive to make a difference, not only for the patient and their loved ones but others in the future, can be a very positive, therapeutic practice for families both during illness and following loss. For the patient themselves, advocacy often becomes part of their personal legacy. For many families, participating in these activities helps to keep the memory of their loved ones alive and recognizes their suffering as a contribution to a greater good in the future. A recent example of this, which became a viral, worldwide phenomenon, was the "Ice Bucket Challenge" to contribute funding for research on Amyotrophic Lateral Sclerosis (ALS), or Lou Gehrig's disease.[11] This initiative alone raised millions of dollars in the summer of 2014 in the United States, the United Kingdom, and worldwide.

As healthcare providers, our role can be to facilitate these advocacy opportunities for families, and/or to participate individually for the benefit of our patients and the community. For clinicians specifically, participating in positive events surrounding advocacy and awareness can help to offset some of the stressors of providing day-to-day care for individuals with life-threatening illnesses. Specific fundraisers providing contributions directly to patient-related programs can be both a day of celebration and remembrance that collaboratively brings patients, family members, and caregivers together for one positive, unifying cause.

Caregiver Burnout and Compassion Fatigue

For both paid and unpaid caregivers, *burnout* can be a substantial problem, manifested by emotional, physical, and mental exhaustion. Rates of burnout are particularly high in healthcare, especially for those caring for individuals at the EoL who present with multiple, complex needs in often challenging settings. According to the results of an electronic survey regarding the predictors and prevalence of burnout of hospice and PC clinicians by Kamal et al.,[12] respondents (n = 1,357) demonstrated an overall burnout rate of 62%. The majority of burnout in this study was associated with emotional exhaustion.[12] For paid caregivers, poorly managed burnout can ultimately pose limitations within one's chosen field and/or their career trajectory due to poor job satisfaction, which can ultimately reduce the quality of job performance. If left unchecked, burnout can result in multiple detrimental effects across many facets of both professional and personal life. *Compassion fatigue* is a phenomenon associated with a reduced capacity for empathy due to repeated exposures to witnessing patients' suffering.[13] Peters[13] theorized that compassion fatigue can result in unsatisfactory outcomes for providers, the patients receiving their care, and healthcare organizations.

Preventative and restorative measures are recommended to mitigate the effects of compassion fatigue in healthcare, including professional boundaries, self-care, self-awareness, and education at the individual and organizational levels.[13] Professional and peer-to-peer counseling and intervention are often necessary for employees to maintain high functioning in their work setting. As a profession, social work is superior in their mandated, routine counseling of their colleagues; however, other healthcare disciplines are unfortunately not as deliberate with their preventative and restorative interventions.

Clinician rounds such as *The Schwartz Rounds*, founded at Massachusetts General Hospital (Boston, MA, USA) by the late Dr. Ken Schwartz, can be helpful in providing colleague support in difficult situations facing healthcare providers.[14] Offered internationally in the United States, Canada, the United Kingdom, Ireland, Australia, and New Zealand, the Schwartz Rounds provide a brief case presentation by an interdisciplinary panel of clinicians, followed by discussions and different perspectives offered by those in attendance, usually as a monthly gathering. Different topics are covered in each session in a supportive and positive environment in order to promote caring and understanding among colleagues.[14] Regular attendance at IDT meetings held by hospice providers can be another avenue of support as each death is discussed, with an opportunity to share one's experience around the care.

Summary

Regardless of the actual mechanisms dedicated to providing care for the caregivers, close attention should be paid to regular needs assessments, early identification of issues, routine interventions to address issues identified, creative and effective ways to offer support, and assessments of effectiveness. Caregivers are the heart of what makes PC and hospice work; therefore, every effort needs to be made to deliberately and intentionally hardwire in proactive strategies to maintain this extremely valuable asset. Caregiver support should not be an afterthought in system and process design but rather at the forefront of what we do in healthcare.

References

1 Ornstein KA, Kelley AS, Bollens-Lund E, Wolff JL. A national profile of end-of-life caregiving in the United States. *Health affairs (Project Hope).* 2017;36(7):1184–1192. https://www.ncbi.nlm.nih.gov/pubmed/28679804. doi:10.1377/hlthaff.2017.0134.

2 Rich E, Lipson D, Libersky J, Parchman M. Coordinating care for adults with complex care needs in the patient-centered medical home: Challenges and solutions. White paper (Prepared by Mathematica Policy Research under Contract No. HHSA290200900019I/HHSA29032005T). AHRQ Publication No. 12-0010-EF. Rockville, MD: Agency for Healthcare Research and Quality. January 2012.

3 National Institute for Occupational Safety and Health. Safe Patient Handling and Mobility. https://www.cdc.gov/niosh/topics/safepatient/. Updated August 2, 2013. Accessed August 22, 2020.

4 Waters T, Putz-Anderson V, Garg A, Fine LJ. Revised NIOSH equation for the design and evaluation of manual lifting tasks. *Ergonomics.* 1993;36(7):749–776. https://www.cdc.gov/niosh/docs/94-110/pdfs/94-110.pdf.

5 Waters, T. When is it safe to manually lift a patient. *Am J Nurs.* 2007;107(8):53–58.

6 Caregiver Support Offering Hands-On Skills 'Boot Camp' For Family Caregivers. https://www.well-springsolutions.org/event/hands-skills-boot-camp-family-caregivers-2/. Published 2018. Accessed August 22, 2020.

7 Caregiver Bootcamps. UCLA Division of Geriatrics. https://icared.med.ucla.edu/caregiver-bootcamp/. Published 2015. Accessed January 30, 2020.

8 Smith S, Wilson CM, Lipple C, et al. Managing palliative patients in inpatient rehabilitation through a short stay family training program. *Am J Hosp Palliat Med.* 2020;37(3):172–187. doi:10.1177/1049909119867293.

9 Ability Tools: Device Lending and Demonstration Centers. https://abilitytools.org/services/natads-public-access.php. Published 2015. Accessed August 22, 2020.

10 Wilson CM, Stiller CH, Doherty DJ, et al. Physical therapists in integrated palliative care: A qualitative study. *BMJ Support Palliat Care.* Published Online First: February 20, 2020. doi:10.1136/bmjspcare-2019-002161.

11 ALS Association. Ice bucket challenge. http://www.alsa.org/fight-als/ice-bucket-challenge.html. Published 2020. Accessed February 25, 2020.

12 Kamal AH, Bull JH, Wolf SP, et al. Prevalence and predictors of burnout among hospice and palliative care clinicians in the U.S. *J Pain Symptom Manage*. 2016;51(4):690–696. doi:10.1016/j.jpainsymman.2015.10.020.

13 Peters E. Compassion fatigue in nursing: A concept analysis. *Nurs Forum*. 2018;53(4):466–480. doi:10.1111/nuf.12274.

14 Schwartz Rounds and membership. https://www.theschwartzcenter.org/programs/schwartz-rounds. Published 2020. Accessed August 22, 2020.

6 Integration with the Interdisciplinary Care Team

Christopher M. Wilson and Amy J. Litterini

Introduction

A key strength of the palliative care (PC) approach is bringing a variety of team members together in a cohesive and coordinated manner, each of whom has a unique skill set and knowledge base to provide expert care and symptom management for the individual with life-threatening illness. When done right, the team can work like a well-oiled, efficient, effective machine that complements each other's skills and collaborates and refers openly and proactively. Conversely, when there is unclear communication or there is role confusion, care can be inefficient, counterproductive, and even could cause harm. A clear understanding of the interdisciplinary team (IDT) within PC and the myriad individuals who provide care or supportive roles across the disease journey is essential to achieve optimal outcomes.

Importance of Integration into the Interdisciplinary Team

A person with a life-threatening illness will experience a variety of physical, psychosocial, emotional, and spiritual challenges and opportunities across the disease spectrum. Oftentimes, these changes will require the support of the entire IDT and the family/caregivers. Although not detailed specifically in this chapter, the individual facing the illness and their family are critically important members of the IDT, and nuances of their roles are highlighted in Chapter 5. For the care team to best provide patient/family-centered care, it is imperative that all team members actively seek opportunities to collaborate and complement each other's skills. No member of the team can be an expert in everything, and when an issue is identified, it is important that the expert of that domain is promptly consulted.[1] In order to accomplish this goal, the therapist should strive to understand each professional's role and develop a collegial, personal relationship.[1]

In 2013, Nancarrow et al.[2] described key reasons for the need for IDT care as follows:

1   An aging population with frail older people and larger numbers of patients with more complex needs associated with chronic diseases;

2   The increasing complexity of skills and knowledge required to provide comprehensive care to patients;
3   Increasing specialization within health professions and a corresponding fragmentation of disciplinary knowledge resulting in no [individual] healthcare professional being able to meet all the complex needs of their patients;
4   The current emphasis in many countries' policy documents on multi-professional teamwork and development of shared learning;
5   The pursuit of continuity of care within the move toward continuous quality improvement.[2]

For the therapist, there may be competing demands for full integration with the care team.[3] Table 6.1 highlights common barriers to therapist integration with suggestions to navigate or manage these challenges.

Case Study: NG was a 53-year-old male with a history of metastatic colon cancer. His past medical history was otherwise unremarkable. He was married with a very supportive family. He had been in the hospital multiple times for chemotherapy and complications of cancer. Recent scans demonstrated progressive disease with abdominal carcinomatosis. He had several rounds of chemotherapy and presented to the emergency department with intractable nausea and vomiting. A nasogastric tube was placed to address his bowel obstruction. Initially, his goal was to receive more chemotherapy and get better in order to achieve his personal goal of being able to walk his daughter down the aisle for her upcoming wedding.

It was over several meetings with the PC nurse practitioners (NP) that NG mentioned another goal when it was becoming evident that curative care may not be achievable. He and his wife had just closed on a cottage on Lake Huron in northeast Michigan, USA. He wanted to spend time there, to dangle his feet in the water. It became evident that both of his goals were logical and reasonable but that one would have to come at the expense of the other.

Once this new achievable care goal was identified, the entire IDT united to assist in pursuing this goal. The PC physician coordinated the PC IDT via team meetings. In addition, he was the point of contact with NG's attending physician and other consultants, including NG's medical oncologist and gastroenterologist to keep them all appraised of the NG's new goal. The PC NPs conducted daily rounds in the acute hospital setting to assure optimal pain control and that tests, procedures, and other medical interventions would contribute toward his goal of discharge. A key role of the PC NP was to carefully examine if an ordered medical procedure was necessary to assure safe discharge or improve quality of life (QoL) and open a dialogue with the ordering provider. The nursing team organized and administered the care plan within the context of the patient's daily status. The social worker facilitated discharge planning and provided coping strategies during this difficult time. Although the patient was not overtly religious, the pastoral care chaplain let NG and his family know that he was available and could provide another 'non-medical'

Table 6.1 Barriers to Therapist Integration and Suggestions to Address Them

Administrative Barriers to IDT Integration	Potential Impact If Not Addressed	Possible Solution	Positive Outcomes
Productivity demands	Therapists not able to participate in "non-billable" time like rounds and team meetings	Closely track key healthcare metrics to contextualize the value and quality of PC-focused therapists	Reducing length of stay or readmissions and more referrals from new referring providers
Non-PC patient care priorities (e.g. orthopedics prioritized over PC)	Delayed hospital discharge, increased length of stay	Attend IDT meetings to determine which palliative patients are highest priority	Reduction in falls and optimum discharge recommendations
Resource or payment issues limiting therapist care with PC patients	Not enough therapist hours or resources to cover palliative patients and non-palliative patients	Strategically dose visit frequency as some palliative patients do not require daily visits	Reduced overall cost of hospital stay as an indirect value of therapist services to the health system
Not integrated as a member of the PC IDT team	Therapists consulted too late to be impactful on discharge planning or not able to provide care	In collaboration with his/her manager, the therapist should invite self to IDT meetings	Consulted on PC patients earlier during hospital stay for more effective, timely treatments
Practicing in a separate physical location or institution than the IDT (e.g. outpatient clinic)	Disjointed care and feeling 'out of the loop' and not being able to align therapy goals to overall goals and medical status	Most PC teams have a conference call option for offsite members to participate	Improved coordination of care and remaining connected with the patient's overall care goals and disease trajectory

IDT = Interdisciplinary Team, PC = Palliative Care.

person to talk to during this difficult time, of which NG's family verbalized appreciation. In this institution, the chaplain also helped to facilitate completion of the advance care directive.

The occupational therapist (OT) discussed safe performance of activities of daily living (ADL), especially as his physical capabilities changed due to the advancing disease process. In addition, NG was coached in energy conservation and pacing techniques to allow him to conserve energy for important or life-enriching activities. As NG was ambulatory without any significant strength or balance deficits, the physical therapist (PT) initiated an exercise prescription to build up his endurance and functional capacity in anticipation of his future disease trajectory. Although not consistently part of the PC rounds, there were several other disciplines that played key roles in facilitating achievement of NG's care goals. With this coordination of care, NG was able to travel to his cottage after the hospital admission and he was also able to get to his cottage several more times with his family during the subsequent months.

Multidisciplinary Palliative Care Meetings or Rounds

There are a substantial and varied number of healthcare professionals who may be assisting with various aspects of care of an individual with a chronic, life-threatening, or terminal illness. Within this care team are medical and nonmedical professionals and individuals at a variety of educational levels and specialty training. In order to provide individualized, person-centered care, it is imperative that the IDT work as a cohesive, synchronized unit. Currently, within PC teams, therapists are not consistently integrated as core IDT members.[3,4] However, when they are integrated, they provide a unique, skilled, and valued perspective that would not otherwise be provided.[5] It is a beneficial opportunity for the therapist to receive critical information about the patient's disease prognosis as well as internal and environmental/contextual factors that will help the therapist in their provision of patient- and family-centered care.[6] Many healthcare systems that have PC IDTs will also have some form of interdisciplinary PC meetings to discuss the care of individuals with chronic or life-threatening issues. In addition, healthcare systems that care for individuals with cancer will also have regularly recurring tumor boards and multidisciplinary clinics.

Within the healthcare system, many hospitals have convened these PC IDT meetings on a regular basis to facilitate the exchange of information and discuss beneficial next steps. Although it behooves the palliative therapist to participate in these meetings to get an overall understanding of a variety of disease trajectories and learn more about the navigation and care of the patient with a life-threatening illness, there are also valuable pieces of information that a therapist can convey to provide immediately applicable care improvements.[3] For example, the odds of 30-day readmissions were 3.78 times greater when a physical therapist was absent from the interdisciplinary team compared with the odds of 30-day readmissions when a physical therapist participated in the interdisciplinary team. In addition, the odds of 30-day readmission for patients discharged to their home were 2.47 times greater than those who were not discharged to their home.[7]

Although this attendance may not be considered traditionally "productive" or "billable" patient care time, the reduction in readmissions and associated cost savings likely outweigh the revenue produced by a therapist in seeing an additional patient instead of attending the IDT meeting.

In addition, the therapist should strive to be a productive and active participant in this care team meeting in order to provide the best patient/family-centered care.[8] Professional confidence and courage is an essential skill to embody one of the main roles of the therapist within PC, that of advocacy for the patient.[6] In order to best serve in this role, the therapist should strive to be prepared before each meeting by obtaining the list of patients that will be discussed on that day and establish which of them have active therapy services. Of those that do have active therapy services, the therapist should proactively review the health record to understand the patient's diagnosis, contextual factors, therapy progress, participation, motivation, and attempt to glean the current goals of care. In some larger institutions, the therapist who attends the PC IDT meetings may not always be the direct care provider for all the patients discussed, as there may be several different therapists or assistants who provide interventions to these patients. In this case, the therapist who attends these PC IDT meetings should prepare to be a communication conduit with the rest of the therapy team, relaying vital messages about relevant patient nuances to all parties. As this may require additional time, the therapist should allocate a sufficient amount of time after the IDT meeting to complete this critical role properly. This can also improve efficiency of the team members; for example, if the therapist attending the IDT meeting finds out that a patient is not appropriate for therapy services or is undergoing a surgical procedure/diagnostic test, this information can be conveyed to the treating therapist who can now pick up a different patient without losing time trying to see the original patient. Finally, to most efficiently utilize resources, the therapist representative on the IDT meeting may be required to represent several disciplines besides their own. For example, if an OT attends the IDT meetings, she or he may be also conveying messages to and from the PT, speech therapists, recreation therapists, and others. This requires the OT to have not only a strong understanding of the patient's condition but also a clear understanding of the unique roles and skills of their ancillary team colleagues within PC.

In some healthcare systems, patients in PC may be housed throughout the hospital and spread out among many floors and hospital units, while other healthcare systems may have a PC or hospice or EoL ward or unit in their institution.[6] If the patients are centrally located, the PC rounds may be performed in a 'walking rounds' format where the healthcare team as a group may walk from room to room and discuss each patient's status and needed next steps. In different institutions this may occur outside of the patients' rooms or inside the room to integrate the patient and family into the care discussion. Including patients and families in IDT rounds has unique benefits and challenges, which must be considered carefully.[9] It is certainly beneficial because the patient is able to participate in the conversation and understand key information on the nuances of their care provision. Conversely, in larger healthcare systems this may not be feasible if the patients are not centrally located in one ward in the hospital or if there are a large number of patient cases to discuss. In these scenarios, the care team will generally meet in a central location (e.g. conference room) to discuss their thoughts about the patient's case. After the meeting is concluded, one or two providers will follow up with the patient and their family to convey the messages and suggested the next steps of the PC team.[6] This method, although somewhat more disjointed, still allows for patient and family input and participation into care decisions, while still facilitating team input into a unified set of recommendations for care.

Another frequently encountered dilemma by therapists as it relates to the interdisciplinary care team is when a therapist has valuable but negative, news to convey to the care team. Illustrative of this is an example of JP, a 59-year-old male who was an executive at an automobile manufacturing company in metropolitan-Detroit, Michigan. He had been previously diagnosed with lung cancer with spinal metastasis. At the level of the T12 vertebrae, the spinal metastasis began to encroach on the spinal cord causing progressive lower extremity paralysis and an inability to walk. During physical therapy, he was working exceptionally hard to return to his previous ambulatory state, including subjecting himself to a substantial amount of pain. The PT felt that JP was pushing himself harder than what was medically advisable in light of his vertebral body destruction and spinal cord compression. During therapy, JP's pain was rated 10 out of 10 and his rating of perceived exertion (RPE) on the Borg scale[10] was 17/20, despite the PT recommending that JP keep his pain level approximately a 5/10 and his RPE to a 13/20. In discussion with nursing after physical therapy sessions, it was discovered that JP was requiring so much pain medication after PT that he would sleep quite a bit throughout the day and not be able to interact with his family or participate in other care or entertainment activities.

The PT felt, in his professional opinion, that JP was continuing to work toward a goal that was no longer achievable or advisable. During physical therapy, JP would discuss what he would do when he returned to work after he was cured. This information prompted the PT to approach the attending physician (who was a medical oncologist) to have a conversation about whether JP had recently participated in an in-depth discussion about his goals of care, in light of his medical reality. As the PT's conversation was professional, patient-centered, and diplomatic, the attending physician was exceptionally appreciative of this new information. The physician noted that he thought that JP was progressing well, without difficulty in physical therapy, as he had no reason to perceive otherwise based on JP's subjective reports. With this new information from the PT, the attending physician initiated a PC consultation for the care team to discuss the overall goals of care and further clarify that JP's condition was going to worsen as opposed to improve.

Although this was difficult information for JP and his family to digest, the PC IDT was now able to help them to establish new care goals and support them through this challenging time. Regarding his physical therapy sessions, the PT and JP were able to come to a mutually agreeable therapeutic intervention goal. In addition to continuing to incrementally work on ambulation and standing (as this was the patient's long-term goal, so he could maintain hope), JP agreed to stop or rest if his pain was too severe during physical therapy to avoid negatively impacting his remaining QoL and avoid accelerating his spinal cord compression and lower extremity dysfunction. Finally, JP and the PT also agreed to begin working on slide board transfers to a wheelchair and family training in using a mechanical lift for out-of-bed activities. This continued throughout the hospital stay and JP was able to return home. It was anticipated that he would be able to live out the rest of his life in the comfort of his home as he had the equipment, skills, and family support to be successful.

Emotional Needs and Self Care of Interdisciplinary Team Members

One of the most underestimated but important roles of the interdisciplinary care team is to serve as a 'support group' for each other. Burnout syndrome is the chronic long-term emotional distress of healthcare professionals providing care for those in challenging health situations and is a concern in PC (see Chapter 5).[11] An additional concept is compassion fatigue, where providers who are working with those who are suffering often experience emotional consequences to providing care, termed the 'cost of caring.'[12] An inverse term to compassion fatigue is the concept of compassion satisfaction, where healthcare providers experience "emotional rewards of caring for others in a health care context; clinicians feel a sense of return or incentive by seeing a 'change for the better' in patients and families."[12] Best practices for addressing burnout and compassion fatigue include participating in mindfulness, meditation, and creative writing, of which effectiveness was established in a randomized controlled trial.[13] A mixed-methods study in Portugal cited the impactful role of the IDT in protecting against burnout, which may lend credence to the benefit of shared decision-making and the 'support group' concept within the IDT.[14] In addition to the clinical benefit of supporting team members during difficult times, a therapist providing emotional support and encouragement firmly establishes him or her as a valuable member of the team.

Reporting Structure for Therapists in Palliative Care Situations

One of the challenges that therapists might face within the role of PC is identifying who to collaborate with in order to coordinate and optimize patient care. Although it is logical to assume that the referring physician would be the first point of contact in an acute hospital or inpatient setting, this physician may be a consultant, and the therapist may be better served to interact with the patient's attending physician first. In some cases, the PC physician or other PC team member may provide the therapist with a consult to assist with the management of symptoms, physical mobility, and transitions in care planning (a.k.a. discharge planning). Although this referral and information may be discussed in PC IDT meetings, should any action need to be taken, the therapist may need to closely consider to whom to communicate this information. When in doubt, the attending physician is generally an appropriate first contact point. This decision-making process also relies heavily on the personal relationships that the therapist has with the rest of the care team members and the communication culture of the therapist's institution (see Box 6.1).

As with the previously illustrated case of JP, therapists can be an essential component in helping to identify and facilitate when the PC service may be needed to help with coordination of care, management of symptoms, and discussion of long-term care goals. As not every healthcare professional has a full understanding of the services of PC, a therapist abruptly calling the attending physician and saying "I think your patient needs palliative care" would be inadvisable and may damage the therapist-physician relationship. In addition, the well-intentioned therapist may not be privy to certain contextual or medical details, and this recommendation may be misperceived as giving up on the patient or stepping beyond the therapist's clinical role.

Box 6.1 Questions to Consider If a Palliative Care Consultation Would Be Beneficial

When a PC consultation may be warranted:

- The patient is experiencing challenges from pain or symptoms
- You have a feeling that the curative treatment options could do more harm than good
- The patient would benefit from goals-of-care discussions
- The patient and family are distressed at worsening medical news
- There are complex social, economic, or environmental issues
- Would you be surprised to learn this patient died in the next 12–18 months?

As the therapist's primary role, in this case is to be an advocate for the patient's QoL, a tactful, strategic conversation is warranted. Many additional skills and resources can be found in Chapter 7. A better conversation between the therapist and physician may be:

> "Good morning doctor. Thank you for the opportunity to work with your patient JP. He and I have been working towards some very important goals, but during our therapy sessions I noticed that his pain and symptoms were continuing to limit his progress in therapy. In addition, he repeatedly mentions that he is looking forward to being cured and going back to work. I wanted to make sure that you were aware and had all the information to help provide him the best care you can. In your opinion, do you feel that he has a full grasp of his medical situation? Do you think there is any other steps that we need to take to help him understand his disease reality?"

Care Team Members

Attending Physician

As was described earlier, the attending physician is focusing on overall co-ordination of care, consultation with specialists, ordering (or collaborating on) diagnostic tests, procedures, or medications. In the ambulatory or outpatient setting, this may be the patient's general practitioner or family medicine physician. Useful information for the therapist to gather from the attending physician includes the patient's overall understanding of the medical situation, diagnostic decision-making, and disease prognostication. For example, if a therapist suspects that the client/patient may have developed a deep vein thrombosis after observation of new-onset unilateral lower extremity swelling and tenderness, a call to the attending physician would be warranted. The therapist would coordinate with the attending physician to discuss if and when a diagnostic test would be appropriate. One important consideration for the therapist to ponder is that in some cases, diagnostic tests, especially invasive ones, may not be appropriate to order depending on the patient's prognosis.[15] If a new medical condition was diagnosed in an individual with an imminently terminal illness, should the medical team do anything about it? For example, it may not be advisable to aggressively anticoagulate this individual's deep vein thrombosis in light of his imminent death.[15] Another clinical scenario may be when a patient has a large metastatic bone lesion that could potentially result in a pathologic fracture. In an EoL situation, prophylactic internal fixation surgery may not be medically advisable considering the individual's disease trajectory; surgery may actually worsen the person's QoL or shorten their remaining life.[16] The therapist's understanding of this thought process will help to alleviate some professional distress regarding this medical ambiguity; however, some anxiety may be unavoidable when working with an individual with a life-threatening illness that has an untreated medical issue. In this case, the therapist is reminded that their patient is in knowledgeable, professional hands and that all efforts are focusing on optimizing the patient's QoL and autonomy.

Palliative Care Physician

This is often a medical physician who receives postgraduate training or board certification as a PC specialist.[17] This board certification process involves specialized education in advanced, aggressive symptom management, palliative conversations, and EoL care to facilitate hospice admission or to optimize the dying process.[17] This person may be the leader of the PC IDT. When the IDT establishes recommendations for care that would be advisable to convey to other physicians, the message may be best conveyed via a 'peer-to-peer' discussion between physician colleagues. This may be beneficial, as in some institutions there remains a hierarchical system where therapists, nurses, or other ancillary team members may be perceived by some as subordinate to physicians; however, in the 21st-century healthcare environment, this is rapidly changing.[18]

A relatively novel but essential component to PC is the use of physician assistants (PA) or NPs to serve as a care extender to the physician – sometimes these professionals are termed mid-level providers. As with their physician colleagues, specialty training in PC for these team members is available. Oftentimes, these individuals may provide more of the direct care counseling, setting goals of care while providing crucial information for the PC physician to make care recommendations and decisions. Often, these PAs and NPs are trained at the post-baccalaureate level (masters or doctorate) – this is especially relevant when attempting to understand the difference between an NP and a registered nurse. In broad terms, an NP functions more closely to a physician or a PA. The roles of the registered nurse tend to frequently revolve around direct care provision on an ongoing or extended basis, as opposed to the consultant role more often performed by the NP.

Nurses

Therapists will mainly interact with nurses (aka registered nurse) during an acute hospitalization, in an inpatient rehabilitation setting, skilled nursing facility, or in home care; however, nurses will be integral to PC provision in any setting. As most therapists have had some opportunity for interaction with nurses, they will likely be familiar with the fact that the nurses often facilitate the day-to-day care activities of a patient during an inpatient stay or provide care in a home setting. Nurses are an invaluable resource of information exchange with therapists who will be assisting in the physical activity and therapeutic care of individuals in these settings.[4] Prior to the initiation of a therapeutic intervention, it is highly recommended that the therapist review all relevant medical record documents. Before interacting with the patient, collaborate with the nurse to gather the latest and most relevant information, especially things that might not be fully conveyed within the medical record. Valuable information that may be exchanged with the patient's nurse includes the patient's current physical status, such as pain, vital signs, mood, or affect. In addition, valuable contextual information should be requested, including the patient's ability or willingness to participate in therapy. Examples include if the patient had recently received bad medical news, was considering transitioning to hospice/EoL care, or a diagnostic test had come back with a disappointing result.

In addition, nurses can provide contextual information about the social and family situation, as it would be valuable for the therapist to know whether he or she was walking into an intense family argument or emotional moment. This might be a case where the therapist may elect to schedule a different time for therapy for the benefit of all involved. Finally, nurses will also be the coordinator and/or supervisor for healthcare assistants.[19] In different nations, practice settings, roles, or institutions, these individuals may be called home health aides, nursing assistants, or nurse technicians. On many occasions, this individual will report directly to the nurse to provide direct care activities that do not require the skill of a licensed or registered nurse. In addition, these healthcare assistants can be a valuable source of information on the patient's physical or ADL status as they often perform or assist with many of these activities throughout the day. Conversely, a collegial relationship between nursing personnel and therapy is imperative and is strengthened by the therapist reporting back to the nursing team about how the patient did with therapy. This might include any follow-up care needs and recommendations or training to the nursing team as to how best to assist with care activities based on the patient's current functional status. In 2020, Campbell, Trojanowski, and Smith[20] described an EoL simulation involving both nursing students and PT students and found that participating in EoL simulations helped students understand their own roles in this area as well as the importance of interprofessional team collaboration. Additional simulations and activities such as this one may help to further reinforce the integral relationship between PC and EoL care.

Chaplain/Spiritual Leader/Religious Counselor

One notable difference from PC teams as opposed to other interdisciplinary care teams is the presence of a spiritual or religious advisor. Even in the cases where the patient, family, or even the therapists do not hold to specific religious beliefs, there is an essential and integral role of the spiritual care professional.[21] As would be expected when facing the EoL, those who follow certain spiritual or religious beliefs will place an increasingly heavy emphasis on participating in religious or spiritual ceremonies and conferring frequently on medical decisions with a religious or spiritual advisor.[22] One of the domains that Cicely Saunders discussed in her definition of Total Pain (as discussed in Chapter 1) was the concept of spiritual pain or distress.[23] As with other forms of psychosocial distress, spiritual pain may also amplify or increase a person's perception of physical pain or symptoms (see Chapter 17). A potentially impactful pain management intervention for a therapist is to recognize spiritual or existential distress and initiate a referral to a spiritual care provider; this is not a first-line pain intervention commonly taught to therapists in entry level training.

In some areas where there is a homogeneous religious population, the spiritual care professional may be a pastor from the dominant religion. For example, in Ireland, where Roman Catholicism is practiced by a substantial number of individuals, the spiritual care representative on the IDT may be a Catholic priest, or in predominantly Muslim locales, this may be an Imam/Islamic religious leader. In other more heterogeneous populations with many diverse religious or spiritual affiliations for the patient population, the spiritual care chaplain may not be of a specific religious denomination but serve as an overall spiritual care supporter.[24] He or she may also focus on facilitating communication between an individual's personal religious leader during a hospitalization or other inpatient stay.

In 2016, Lebaron et al.[24] examined the ways that community clergy members provide EoL care via a qualitative study. They proposed three main focuses of these individuals' care provision – the concepts of *being*, *doing*, and *believing*.

Being: The clergy member "listen[s] carefully to patients, families, and health-care providers to understand more deeply the difficult medical choices under consideration."[24]

Doing: In this role the clergy can serve by "praying for wisdom as patients face medical choices and direct facilitation of spiritual practices that remove anxiety, fear, and anger and help the patient look beyond their death to faith and hope in God."[24]

Believing: In this capacity, a clergy member would help an individual identify "doctrines within their faith tradition that most appropriately apply to the medical context and specific choices that must be made."[24]

One of the additional benefits of the spiritual care professionals, even if the individual or family is not religious or spiritual, is that the spiritual care professional is not a medical professional and is generally perceived to be a neutral mediator between the physician/medical team and the patient to discuss non-medical implications of medical decisions.[21,24] Therapists working with individuals with life-threatening illnesses should be screening for spiritual or emotional distress, and proactively offer the services of a spiritual care professional if needs are identified or if the person simply needs someone to talk to and the therapist is limited in time, topic proficiency, or comfort level.

Useful information regarding therapist care from the spiritual care professional includes the individual's spiritual perception, traditions, family support, and also general psychosocial and family dynamics.[25] Even though conversations related to family dynamics or psychosocial/emotional issues are not explicitly religious, these issues often come up during therapist interventions. Preemptive conversations with the spiritual care professionals will provide the therapist with useful information during these forthcoming conversations. This contextual information will help the therapist to provide the best patient- and family-centered care.[25] Finally, if there are certain times or days where sacred ceremonies or prayer may occur, this knowledge will help the therapist to coordinate around these times to avoid interrupting these important activities.

Social Worker or Counselor

Another integral member of the PC team is the social worker or counselor. In different institutions, this person may have formal social work training or be a trained counselor. A key role of social workers or counselors is to help identify and assist with psychosocial, emotional, and logistical issues during a disease process or hospital stay. In non-PC situations, these issues are often handled by the medical and nursing team members without integrated need for social work or counselors; however, as these issues take on an increasingly dominant role when approaching the EoL, a specific, dedicated professional to assist with this is imperative. There are a wide variety of roles that the social worker serves on the PC team and it generally depends on the needs of the institution and who else is available to also perform some of these roles.[26] In some occasions, the social worker is the person to facilitate and document the advance care directive or advance care planning document (see Appendix 1). This individual can also help to provide counseling services or recommendations for coping strategies. This may include meditation, reflective journaling, and advice on navigating family dynamics.

The therapist's interaction with the social worker/counselor is a very valuable relationship, as the therapist can provide information that they have learned to help the social worker/counselor perform their job to the best of their abilities, and vice-versa. If the social worker was only peripherally monitoring the patient's case due to minimal needs, the therapist would be able to communicate new or evolving needs, distress, or anxiety and proactive interventions could be administered. Conversely, the therapist can gather a significant amount of useful contextual information about the individual's living environment, prior functional level, life goals, key family relationships, and current goals of care. Likewise, the social worker can relay information to the therapist regarding a patient's fears or anxieties related to their condition and any potential goals relating to physical function. An astute therapist can then integrate all these concepts into their physical activity or therapeutic interventions to provide the most optimum patient-centered care to facilitate QoL.

Integrative Medicine Practitioners and Interventions

A holistic approach to care aims to consider the whole person within a patient-practitioner partnership. Integrative medicine combines *complementary*, non-mainstream approaches with conventional medicine. *Alternative* therapies are considered non-mainstream approaches that occur in place of conventional medicine.[27] Integrative medicine and its practitioners, as a representative part of the interdisciplinary care team, may enhance many of the innate goals of skilled rehabilitation, including improved QoL and reduced pain. Techniques such as guided imagery, progressive relaxation, yoga, massage, the use of herbal and botanical supplements, Pilates, tai chi, acupressure/acupuncture, chiropractic medicine, creative arts, music therapy, aromatherapy, and cranial-sacral therapy are examples of commonly used approaches within integrative medicine.

According to the Centers for Disease Control and Prevention National Health Interview Survey, adult use of complementary and alternative medicine (CAM) has increased in the United States between the years 2012 and 2017 (e.g. yoga: from 9.5% to 14.3%; meditation: from 4.1% to 14.2%).[28] With an increased interest in CAM utilization in the general population, and the frequent use of Traditional Medicine internationally (see Chapter 10), there is an increased need for awareness of use, available evidence, and appropriate referrals within hospice and PC. The Hospice and Palliative Nurses Association recommends only licensed and/or certified therapists deliver complementary health approaches.[29]

The available literature of well-designed studies on the use of CAM in hospice and PC is lacking, and/or outcomes often demonstrate mixed results or inadequate evidence to make appropriate generalizable recommendations where benefits outweigh risks for all diagnoses and patients.[30,31] However, Zeng et al.[32] completed a systematic review of 4,682 CAM studies for the management of symptoms in patients receiving hospice and PC, including anxiety, pain, dyspnea, cough, fatigue, insomnia, nausea, and vomiting. Seventeen studies were included for further analysis. Although they concluded that all the studies had significant limitations, they determined that music therapy, massage therapy, and Reiki had the most potential benefit for individuals receiving PC or hospice. Evidence of short-term benefit was noted, with minimal adverse events reported.[32]

Regarding formal rehabilitation, there are several interventions that provide therapy from the perspective of the philosophy of integrative medicine. Art therapy and music therapy are specializations within rehabilitation which perform skilled evaluations, develop plans of care, and perform goal-setting, such as those created by PTs, OTs, and speech therapists, with the use of art media/techniques and music as the intervention modalities. For individuals at the EoL, the use of creative expression can be therapeutic and cathartic in a variety of ways, including life reflection, symptom management, emotional expression, and social support.

Creative Arts: Art Therapy and Music Therapy

According to the American Art Therapy Association, art therapy is "an integrative mental health and human services profession that enriches the lives of individuals, families, and communities through active art-making, creative process, applied psychological theory, and human experience within a psychotherapeutic relationship."[33]

For many patients facing a terminal diagnosis, the ability to find meaning, and actively reminisce about and document their life story can be very beneficial and transformative. Various programs led by art therapists, and artists, often in collaboration with social workers, can be utilized to allow for activities such as creative writing/journaling, art (e.g. paint, clay, sculpture, Papier-mâché, collage), scrapbooking with photos, and other forms of creative expression. These activities may include helping an individual to develop a piece of art or a memory book illustrating their emotions and/or life story. Programs such as the Center for Cancer Care at Exeter Hospital in Exeter, New Hampshire, USA, have had long-standing art services available to their patients for this purpose.[34] Additionally, organizations such as the Alzheimer's Association and Compassus Hospice have programs to create memory or reminiscence books, and life journals, for their clients which ultimately become treasured gifts for their families when the patient passes.[35,36] Often, the art and writing created by the patient are cherished gifts shared at wakes, funerals, and with extended family members as a very personal and heartfelt remembrance of their loved one.

According to the American Music Therapy Association, music therapy is,

> "the clinical and evidence-based use of music interventions to accomplish individualized goals within a therapeutic relationship by a credentialed professional who has completed an approved music therapy program. Music Therapy is an established health profession in which music is used within a therapeutic relationship to address physical, emotional, cognitive, and social needs of individuals."[37]

Schmid et al.[38] completed a systematic review of the use of music therapy by certified music therapists with adults in the PC setting. Twelve studies from 1978 to 2016, both quantitative (9) and qualitative (3), were analyzed for patient and healthcare provider perspectives and identified themes. In the quantitative studies, pain was the most frequently assessed outcome. Positive effects were found in all of the study outcomes, with patients associating music therapy with emotional expression and improved well-being.[38] A meta-analysis of the literature on music therapy in individuals with terminal illness by Qi He Mabel, Drury, and Hong[39] concluded "that patients experienced improved social interaction and communication with the people around them, and a more holistic care for as their physical, psychological and spiritual needs were met." Regarding the type of music therapy recommended, receptive (i.e. listening to music: patients' favorites or classical music) was superior to interactive (i.e. methods involving active participation: singing, playing an instrument) in a systematic review and meta-analysis of 38 trials with 1,418 participants with a diagnosis of dementia. Positive effects were seen in a significant reduction of agitation (Cohen-Mansfield Agitation Inventory: MD = -7.99, 95% CI -5.11 to -0.87) and behavioral problems (Neuropsychiatric Inventory: MD = -3.02 95% CI -5.90 to -0.15) in participants receiving receptive music therapy when compared to usual care.[40]

As the majority of published literature on utilization of CAM pertains to cancer survivors, greater confidence in appropriate recommendations is provided from the volume of published studies. A systematic review of integrative medicine strategies for supportive care of breast cancer survivors was conducted by Greenlee et al.[41] for the development of a clinical practice guideline. Of the 4,900 studies found in their literature search from 1990 to 2013, 203 were eligible for analysis. The authors determined that (1) meditation, yoga, and relaxation with imagery are recommended for routine use for anxiety and mood disorders; and (2) stress management, yoga, massage, music therapy, energy conservation, and meditation are recommended for reducing stress, anxiety, depression, fatigue, and improving QoL.[41]

Additional descriptions and available evidence for the use of Integrative Medicine interventions follow for several types of methods and approaches.

Yoga: For medically compromised patients, yoga practice provides emphasis on flexibility, posture, deep breathing, strength, and relaxation. A systematic review of the effects of yoga on health-related quality of life (HRQoL), mental health, and cancer-related symptoms for female breast cancer survivors was conducted on 24 studies by Cramer et al.[42] Moderate quality evidence was found to recommend yoga as an intervention to address HRQoL, sleep disturbances, depression, anxiety, and fatigue.

Acupuncture: According to a systematic review by Garcia et al.[43] acupuncture is an appropriate intervention for chemotherapy-induced nausea and vomiting. A meta-analysis by Tao et al.[44] found acupuncture to result in small-to-large effects on improving pain, fatigue, sleep disturbance, and gastrointestinal distress. Specific to cancer survivors referred for PC (n = 68), Miller et al.[45] found statistically significant reductions in the symptoms of pain, anxiety, depression, drowsiness, dyspnea, fatigue, nausea, and well-being after the first, and across all subsequent acupuncture treatments ($P < 0.001$).

Massage Therapy: In a review of meta-analyses and systematic reviews, Field[46] documented the benefits of massage in breast cancer survivorship to include pain reduction and immune system benefits, including increased natural killer cells and improved natural killer cell activity.

Guided Imagery or Visualization Exercises: This mind-body therapeutic technique uses the senses, imagination, memory, and sometimes music to decrease stress, alleviate pain, and increase feelings of well-being.[47,48]

Progressive Muscle Relaxation (PMR): This guided approach involves slowly and sequentially tensing and releasing muscles to bring about feelings of relaxation. Studies have indicated that PMR has assisted individuals with breast cancer by reducing nausea, vomiting, anxiety, and depression.[49,50]

Tai chi: A type of martial art that combines low-impact movement, meditation, and breathing and is known to decrease cancer-related fatigue.[51] A systematic review by Pan et al.[52] determined tai chi to be effective in improving upper extremity function (handgrip strength via dynamometry and strength in elbow extension, abduction, and horizontal adduction) in 322 breast cancer survivors when compared to controls.

Reiki: A Japanese healing technique based on the principle of channeling energy via touch to activate natural healing processes, which is known to bring about feelings of deep relaxation, decreased stress, and an increased sense of calm, peace, and well-being.[53] The International Center for Reiki Training indicates that Reiki therapy should be provided only by practitioners who have received a certificate of training in Reiki.[54]

Herbals and Botanicals: Products made from plants, or *botanicals*, when used for the purpose of maintaining health or to treat disease, are considered herbal products. When used solely for internal use in various forms (e.g. powdered, dried, chopped, liquid, or capsule), they are considered *supplements*. Although they are commonly used across the world in Traditional Medicine, they are considered foods rather than drugs by the US Food and Drug Administration and are, therefore, not tested, manufactured, labeled, or regulated in the same ways as medications. Because of this, caution should be taken due to the risk of interaction with conventional medicine, and use should always be discussed with the attending medical provider.[55]

Rehab practitioners are trained to use a variety of techniques, interventions, and approaches to holistically address concerns and symptoms across the continuum of care for individuals at the EoL. Due to the medically compromised nature of these patients and the need to consider contraindications by diagnosis and treatment regimen, an evidence-based approach is necessary to make safe recommendations for the right technique, for the patient, at the right time. Additionally, cultural awareness and humility are required by the IDT to consider the influence of cultural and spiritual beliefs on patient and family choices at the EoL. Insurers are slowly realizing the benefits of covering strategies such as integrative medicine; however, it is important for rehab practitioners to recognize that the use of specific integrative therapy techniques may be subject to federal, state, and often local municipal regulations that govern the scope of practice, advertising, ethics, professional terminology, and training.

Clinicians who have demonstrated competency following proper training with certification/licensure can utilize various integrative medicine approaches, which may increase well-being, physical and psychological health, and QoL for individuals at the EoL. Ideally, rehabilitation practitioners who do not themselves provide integrative therapies as part of their own individualized training background would collaborate with, and refer to, local and regional integrative therapy practitioners experienced in treating medically complex individuals. Collegial discussions about indications and contraindications help to ensure the safe application of these interventions, and smooth handoffs in PC and hospice. In addition to addressing the long-term side effects of progressive disease and ongoing treatments, by embracing the potential benefits of integrative medicine, clinicians may also help to address the social, spiritual, and emotional domains for individuals receiving PC and hospice.

Summary

The interdisciplinary PC team is a unique, complex, and valuable resource. Therapist involvement in these interdisciplinary care teams can improve care, reduce readmissions, facilitate care planning, and optimize QoL. In order to be an effective care team member, the therapist must understand the roles of each of the team members, participate actively in team meetings, advocate for the patient, and serve as an equal partner for the betterment of the individual's long-term outcomes. Finally, the care team can be a source of emotional support for each other, as caring for those at the EoL is emotionally taxing and burnout is a frequent concern. An important role of the therapist is to support PC colleagues during emotional difficulties and seek out their support as well.

References

1 O'Connor M, Fisher C. Exploring the dynamics of interdisciplinary palliative care teams in providing psychosocial care: "Everybody thinks that everybody can do it and they can't." *J Palliat Med.* 2011;14(2):191–196. doi:10.1089/jpm.2010.0229.
2 Nancarrow SA, Booth A, Ariss S, Smith T, Enderby P, Roots A. Ten principles of good interdisciplinary teamwork. *Human Resour Health.* 2013;11(1):19. doi:10.1186/1478-4491-11-19.
3 Wilson CM, Barnes C. Physical therapy in interdisciplinary palliative care and hospice teams. *Rehabil Oncol.* 2018;36(2):143–145. doi:10.1097/01.REO.0000000000000109.
4 Wilson C, Mueller K, Briggs R. Physical therapists' contribution to the hospice and palliative care interdisciplinary team: A clinical summary. *J Hosp Palliat Nurs.* 2017;19(6):588–596.
5 Harding Z, Hall C, Lloyd A. Rehabilitation in palliative care a qualitative study of team professionals. *BMJ Support Palliat Care.* 2019. doi:bmjspcare-002008.
6 Goldsmith J, Wittenberg-Lyles E, Rodriguez D, Sanchez-Reilly S. Interdisciplinary geriatric and palliative care team narratives: Collaboration practices and barriers. *Qual Health Res.* 2010;20(1):93–104. doi:10.1177/1049732309355287.
7 Kadivar Z, English A, Marx BD. Understanding the relationship between physical therapist participation in interdisciplinary rounds and hospital readmission rates: Preliminary study. *Phys Ther.* 2016;96(11):1705–1713.
8 Sims S, Hewitt G, Harris R. Evidence of collaboration, pooling of resources, learning and role blurring in interprofessional healthcare teams: A realist synthesis. *J Interprof Care.* 2015;29(1):20–25. doi:10.3109/13561820.2014.939745.
9 Hui D, Bruera E. Integrating palliative care into the trajectory of cancer care. *Nat Rev Clin Oncol.* 2016;13(3):159–171. Accessed November 3, 2019. doi:10.1038/nrclinonc.2015.201.
10 Ritchie C. Rating of perceived exertion (RPE). *J Physiother.* 2012;58(1):62. doi:10.1016/S1836-9553(12)70078-4.
11 Martins Pereira S, Fonseca AM, Sofia Carvalho A. Burnout in palliative care: A systematic review. *Nurs Ethics.* 2011;18(3):317–326.
12 Slocum-Gori S, Hemsworth D, Chan WW, Carson A, Kazanjian A. Understanding compassion satisfaction, compassion fatigue and burnout: A survey of the hospice palliative care workforce. *Palliat Med.* 2013(27):172–178.
13 Baird K, Kracen AC. Vicarious traumatization and secondary traumatic stress: A research synthesis. *Couns Psychol Q.* 2006;19(2):181–188. doi:10.1080/09515070600811899.
14 Hernández-Marrero P, Pereira SM, Carvalho AS. Ethical decisions in palliative care: Interprofessional relations as a burnout protective factor? Results from a mixed-methods multicenter study in Portugal. *Am J Hosp Palliat Care.* 2016;33(8):723–732. doi:1210.1177/1049909115583486.
15 Schouten HJ, Koek HL, Kruisman-Ebbers M, et al. Decisions to withhold diagnostic investigations in nursing home patients with a clinical suspicion of venous thromboembolism. *PloS one.* 2014;9(3):e90395.
16 Cheung FH. The practicing orthopedic surgeon's guide to managing long bone metastases. *Orthop Clin North Am.* 2014;45(1):109–119. doi:10.1016/j.ocl.2013.09.003.

17 Gunten CFv, Sloan PA, Portenoy RK, Schonwetter RS. Physician board certification in hospice and palliative medicine. *J Palliat Med*. 2000;3(4):441–447. doi:10.1089/jpm.2000.3.4.441.

18 Kaplan K, Mestel P, Feldman DL. Creating a culture of mutual respect. *AORN J*. 2010;91(4):495–510.

19 Ingleton C, Chatwin J, Seymour J, Payne S. The role of health care assistants in supporting district nurses and family carers to deliver palliative care at home: Findings from an evaluation project. *J Clin Nurs*. 2011;20(13–14):2043. doi:10.1111/j.1365-2702.2010.03563.x.

20 Campbell D, Trojanowski S, Smith LM. An interprofessional end-of-life simulation to improve knowledge and attitudes of end-of-life care amongst nursing and physical therapy students. *Rehabil Oncol*. 2020;38(1):45–51. doi:10.1097/01.REO.0000000000000192.

21 Cooper RS. The palliative care chaplain as story catcher. *J Pain Symptom Manage*. 2018;55(1):155–158. doi:10.1016/j.jpainsymman.2017.03.035.

22 Perkins HS. *A Guide to Psychosocial and Spiritual Care at the End of Life*. 1st ed. New York, NY: Springer; 2016. 10.1007/978-1-4939-6804-6.

23 Clark D. Total pain: The work of Cicely Saunders and the hospice movement. *Am Pain Soc Bull*. 2000;10(4):13–15.

24 Lebaron VT, Smith PT, Quiñones R, et al. How community clergy provide spiritual care: Toward a conceptual framework for clergy end-of-life education. *J Pain Symptom Manage*. 2016;51(4):673–681. doi:10.1016/j.jpainsymman.2015.11.016.

25 Sargeant MD, Newsham RK. Physical therapist students' perceptions of spirituality and religion in patient care. *J Phys Ther Ed*. 2012;26(2):63–73. doi:10.1097/00001416-201201000-00010.

26 Weisenfluh SM, Csikai EL. Professional and educational needs of hospice and palliative care social workers. *J Soc Work End Life Palliat Care*. 2013;9(1):58–73.

27 Complementary, Alternative, or Integrative Health: What's in a Name? National Center for Complementary and Integrative Health website. https://nccih.nih.gov/health/integrative-health. Updated June 2016. Accessed June 17, 2020.

28 Centers for Disease Control and Prevention. NCHS, National Health Interview Survey, 2012 and 2017. https://www.cdc.gov/nchs/data/databriefs/db325-h.pdf. Published November 2018. Accessed June 16, 2020.

29 Hospice and Palliative Nurses Association. HPNA position statement: Complementary therapies in palliative nursing practice. 2015. https://advancingexpertcare.org/position-statements. Published 2015. Accessed June 17, 2020.

30 Anandarajah G, Mennillo HA, Rachu G, Harder T, Ghosh J. Lifestyle medicine interventions in patients with advanced disease receiving palliative or hospice care. *Am J Lifestyle Med*. 2019;14(3):243–257. doi:10.1177/1559827619830049.

31 Coelho A, Parola V, Cardoso D, Bravo ME, Apóstolo J. Use of non-pharmacological interventions for comforting patients in palliative care: A scoping review. *JBI Database System Rev Implement Rep*. 2017;15(7):1867–1904. doi:10.11124/JBISRIR-2016-003204.

32 Zeng YS, Wang C, Ward KE, Hume AL. Complementary and alternative medicine in hospice and palliative care: A systematic review. *J Pain Symptom Manage*. 2018;56(5):781–794.e4. doi:10.1016/j.jpainsymman.2018.07.016.

33 American Art Therapy Association. About art therapy. https://arttherapy.org/about-art-therapy/ Published 2017. Accessed August 22, 2020.

34 Exeter Hospital, Cancer Wellness Services: Healing Arts Program. https://www.exeterhospital.com/Services/cancer-care/cancer-wellness. Exeter Hospital website. Published 2016. Accessed August 22, 2020.

35 Alzheimer's Association. https://www.alz.org/. Published 2020. Accessed August 22, 2020.

36 Compassus Hospice. https://campaigns.compassus.com/. Compassus Hospice website. Published 2020. Accessed February 25, 2020.

37 American Music Therapy Association. What is music therapy. https://www. musictherapy.org/about/musictherapy/. Published 2020. Accessed February 25, 2020.

38 Schmid W, Rosland JH, von Hofacker S, Hunskår I, Bruvik F. Patient's and health care provider's perspectives on music therapy in palliative care - an integrative review. *BMC Palliat Care*. 2018;17(1):32. Published February 20, 2018. doi:10.1186/s12904-018-0286-4.

39 Qi He Mabel L, Drury VB, Hong PW. The experience and expectations of terminally ill patients receiving music therapy in the palliative setting: a systematic review. *JBI Libr Syst Rev*. 2010;8(27):1088–1111. doi:10.11124/01938924-201008270-00001.

40 Tsoi KKF, Chan JYC, Ng YM, Lee MMY, Kwok TCY, Wong SYS. Receptive music therapy is more effective than interactive music therapy to relieve behavioral and psychological symptoms of dementia: A systematic review and meta-analysis. *J Am Med Dir Assoc*. 2018;19(7):568–576.e3. doi:10.1016/j.jamda.2017.12.009.

41 Greenlee H, Balneaves LG, Carlson LE, et al. Clinical practice guidelines on the use of integrative therapies as supportive care in patients treated for breast cancer. *J Natl Cancer Inst Monogr*. 2014;2014(50):346–358. doi:10.1093/jncimonographs/lgu041.

42 Cramer H, Lauche R, Klose P, Lange S, Langhorst J, Dobos GJ. Yoga for improving health-related quality of life, mental health and cancer-related symptoms in women diagnosed with breast cancer. *Cochrane Database Syst Rev*. 2017. doi:10.1002/14651858.CD010802.pub2.

43 Garcia MK, McQuade J, Haddad R, et al. Systematic review of acupuncture in cancer care: A synthesis of the evidence. *J Clin Oncol*. 2013;31:952–960.

44 Tao WW, Jiang H, Tao XM, Jiang P, Sha LY, Sun XC. Effects of acupuncture, Tuina, tai chi, Qigong, and traditional Chinese medicine five-element music therapy on symptom management and quality of life for cancer patients: A meta-analysis. *J Pain Symptom Manage*. 2016 April 1;51(4):728–747. doi:10.1016/j.jpainsymman.2015.11.027.

45 Miller KR, Patel JN, Symanowski JT, Edelen CA, Walsh D. Acupuncture for cancer pain and symptom management in a palliative medicine clinic. *Am J Hosp Palliat Care*. 2019;36(4):326–332. doi:10.1177/1049909118804464.

46 Field, T. Massage therapy research review. *Complement Ther Clin Pract*. 2014;20(4): 224–229. doi:10.1016/j.ctcp.2014.07.002.

47 Adeola MT, Baird CL, Sands LP, et al. Active despite pain: Patient experiences with guided imagery with relaxation compared to planned rest. *Clin J Oncol Nurs*. 2015;19(6):649–652.

48 Chen SF, Wang HH, Yang HY, Chung UL. Effect of relaxation with guided imagery on the physical and psychological symptoms of breast cancer patients undergoing chemotherapy. *Iran Red Crescent Med J*. 2015;17(11):1–8.

49 Song QH, Xu RM, Zhang QH, Ma M, Zhao XP. Relaxation training during chemotherapy for breast cancer improves mental health and lessens adverse events. *Int J Clin Exp Med*. 2013;6(10):979–984.

50 Zhou K, Li X, Li J, et al. A clinical randomized controlled trial of music therapy and progressive muscle relaxation training in female breast cancer patients after radical mastectomy: Results on depression, anxiety and length of hospital stay. *Eur J Oncol Nurs*. 2015;19(1):54–59.

51 Larkey LK, Roe DJ, Weihs KL, et al. Randomized controlled trial of qigong/tai chi easy on cancer-related fatigue in breast cancer survivors. *Ann Behav Med*. 2015;49(2):165–176.

52 Pan Y, Yang K, Shi X, Liang H, Zhang F, Lv Q. Tai chi chuan exercise for patients with breast cancer: A systematic review and meta-analysis. *Evid Based Complement Alternat Med.* 2015, 535237. doi:10.1155/2015/535237.

53 Kirshbaum MN, Stead M, Bartys S. An exploratory study of reiki experiences in women who have cancer. *Int J Palliat Nurs.* 2016;22(40):166–172.

54 International Center for Reiki Training. 2016. *Reiki classes.* http://www.reiki.org/. Published date unknown. Accessed June 17, 2020.

55 Johns Hopkins Medicine. Herbal medicine. https://www.hopkinsmedicine.org/health/wellness-and-prevention/herbal-medicine. Published 2020. Accessed August 22, 2020.

7 Communication Strategies

Christopher M. Wilson and Amy J. Litterini

Introduction

Communication has evolved to be the linchpin in the provision of modern healthcare. In the past, the paternalistic model of care did not consistently require a thorough explanation of care and options and rationale. Clear and effective communication is especially important in caring for those with chronic or life-threatening illnesses. Unfortunately, communication in these scenarios is fraught with emotion, anxiety, misguided hopes, and unclear care goals in an evolving or worsening medical situation. Even veteran therapists with decades of experience have voiced anxiety and concern when caring for these individuals as they do not want to say the wrong thing or provide an inappropriate or mixed message. Fortunately, with deliberate practice, mentoring, and utilizing evidence-based communication strategies, a therapist can learn and proficiently apply these skills.

The Critical Therapist Skill of Communication

The first skill of communication that is essential to palliative care (PC) and hospice practice is that of listening. While the therapist may have much to share, the basis for that comes from understanding the patient's perspective, what they have experienced, what is going on now, and perhaps, their emotions related to what the future will hold. Open-ended and patient-centered questions such as "How have things been going for you?", "How have you been feeling with all of this?", or even "Can you give voice to those tears?" are not presumptive of their experience and may guide the discussion, even with one's prior knowledge of medical history. Open, reflective listening allows the therapist to build trust and provide opportunities for meaningful exchange.[1] In the authors' experience, some therapy sessions with this patient population may consist of sitting and listening to the patient's needs, emotions, and concerns. Although not likely to be a substantial portion of the therapist's entry-level training, this skill of listening and being present, may prove to be more therapeutic and helpful than physical activity measures.

In traditional therapist clinical practice with individuals without a life-threatening illness, conversations that are exceptionally difficult, existential, or spiritual in origin are uncommon; however, these types of conversations occur quite often in PC and are often invited by the more intimate patient-therapist relationship as suggested earlier. As the individual begins to have more anxiety and is progressively facing their own mortality, questions or topics may occur organically during therapy or physical activity session. As therapists often build long-term, close relationships with individuals as a result of their series of longer-duration visits over weeks and months, the therapist is perceived to be a trusted, knowledgeable, moral professional by the person. This may result in the therapist facing questions like "What do you think happens after you die?", "Do you think there is a God?", and asking the therapist their opinion about the individual's very personal family dynamic issues. In the authors' experience, these are not lines of inquiry that therapists are fully prepared to address in their entry-level training. Some experienced therapists acquire this critical skill set by trial-and-error, observing others, or sharing among the IDT; however, there are a wide variety of training options and strategic approaches that can assist all PC providers to feel more equipped and empowered to communicate effectively with persons with a life-threatening illness.

The Therapist as a Beacon of Hope

One of the primary challenges facing therapists when working with individuals with a life-threatening illness includes balancing the role of an advocate for the patient while maintaining some semblance of hope that "life is still worth living." A core facet of the human living experience is optimism, hope, and excitement for what the future brings.[2] If this is taken away or not carefully kindled, a person is merely existing, not living. However, the therapist's role in enkindling hope, if not approached carefully, can result in increased confusion and distress. The challenge is to foster hope *in the context of reality*, while acknowledging that hope changes over time throughout the disease trajectory.

With a life-threatening disease process, the individual and their family will inevitably receive more increasingly negative news about their disease process and overall prognosis. It is in these moments of vulnerability that these individuals and families will actively seek out any signs of positive news that may contradict or devalue the negative news. Physical performance, pain, and activity of daily living (ADL) performance are extremely tangible, visible, and understandable measures for patients and families to consider. As described by Kubler-Ross,[3] one of the stages of loss and grief is denial; if a patient and family have not accepted the truth of the medical reality or are hoping for a "miracle," improved gait, decreased pain, and new physical capabilities can result in confusion and could potentially provide false or inappropriate hope. Although it is often a tendency of the therapist to embrace this perception and maintain the highest level of hope possible, it is generally not in the best interest of the patients and families who are facing a progressive, ongoing disease process. Useful messaging may include,

> It is good that you are now able to perform this task and we should focus on what new things you wish to do with this new task that you were not able to previously accomplish. These gains may be temporary because of your progressive disease process, but you have worked very hard to achieve this and you should be proud. Let's discuss how to utilize this to help with your quality of life.

This messaging honors and acknowledges the person's hard work, reminds them of the inevitable disease process, and yet strives to leverage new functional gains, however temporary, into improving patient-centered tasks that they may wish to accomplish.

Transtheoretical Model

Within wellness and health promotion coaching is the concept of the transtheoretical model of behavior change (Figure 7.1).[4] This model is often used for making healthy behavior changes. It has been frequently employed in areas such as substance use disorder rehabilitation, smoking cessation, and weight loss.[5] Similarly, it is important for individuals with a terminal illness to come to a realization that their behaviors and thought processes may necessitate change to be able to focus on quality of life (QoL) and adapt around this evolving disease state and physical status. This recognition by the therapist, and identification of the individual's state of mind, will help facilitate conversations and provide efficacious treatment. For example, if the therapist is advocating for use of a mechanical lift for transfers out of bed into a wheelchair, and the individual with the illness is determined to walk again, then a successful therapeutic outcome is not likely. This malalignment of goals should be a higher priority for the therapist to address than the conveying of educational information on using the mechanical lift.

Application of the concepts of the transtheoretical model will be outlined using the case of LM, a 59-year-old male with stage IV metastatic prostate cancer. He had not gone to the doctor for years until he reported difficulty

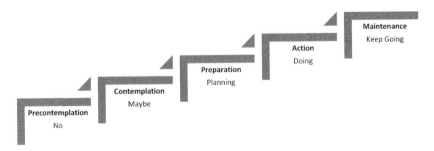

Figure 7.1 Transtheoretical Model of Behavior Change.

initiating a urine stream. He was an automotive worker and had his own shop repairing vehicles, which was very time-consuming and stressful. He smoked a pack of cigarettes a day and other than his job, led a relatively sedentary lifestyle. He had quite limited health literacy and lived alone, but his elderly parents and one sibling lived nearby.

Precontemplation

Within this stage of the transtheoretical model, the individual does not acknowledge or understand that there is a problem or dilemma. Within the precontemplation stage, without the understanding that a change needs to be made, any suggested plans or strategies introduced will be unsuccessful as the care team is assisting the individual to address a "non-existent" problem.

Case example: LM was subsequently admitted to the hospital and is very weak and not able to get out of bed. The doctors have not been able to stabilize or slow the metastatic spread and growth of his prostate cancer, despite administering the relevant first-line interventions. LM is still focused on a cure and feels that his strength and walking status will "work itself out" when he gets home. The acute care physical therapists (PTs) and occupational therapists (OTs) feel that he is not safe to return home alone as he requires maximum assistance of one to two people to get out of bed and onto a chair. He is not interested in participating in any rehabilitation at this time because he has always been able to rehabilitate himself through other sports and work-related injuries.

Contemplation

This stage is characterized by a person's understanding that they have a problem or dilemma but have not made any concrete steps to impact or address this problem nor are they developing a plan or strategy to address the issue.

Case example: After initial frustration and aggravation with his care team members, LM has voiced that he is beginning to recognize that his strength and walking ability are not going to be able to "snap back" as he thought they might. He continues to pressure his doctors into pursuing aggressive medical care, such as chemotherapy, and wants surgery for his bone and liver metastases to "take the tumors out." In discussions, he is beginning to come to an understanding that he may need to participate in a round of inpatient rehabilitation (IPR) before going home. In IPR, he will learn how to modify his ADLs in order to perform self-care at home due to the increasing realization that he may require some assistance at home. He has taken no action steps toward this and is not yet actively participating in physical therapy or occupational therapy.

Preparation

The individual has recognized the problem or dilemma and has begun to develop a strategy or a plan but has not made significant steps toward executing this plan. In this stage, it is important for the plan to be achievable and realistic. Achievement of these goals may require the skills and professional insights of the care team, including therapists.

Case example: LM has begun working more regularly with his PT and OT in the hospital to accept assistance in getting stronger to get home. LM is beginning to consider how he will begin to do specific tasks in his home environment like getting to the bathroom, dressing himself, and bathing himself. He is now strongly considering admission to the hospital's IPR unit for a more thorough series of training sessions. This would include instruction on using assistive devices and durable medical equipment (DME) like a walker, bedside commode, mechanical lift, and wheelchair. He notes that he is getting the feeling that he may not be able to get back to work.

Action

After acknowledging and preparing to address the problem or dilemma, in the action phase the individual begins to take concrete and progressive steps to mitigate or address the entire problem, or strategic components of the problem. For example, this might include integrating healthy eating as a lifestyle change, scheduling and executing regular exercise into their routine, or attending a support group for substance use disorder. As these behaviors are not yet fully integrated into a routine, steps should be taken by the healthcare provider or coach to assist with transitioning these actions steps into long-term maintenance for sustainability.

Case example: LM has, with the coaching and support of his healthcare team, accepted that his strength and personal mobility via ambulation may not be an attainable short-term goal. He continues to have hope for a dramatic improvement; however, with the support and coaching of his healthcare team and family, he has begun to understand that 'hope is not a plan.' He realizes that his focus should currently be on getting home safely, which may require an adaptation to his previous thought process of being able to walk. He has accepted his change in mobility status and agreed to admission into the hospital's IPR unit. There, they will focus on teaching him and his family caregivers how to do slide board transfers and use a mechanical lift and other DME to accomplish daily functional tasks.[6] He is also continuing to request home physical therapy and occupational therapy after discharge to continue to work on his personal goals. He has also participated in recreational therapy to begin to modify his participation in recreational and diversionary activities during his IPR stay.

Maintenance

After the behavior change has occurred, efforts should focus on establishing behaviors to sustain these action items for the long-term. This might include things like periodic follow-up telephone calls, regular home visits by a therapist, and identification and mitigation of the individual's contextual vulnerabilities that may imperil sustainability of the behavior changes. Without this important step, there is an increased likelihood that the behavior change momentum is lost and a person can fall back into previously established poor health decisions, behaviors, or patterns.

Case example: LM has completed his IPR with a short length of stay of six days. He participated in training and education on safe movement techniques with his new physical capability status. The PT and OT in IPR have assisted in the procurement of the needed DME, mobility aids, and mechanical lifts to help him complete his physical mobility at home with his familys. The therapists also trained the family and caregivers in safe patient-handling and mobility techniques and assistance with all aspects of ADLs. In order to maintain this challenging set of tasks, the therapists have scheduled a weekly telephone call with LM and his family to troubleshoot any concerns, issues, or unexpected problems that may have arisen after leaving IPR. In addition, LM will also receive home care physical therapy and occupational therapy to continue to work on optimizing strength and physical status and strategies to maintain or slow the decline of physical capabilities in the presence of his disease process. With this support system in place, LM was able to optimize his physical mobility to address his primary concern of sustaining his personal autonomy and dignity and not being a burden to his family with his new disease state.

Motivational Interviewing

Within the realm of prevention, wellness, and health coaching, a useful communication and behavior-change technique is motivational interviewing (MI).[7] This technique, when employed in a healthcare setting, is a "skillful clinical style for eliciting from patients their own good motivations for making behavior changes in the interest of their health. It involves guiding more than directing, dancing rather than wrestling, listening at least as much as telling."[8] This technique has established a substantial body of knowledge behind its success in helping individuals achieve a number of different behavioral changes. In *A Meta-analysis of Motivational Interviewing: Twenty-five Years of Empirical Studies*, the authors examined 119 articles over 25 years on a variety of topics including substance use (tobacco, alcohol, drugs, marijuana), health-related behaviors (diet, exercise, safe sex), and gambling, and found statistically significant improvements in behavior changes using MI.[7] In a systematic review of ten studies related to physical activity performance in those with chronic illnesses, MI demonstrated a moderate but statistically significant effect as compared to traditional advice or interventions in improving physical activity.[9]

A key component of MI is facilitating and emphasizing a conversation to help an individual to self-recognize a problem and self-identify the issues and barriers or problems that need to be addressed in their own lives. Instead of a healthcare provider telling the individual what the problem is and how to solve it, the motivational interview coach will initiate a non-threatening, productive conversation to assist the individual to think deeply about what their current health issues are, and what they believe the long-term and short-term consequences might be to their health choices. Within this initial conversation, the MI coach will seek to identify what transtheoretical model stage this individual is in and begin to facilitate what will help them to transition from one stage to the next stage. This is an exceptionally important step because if the individual is in the precontemplation stage and has not recognized the problem, a conversation of how to implement and systematize new health behaviors into their life would be premature and likely not the best use of either individual's time or efforts. Instead, a conversation about establishing and recognizing the health-change behaviors will be a logical next step in the conversation.

A related concept to the transtheoretical model is the approach of wellness coaching or health coaching. Although not thoroughly examined in the domain of those with a life-threatening illness, wellness in the presence of chronic disease has many similarities to wellness in the absence of such diseases, and behavior change can be elicited strategically in both scenarios. Wolever et al.[10] conducted a systematic review of wellness coaching and examined 284 articles to establish best practices for wellness coaching and to attempt a unified definition of the approach. Based on the results, they defined wellness coaching as

> "a patient-centered process that is based upon behavior change theory and is delivered by health professionals with diverse backgrounds. The actual coaching process entails goalsetting determined by the patient, encourages self-discovery in addition to content education, and incorporates mechanisms for developing accountability in health behaviors."[10]

Linden, Butterworth, and Prochaska[11] examined the health outcomes of chronically ill individuals who were health coached as compared to those who did not receive health coaching; however, it should be noted that these individuals were not near the end of life (EoL) and did not appear to have severely advanced disease. Those who received health coaching demonstrated better self-efficacy ($p = 0.01$), patient activation (e.g. empowered to develop partnerships with healthcare professionals to improve their health) ($p = 0.02$), lifestyle change score ($p = 0.01$), and perceived health status ($p = 0.03$). This provides evidence that therapists working with chronically ill individuals should endeavor to improve their skills in MI and wellness coaching within the context of the transtheoretical model to optimize and sustain physical activity and rehabilitation outcomes.

Communication Strategies in Advanced Disease and Near the End of Life

An exceptionally well-established area of PC is the concept of having difficult conversations and delivering difficult news; however, therapists generally do not receive much education in this area in their entry-level training. There are several useful resources available to guide the clinician which can be found in Appendix 4. During therapy interventions or consultations in palliative or end-of-life care, emotional responses are common and should be expected. Anger, denial, sadness, fear, and detachment may all be encountered and should be addressed by therapists. In some cases, simply listening and offering to talk allows the person to convey their fears and emotions. Facilitating these difficult conversations is a tangible, skilled role of the therapist.[13] Due to the challenging and important nature of these discussions, utilizing distinct and purposeful strategies will help a therapist to respond to emotion. A commonly used tool to help facilitate conversations include employing "*I wish...*" statements.[14] Some examples of *I wish* statements are "I wish that your strength was returning like we hoped it would" or "I wish you were able to return directly home as opposed to needing to go to a subacute rehabilitation facility first." A conversational format that is beneficial throughout healthcare is the *Ask-Tell-Ask* format.[15] The first *Ask* is a prompt for understanding what the person knows about the current situation. *Tell* includes the delivery of the key medical information. The second *Ask* is another open-ended inquiry about what questions the person might have or what their thoughts or next steps are after receiving this information. Although by their very nature, difficult conversations will always be challenging but with practice and preparation therapists will be able to navigate these situations to help improve outcomes, QoL, and dignity of persons with terminal illnesses.

Communication in the Presence of Confusional States

At death, one out of every three people will have Alzheimer's disease or some other form of dementia.[16] Therapists and families often experience frustration and ineffective care as they attempt to utilize the same communication strategies to those with advanced cognitive impairment as they do for cognitively unimpaired individuals.[17] In an observational study of 18 individuals with dementia and their caregivers, Small et al.[18] identified some communications strategies employed during ADL performance (Box 7.1).

Box 7.1 Communication Strategies for Those with Dementia

- Minimize external distractions (e.g., televisions, phones, distracting crowds, pets)
- Interact in a slow, calming, friendly manner, sit rather than stand; maintain eye contact
- When speaking, use clear, concise sentences and talk slowly
- Try to avoid open ended questions; yes or no questions are preferred
- Avoid asking more than one question at a time
- Allow the person time to consider and answer the question; avoid interrupting or rushing them
- If needed, repeat a question or instruction using the same phrasing or paraphrase your sentence
- Prompt the person to try to 'find' the word or describe the word they are seeking

---

Those with dementia (especially Alzheimer's dementia) may demonstrate communication deficits with memory loss.[16] This may include symptoms such as problems finding the right words, a lack of coherence or logic in speech, or repeating ideas. In addition, decreased attention span and regularly forgetting recent events, names, and faces are characteristics of Alzheimer's dementia (see Chapter 13). Compounding this issue, many older adults with dementia may also have hearing or vision loss further impeding effective communication.

Therapist Interventions for Individuals with Dementia: Facilitating Success

As was noted previously, therapists often get frustrated when treating individuals with dementia because they continue to use strategies for cognitively intact older adults. Some initial recommendations include setting up strategies to facilitate indirect performance of a physical activity task. The therapist should establish an environment that demands performance of the skill without substantial cognitive demands. For example, instead of demanding an unpleasant and fearful complex balance task, the therapist would set up an obstacle course and have the person retrieve a desired item from across the room. If aerobic exercise is desired, consider stationing colleagues around the facility and prompt the individual to rush to visit each individual to shake their hand or give them a prize. As these tasks are still challenging balance and strength, close guarding and other safety measures (e.g. gait belt, following with a chair) are necessary.

Other examples of engaging or pleasant events that may facilitate physical activity include dancing (ideally with familiar music), swimming, water aerobics, tennis, tossing or kicking a ball, or races.[19] Modification of certain tasks to make them fun, silly, or pleasant may facilitate physical activity. For example, in order to initiate a quadriceps-strengthening exercise, Teri, Logsdon, and McCurry[20] suggested instructing "participants to stand and sit very slowly, like a mother hen sitting on her eggs, urging everyone to be careful not to break the eggs." In addition, group activities, games, or obstacle courses are also advocated.[20]

Another useful skill in assisting those with dementia or memory impairment is errorless learning. Werd[21] described errorless learning as "an instructional method for individuals with compromised memory and executive functions and may involve any intervention aimed at reducing the number of errors throughout the various stages of learning." Best practices for errorless learning include breaking down a task into small, achievable steps that should be modeled by the therapist before an attempt. If a person makes an error, correction should be made immediately but not punitively, and efforts should be made to avoid embarrassment. Also, spaced retrieval can be utilized which is rehearsing the task with increased rest breaks or longer time intervals between tasks.

Vanishing Cues

In order for therapists to have an individual with dementia or confusion perform or learn a new task, the concept of vanishing cues can be applied. An example of this would be an OT who aims to teach a person with cognitive impairment an important task such as reaching for an armchair before sitting down. See Box 7.2 for this sequence of vanishing cues.

Box 7.2 Vanishing Cues

1 Reach back for the armchair when you sit down. (OT demonstrates with a visual cue)
2 What do you do with your arms when you sit down? (OT demonstrates with a visual cue)
3 What do you do with your arms to sit down? (without a visual cue)
4 What do you do with the armchair when you sit down? (with visual cue)
5 What do you do with the armchair when you sit down? (without visual cue)
6 When you sit down you… (with visual cue)
7 When you sit down you… (without visual cue)

To best facilitate success in providing physical activity to those with dementia, Murphy, Nash, and Ross[22] provided a series of recommendations for successful therapist sessions. They recommended that a therapist not attempt to argue or repeatedly attempt to orient the individual to reality; instead, work within their reality. In addition, therapists should carefully observe for pain behaviors including anxiety and monitor vital signs or sympathetic responses to noxious stimulus. Other recommendations included varying activity experiences, engaging and collaborating with families or caregivers, incorporating likes (and avoiding dislikes), and slowly increasing the cognitive load, but not to failure.[22]

Therapists are encouraged to emphasize creativity, flexibility, and fun into physical activity tasks. One example that may be useful is engaging in dynamic balance and weight shifting activities via a game "Red light, green light." Many people played this game as a child, which leverages the individual's long-term intrinsic memory, familiarity, and nostalgia. The participant stands at a distance from the game facilitator and awaits a verbal cue to start ambulation with a "green light" command. After ambulation is started, the facilitator then states "red light" which prompts immediate stopping of ambulation. This facilitates balance reactions, engagement of fast-twitch muscle fibers, and dynamic balance. As this may be a challenging, impulsive task, close guarding by another clinician and a gait belt are highly recommended.

As the patient's caregivers may be experiencing significant frustration and distress, a key role of the therapist should be to educate the spouse, family, and others in the "new" way that their loved one's brain works. It is often difficult for the family to separate the new disease process from the memory of their loved one and their previous mental state. This will help sustain the caregivers to maintain their own self-care techniques to help their loved one with these key tasks. In these cases, therapists may note responses similar to grieving the loss of a loved one such as denial, anger, betrayal, or sadness. This initially seems paradoxical; however, upon further reflection, this bereavement process is natural and should be acknowledged because, in fact, the person that they knew and loved is no longer fully present.

Saying Goodbye as a Healthcare Provider

One of the most relevant and anxiety-producing topics when working with individuals near death is *if, how,* and *when* to acknowledge that further interactions may not be possible due to the EoL. Some common concerns by the therapist might include, "What if I say goodbye and I see the patient again?", "Will my acknowledgment of this scenario cause the patient (or me) to become upset?", or "If I say goodbye, will the patient think that I am abandoning them?" As with other unconscious biases, it is important for the clinician to recognize these concerns and acknowledge their existence in order to consciously deal with this issue. Although this topic has not been studied extensively in the medical literature, Back et al.[23] contended that patients and families may experience feelings of stress, confusion, and abandonment when a trusted healthcare provider ends a relationship without saying goodbye. "By saying goodbye, a physician can acknowledge the end of the relationship and at the same time underscore its importance, leaving the patient with a sense of feeling valued and cared for rather than abandoned."[23]

Although saying a last goodbye is an important step in the therapeutic relationship and can be a healing catalyst for the family and the healthcare provider, it likely requires conscious effort, practice, and reflection. Mott and Marcus[24] described that the expert clinician should be prepared to have this conversation and carefully consider what to say and, more importantly, what not to say. They noted that platitudes should be avoided including statements like "see you later," "take care," "see you soon," as they may seem superficial or even insensitive. Mott and Marcus also contended that "Patients must understand that even when further treatment is not effective, relief of suffering in all forms is still available from the healthcare provider."[24] Back et al.[23] described a series of steps to help facilitate the healthcare provider to say a thankful and meaningful goodbye to their patient (Box 7.3).

Clinicians may be asked to visit with a patient for a final time, either by the patient themselves or by the family. These opportunities can be beneficial for everyone involved to leave no words left unsaid. Even though these final meetings may be difficult and sometimes emotional, they should be considered as a positive way to receive closure to the relationship. Finding a ritual that works

Box 7.3 Saying Goodbye as a Healthcare Provider

Adapted from Back et al. (2005).[23]

1   **Choosing a Time and Place** – the setting and environment should be private and calming to allow for longer, meaningful discussions.

2   **Acknowledge the End of Routine Contact or Uncertainty about Future Contact** – This allows for closure and a transition to a different conversation. "I am not sure when we will see each other again but I was hoping to say something about our relationship."

3   **Ask Permission or Request a Response** – "Would it be okay if I talked about that?" or "How would you feel about that?" allows the patient to have some control and 'buy in' to the conversation

4   **Framing the Goodbye with Your Gratitude** – acknowledging that the relationship was a meaningful one to you. "I wanted to thank you for your kindness, humor (or individual qualities that the patient has) and I will miss our time together."

5   **Acknowledge the Difficulty and Awkwardness** – "I imagine this might feel awkward but I wanted to make sure you knew how I felt about our time together."

6   **Explicitly Reassure of Your Ongoing Support** – "Of course, I will be available if you need anything else or if any questions come up." Provide a means to contact you if there is not one clearly established.

7   **Reflection, Self-care, and Bereavement** – Be sure to find time to reflect on this loss, seek support of friends, families, and colleagues, and maintain mindfulness and healthy behaviors for self-care

can be helpful to ease the transition of loss, and it may vary from person to person. After the person passes away, attending a wake or a funeral service, or sending a card to the family, can promote the closure of this natural cycle. The therapist may encounter the individual's family or friends in the community, which provides additional opportunities to help facilitate bereavement and reflection. Useful messages may include, "It was such an honor to work with your mother. She had such a kind and gentle soul. You and your family took such good care of her. How are you doing these days?" This discussion can facilitate reassurance that the family made appropriate choices during an exceptionally difficult time and helps them to remember that there was meaning and purpose to this life transition. Even beyond death, the therapist can help with healing and recovery – truly the definition of a therapeutic relationship. For more information on grief and bereavement, see Appendix 3.

Summary

As there is growing evidence of the role of physical activity in affecting health and QoL, therapists will be further integrated into the care team of those with a life-threatening illness. With this integration comes the inevitability of challenging conversations. As therapists do not consistently receive training in conversations about life-and-death circumstances, this may be a barrier to therapists' motivation to participate in the care of an individual with a life-threatening illness. With the use of our listening skills, proper preparation, and advanced training, a therapist can turn an anxiety-ridden, emotional conversation into a positive experience that improves the QoL of an individual with a terminal illness and the loved ones they leave behind.

References

1   Briggs RW. Clinical decision making for physical therapists in patient-centered end-of-life care. *Top Geri Rehabil.* 2011;27(1):10–17.

2   DeFord B. Reflections on the betrayal of the body and other common spiritual wounds of people dying from cancer receiving hospice care. *Rehabil Oncol.* 2020;38(1):39–44. doi:10.1097/01.REO.0000000000000198.

3   Kubler-Ross E. *On Death and Dying.* London, England: Macmillan; 1969.

4   Prochaska JO. Transtheoretical model of behavior change. In: Gellman MD, eds. *Encyclopedia of Behavioral Medicine.* 2nd ed. New York, NY: Springer; 2020:2266–2269.

5   Prochaska JO, Redding CA, Evers KE. The transtheoretical model and stages of change. In: Glanz K, Rimer BK, Viswanath K, eds. *Health Behavior: Theory, Research, and Practice.* San Francisco, CA: Jossey-Bass; 2015:125–148.

6   Smith S, Wilson CM, Lipple C, et al. Managing palliative patients in inpatient rehabilitation through a short stay family training program. *Am J Hosp Palliat Med.* 2020;37(3):172–178.

7   Lundahl BW, Kunz C, Brownell C, Tollefson D, Burke BL. A meta-analysis of motivational interviewing: Twenty-five years of empirical studies. *Res Soc Work Pract.* 2010;20(2):137–160.

8   Rollnick S, Miller WR, Butler CC. *Motivational Interviewing in Health Care Helping Patients Change Behavior.* New York, NY: Guilford Publications; 2007.

9   O'Halloran PD, Blackstock F, Shields N, et al. Motivational interviewing to increase physical activity in people with chronic health conditions: A systematic review and meta-analysis. *Clin Rehabil.* 2014;28(12):1159–1171.

10 Wolever RQ, Simmons LA, Sforzo GA, et al. A systematic review of the literature on health and wellness coaching: Defining a key behavioral intervention in healthcare. *Glob Adv Health Med.* 2013;2(4):38–57.

11 Linden A, Butterworth SW, Prochaska JO. Motivational interviewing-based health coaching as a chronic care intervention. *J Eval Clin Pract.* 2010;16(1):166–174. doi:10.1111/j.1365-2753.2009.01300.x.

12 Mueller K, Wilson CM, Briggs R. Chapter 27: Hospice and end of life. In: Avers D, Wong R, eds. *Guccione's Geriatric Physical Therapy.* 4th ed. St. Louis, MO: Mosby; 2019:612–645.

13 Quill TE, Arnold RM, Platt F. "I wish things were different": Expressing wishes in response to loss, futility, and unrealistic hopes. *Ann Intern Med.* 2001;135(7):551–555.

14 Shannon SE, Long-Sutehall T, Coombs M. Conversations in end-of-life care: Communication tools for critical care practitioners. *Nurs Crit Care.* 2011;16(3):124–130.

15 Vital Talk. Establishing Rapport. Vital Talk website. www.vitaltalk.org/topics/establish-rapport/. Accessed July 12, 2020.

16 Alzheimer's Association. 2020 Alzheimer's disease facts and figures. *Alzheimer's Dement.* 2020;16(3):391–460. doi:10.1002/alz.12068.

17 Ries JD. Rehabilitation for individuals with dementia: Facilitating success. *Curr Geriatr Rep.* 2018;7(1):59–70.

18 Small JA, Gloria G, Saskia M, Beth H. Effectiveness of communication strategies used by caregivers of persons with Alzheimer's disease during activities of daily living. *J Speech Lang Hear Res.* 2003;46(2):353–367. doi:10.1044/1092-4388(2003/028).

19 Alzheimer's Association. 10 early signs and symptoms of Alzheimer's. Alzheimer's Association website. https://alz.org/alzheimers-dementia/10_signs. Accessed November 9, 2019.

20 Teri L, Logsdon RG, McCurry SM. Exercise interventions for dementia and cognitive impairment: The Seattle protocols. *J Nutr Health Aging.* 2008;12(6):391–394.

21 Werd MME. Errorless learning in dementia. *Clin Interv Aging.* 2017;8:1177–1190.

22 Murphy M, Nash J, Ross C. A skilled physical therapist's approach to Alzheimer's disease [conference proceedings]. American Physical Therapy Association's Combined Sections Meeting. Indianapolis, IN. February 6, 2015.

23 Back AL, Arnold RM, Tulsky JA, Baile WF, Fryer-Edwards KA. On saying goodbye: Acknowledging the end of the patient–physician relationship with patients who are near death. *Ann Intern Med.* 2005;142(8):682–685.

24 Mott FE, Marcus JD. The final goodbye. *Palliat Support Care.* 2013;11(3):277–279. doi:10.1017/S1478951512000223.

Part II
Diagnoses and Conditions in Life-threatening Illness

8 Diseases of the Heart

Amy J. Litterini and Christopher M. Wilson

Introduction

The leading cause of death in the United States, and worldwide, is cardio-vascular disease.[1,2] Several mechanisms can lead to morbidity and mortality from heart disease including heart failure, cardiomyopathy, coronary artery disease, and myocardial infarction, with coronary artery disease being the most prevalent.[2] Primary risk factors for the development of heart disease include hypertension, high cholesterol, and tobacco use disorder, while additional secondary risk factors include a history of diabetes, elevated body mass index (BMI), and lifestyle choices including suboptimal diet, physical inactivity, and excessive alcohol use.[2,3] Health disparities associated with socio-economic status and cardiovascular disease worldwide have been identified, and the majority of deaths, specifically premature deaths under the age of 70, occur in low to middle-income countries (Table 8.1).[4]

Heart failure (HF), previously referred to as congestive heart failure, is most often associated with cardiac muscle dysfunction, or *cardiomyopathy*, and results in approximately 250,000 deaths annually in the United States.[2] Alterations in systolic or diastolic activity, as a result of dysfunction of the myocardium,

Table 8.1 Incidence Rates and Mortality in Heart Disease

Type of Heart Disease	United States		Worldwide	
	Incidence	Mortality	Incidence	Mortality
Total: Cardiovascular diseases	92.1 million	647,457		17.9 million
Heart failure	6.2 million	379,800	26 million	
Myocardial infarction	805,000			
Coronary artery disease	18.2 million	365,914		
Sudden cardiac arrest		366,494		

Sources: Centers for Disease Control and Prevention. Heart disease facts. https://www.cdc.gov/heartdisease/facts.htm. Updated December 2, 2019. Accessed January 30, 2020, and The World Health Organization. Cardiovascular diseases. https://www.who.int/en/news-room/fact-sheets/detail/cardiovascular-diseases-(cvds). Updated May 17, 2017. Accessed March 12, 2020.

can cause changes in normal heart structure and function to develop. For individuals with a known diagnosis of heart failure, several mechanisms can also cause electrical irregularities that predispose them to potentially fatal cardiac arrhythmias, or sudden cardiac death (SCD). Abnormalities of atrial or ventricular electrophysiology can also alter the signaling cascades, resulting in an electrically unstable heart.

HF is generally diagnosed by measuring ejection fraction (EF), or the percentage of blood moved from the left ventricle with each cardiac contraction. Diagnostic techniques including echocardiogram, multiple-gated acquisition (MUGA) scan, cardiac catheterization, and nuclear stress testing are most commonly utilized in the diagnosis of heart failure. A normal EF is 50–70%, although some individuals have heart failure without an abnormally low EF (preserved ejection fraction [HFpEF]). An EF >75% can be indicative of hypertrophic cardiomyopathy. A borderline EF is 41–49%, while evidence of HF is considered at an EF <40% (reduced ejection fraction [HFrEF]).[5] HF is also categorized into subtypes based on both structural and functional abnormalities. HF is staged by the American Heart Association based on the progressive nature of the severity of the disease from stage A to stage D.[3] Stage A represents a high risk of developing heart disease with no manifestations, and Stage D represents advanced structural abnormalities with symptoms at rest. Additionally, the New York Heart Association has classified heart disease in corresponding categories ranging from I (no limitation in physical activity) to IV (unable to perform physical activity without symptoms; symptoms at rest).[5] Patients receiving palliative care and hospice for advanced heart disease will most frequently present with stages C and D (Class III-IV), with symptomatic presentation and progressively worsening limitations in functional mobility. However, clinicians should be cognizant of any cardiac history as a comorbidity, regardless of the primary diagnosis causing terminal illness (see Box 8.1).

Cardiac arrest, defined by the cessation of cardiac mechanical activity, is categorized by either external causes (e.g. drowning, electrocution, trauma)

Box 8.1 Common Symptoms of Advanced Heart Disease

Unrelieved shortness of breath or at rest	Need to sit in a chair to sleep, difficulty sleeping
Unrelieved angina	Weight gain or loss of five pounds in two days
Frequent dry, hacking cough	Discomfort of swelling in the lower extremities
Wheezing or chest tightness at rest	New or worsening dizziness or confusion
Loss of appetite	New or worsening sadness or depression

or medical causes.[3] SCD, the unexpected death from cardiac arrest often following unsuccessful attempts at resuscitation, usually occurs within one hour of the onset of new symptoms.[3] Ventricular tachycardia and/or fibrillation increases the likelihood of cardiac arrest, although the precise cause of SCD is often undetermined. Although immediate signs of SCD such as shortness of breath and/or angina may be present, the symptoms exhibited typically include patient collapse, loss of consciousness, and cessation of pulse and respiration.[3] Most episodes of cardiac arrest occur outside of a hospital; although 90% are fatal, there is improved survival for those occurring in public places receiving assistance by emergency medical services. SCD accounts for a significant portion of the annual deaths attributed to heart disease in developed countries. Acute myocardial infarction (MI) may be the definitive cause of SCD upon autopsy, and may be secondary to coronary artery disease.

The Agency for Healthcare Research and Quality (AHRQ) developed an algorithm describing the corresponding signs and symptoms, and defining appropriate precautions and actions for patients with known heart disease.[6] These categories range from the "green zone," or *all clear*, to the "red zone," or *medical alert*, and are intended as a patient education tool and self-awareness strategy for the need for medical management (see Table 8.2).

For patients presenting in the "red zone" with advanced heart disease, several symptoms may be evident (see Table 8.2) and indicative of overt decompensation.[7] Being cognizant of the individual's choices about further medical intervention is critical while in palliative care or hospice, and being able to significantly alter or hold an intervention is key with this patient population.

A recent clinical practice guideline by Shoemaker et al.,[8] published by the American Physical Therapy Association, further delineated clinical responses and physical therapist recommendations for each of the corresponding zones of heart disease. This guideline outlines an algorithm describing the steps in the physical therapist evaluation in response to the individual's clinical presentation.[8]

Early versus Late-stage Disease

For patients with early stage heart disease, lifestyle modification is at the forefront of initial medical management. Addressing issues associated with elevated BMI, physical inactivity, suboptimal nutrition, and smoking cessation are key and often require an intensive educational component frequently provided through comprehensive progressive exercise with close monitoring (often termed cardiac rehabilitation). Successful medical management and pharmacological interventions for comorbidities such as diabetes, hypertension, hypercholesterolemia, and chronic kidney disease are also critical to prevent or slow the progression of known heart disease.

For individuals with confirmed evidence of significant coronary artery disease, arrhythmias, damage to the myocardium, and/or valvular disease,

Table 8.2 Heart Failure Zones for Management[6]

Green zone: All clear
  Your goal weight:
  No shortness of breath
  No swelling
  No weight gain
  No chest pain
  No decrease in your ability to maintain your
  activity level
	Green zone means:
	  Your symptoms are under
	control
	Continue taking your
	medications as ordered
	Continue daily weights
	Follow a low salt diet
	Keep all physician
	appointments

Yellow zone: Caution
If you have any of the following signs and
  symptoms:
  Weight gain of three or more pounds in two days
  Increased cough
  Increased swelling
  Increase in shortness of breath with activity
  Increase in the number of pillows needed
  Anything else unusual that bothers you
  **Call your physician if you are going into
  the YELLOW zone**
	Yellow zone means:
	  Your symptoms may
	  indicate that you need
	  an adjustment of your
	  medications
	  **Call your physician,
	  nurse coordinator, or
	  home health nurse.**
	Name: _____
	Number: _____
	Instructions: _____

Red zone: Medical alert
  Unrelieved shortness of breath: shortness of
  breath at rest
  Unrelieved chest pain
  Wheezing or chest tightness at rest
  Need to sit in a chair to sleep
  Weight gain or loss of more than five pounds in
  two days
  Confusion
  **Call your physician immediately if you
  are going into the RED zone**
	Red zone means:
	This indicates that you
	  need to be evaluated by a
	  physician right away
	  **Call your physician
	  right away**
	Physician _____
	Number _____

Source: Agency for Healthcare Research and Quality. Red-Yellow-Green Congestive Heart Failure (CHF) Tool. https://innovations.ahrq.gov/qualitytools/red-yellow-green-congestive-heart-failure-chf-tool. Published January 2007. Updated April 11, 2008. Accessed January 11, 2020.[6]

surgical interventions followed by cardiac rehabilitation (including lifestyle modification) are the mainstay options for management in most countries. For individuals surviving myocardial infarction(s), with or without cardiac arrest, the above interventions are key to continued survival and recovery of damaged cardiac muscle. Options for surgical interventions to address heart disease are dependent upon the structures and underlying pathology involved (see Table 8.3).[9] International guidelines on cardiac rehabilitation management for individuals with heart disease demonstrate geographical similarities, but also minor discrepancies, in approaches to care.[10] Consensus among most major international societies is observed in high-intensity exercise in combination with resistance training; however, variations are noted in the need for highly technical exercise testing equipment such as electrocardiograph-monitored exercise stress testing.[10] Please see Chapter 3 for additional information on physical activity recommendations.

Table 8.3 Cardiac Surgical Procedures by Structure and Purpose[9]

Procedure	Structure	Purpose
Angioplasty	Coronary artery	Uses a balloon catheter or laser catheter to widen a narrowing in a blocked artery to improve blood flow
Heart valve replacement	Heart valve	Restores valvular function by replacing a diseased valve with an artificial valve
Implantable cardiac defibrillator	Myocardium	Monitors cardiac rhythms and delivers defibrillation in the presence of a dangerous rhythm or cardiac arrest
Pacemaker	Myocardium	Addresses dysfunctional cardiac rhythms with electronic pulses that restore normal rhythms
Atherectomy	Coronary artery	Uses a rotating shaver to clear plaque from a blocked artery
Bypass surgery	Coronary artery	Uses veins resected from the lower extremities to create a bypass for blocked arteries. Also known as coronary artery bypass grafting (CABG)
Stent placement	Coronary artery	Places a wire mesh stent within an artery during angioplasty to maintain an opening
Radiofrequency ablation	Myocardium	Uses a catheter electrode via fluoroscopy to ablate areas of myocardium that create abnormal heart rhythms
Cardiomyoplasty	Myocardium	Resected skeletal muscle, activated by a pacemaker, improves cardiac muscle function.
Transmyocardial revascularization (TMR)	Myocardium	Uses a laser to create channels through the myocardium to relieve severe angina. The healing process results in angiogenesis, and thus, revascularization.
Ventricular assist device (VAD)	Heart organ	A mechanical pump (implanted internally/worn external) and an electronic controller attached to a battery /power source. Blood is diverted from the ventricle of the heart to the pump, which in turn, pumps the blood through additional tubing into the aorta or other major arteries to circulate throughout the body.
Heart transplant	Heart organ	Replaces permanently damaged heart with organ-donated human heart

For individuals with advanced heart disease, symptom burden becomes more significant (see Table 8.1).[11] Initially, pharmacological management is paramount in maintaining cardiac function, appropriate blood pressure levels, heart rate, pain management, and symptom control. Supportive care by an interprofessional team is critical for continued functional mobility and quality of life for as long as possible. As the disease progresses, surgical interventions become less appropriate, and palliative and hospice care become more prominent. Homecare consultations for home safety assessments, caregiver training, and modifications for activities of daily living are indicated, as is adaptive and durable medical equipment to improve functional independence. As the patient declines, certain cardiac medications can often be withdrawn as the goal progresses toward overall symptom palliation. Other pharmacological interventions specific to symptom management, and supplemental oxygen with increasing liters often required over time, become necessary.

As individuals near the end of life, there are several important logistical and referral considerations for the patient and family. Difficult considerations include the deactivation of supportive mechanical devices such as an implantable cardioverter-defibrillator, or the discontinuation of a mechanical heart pump or a ventricular assist device (VAD).[11] In patients with limited life expectancy, these devices can unnecessarily prolong life as the disease takes its natural course. Clearly, a referral to end-of-life care for the appropriate support and guidance in these decisions, and necessary palliation of presenting symptoms, is indicated. Additionally, the treating clinicians should be aware of any such decisions and the patient's wishes including advance directives, do not resuscitate orders (DNR) and Physician's Orders for Life-Sustaining Treatment (POLST). See Appendix 1 for additional information on these options.

References

1 Dobkowski D, Becker RC. CDC: Heart disease, cancer leading causes of death in 2017. *Cardiol Today*. 2019;22(2):1–5. https://search.proquest.com/docview/2225755106.
2 Centers for Disease Control and Prevention. Heart disease facts. https://www.cdc.gov/heartdisease/facts.htm. Updated December 2, 2019. Accessed January 30, 2020.
3 Benjamin E, Salim V, Clifton C, et al. Heart disease and stroke statistics—2018 update: A report from the American Heart Association. *Circulation*. 2018;137: e67–e492. doi:10.1161/CIR.0000000000000558.
4 World Health Organization. Cardiovascular diseases. https://www.who.int/en/news-room/fact-sheets/detail/cardiovascular-diseases-(cvds).   Updated May 17, 2017. Accessed March 12, 2020.
5 American Heart Association. Classes of heart failure. https://www.heart.org/en/health-topics/heart-failure/what-is-heart-failure/classes-of-heart-failure. Published 2020. Accessed January 30, 2020.
6 Agency for Healthcare Research and Quality. Red-Yellow-Green Congestive Heart Failure (CHF) Tool. https://innovations.ahrq.gov/qualitytools/red-yellow-green-congestive-heart-failure-chf-tool. Published January, 2007. Updated April 11, 2008. Accessed January 30, 2020.
7 American Heart Association. Warning signs of heart failure. https://www.heart.org/en/health-topics/heart-failure/warning-signs-of-heart-failure. Updated 2020. Accessed March 10, 2020.
8 Shoemaker MJ, Dias KJ, Lefebvre KM, Heick JD, Collins SM. Physical therapist clinical practice guideline for the management of individuals with heart failure. *Phys Ther*. 2020;100(1):14–43. doi:10.1093/ptj/pzz127.
9 American Heart Association. Cardiac procedures and surgeries. https://www.heart.org/en/health-topics/heart-attack/treatment-of-a-heart-attack/cardiac-procedures-and-surgeries. Updated 2020. Accessed March 5, 2020.
10 Price KJ, Gordon BA, Bird SR, Benson AC. A review of guidelines for cardiac rehabilitation exercise programmes: Is there an international consensus? *Eur J Prev Cardiol*. 2016;23(16):1715–1733. doi:10.1177/2047487316657669.
11 American Heart Association. Planning for advanced heart failure. https://www.heart.org/en/health-topics/heart-failure/living-with-heart-failure-and-managing-advanced-hf/planning-ahead-advanced-heart-failure. Updated 2020. Accessed March 1, 2020.

9   Malignant Neoplasms

Amy J. Litterini and Christopher M. Wilson

Introduction

Care for *cancer survivors*, considered from the day of diagnosis throughout the duration of life, is an area of medicine and rehabilitation which requires advanced knowledge of the treating clinician. Awareness about how the many different types of cancers present, signs and symptoms of primary and metastatic cancers, side effects of the disease and the various treatments utilized, and a firm understanding of needs and prognoses across the cancer survivorship continuum are vital components for individuals wishing to provide oncology rehabilitation. This chapter will provide an overview of these major aspects, particularly pertaining to advanced cancer, but the authors strongly encourage mentorship from experienced oncology clinicians as well as networking and collaboration with local, regional, and national oncology societies and associations.

Malignant Neoplasms: Advanced or Terminal Cancer

Cancer, a group of many diseases which represents over 200 different diagnoses, occurs when cells in the body mutate and proliferate in an uncontrolled manner. Cancers are often categorized as solid, hematological (or liquid), or central nervous system (CNS) types. Solid cancers, most commonly identified as carcinomas or sarcomas, form an abnormal mass called a *tumor* or *lesion*, and are most frequently identified by the tissue of origin. Hematological tumors are considered systemic and include blood and lymphatic cancers such as leukemias, lymphomas, and multiple myeloma, as well as myelodysplastic syndrome. CNS tumors can occur anywhere within the nervous system, including the brain, meninges, or spinal cord. Tumors are generally classified as either *benign,* that is, unable or unlikely to spread to distant parts of the body and considered non-cancerous, or *malignant,* comprised of cancer cells and capable of invading surrounding tissues. Additionally, tumors are considered as either *primary*, or from the anatomical location and tissue of origin, or *metastatic*, referring to distant spread from the original location of origin to other areas of the body.

Cancerous tumors are categorized histologically into grades which indicate the aggressiveness of the cells. The typical histological grades are *low* grade I (well-differentiated cells), *intermediate* grade II (moderately differentiated cells), and *high* grade III (poorly differentiated cells). The factors which determine the tumor grade include the morphology of the cancerous cells (specifically how mutated they appear when compared to a normal cell of the tissue of origin), how rapidly they are dividing (or mitotic activity), and invasive capability. For CNS tumors, which are graded rather than staged, the grading system from the World Health Organization extends to IV by identifying the likelihood of recurrence.[1] The percentage of cells observed in synthesis, or *S-phase*, of cell division are indicative of how rapidly a tumor is growing. The higher the grade, the more aggressive the tumor type, and subsequently, a more aggressive treatment plan is most often prescribed.

Each type of solid cancerous tumor has an elaborate staging system to classify tumor size, nodal involvement, and metastatic spread. The clinical staging of cancer uses the TNM system whereas **T** refers to *tumor* size in centimeters, **N** refers to *nodal* status, or lymph node involvement, and **M** refers to *metastasis* to distant tissues or organs. The TNM staging system is defined by the Union for International Cancer Control (www.uicc.org) which is the most widely utilized staging system. Each cancer type has different tumor sizes and node status to denote the extent of the cancer, and the higher the number means that a tumor has spread more extensively into surrounding tissue or that an increasing number of lymph nodes have detectable disease. For the metastatic category, three options may be found, 0 denotes that distant metastases have not been detected, 1 denotes the presence of any distant metastasis, and X means that staging has not been attempted for this category. In some situations, clinicians may see a lowercase **c** or **p** in front of the traditional staging categorization indicating that this diagnosis was established by clinical examination (c) or histopathologic staging (p). The nodal status in the pathology report includes the total number of lymph nodes removed, the number of nodes found to be positive (+) for cancer cells, as well as the size of any cancerous deposits identified within the nodes (microscopic, gross, and/or extracapsular extension). For tumors often influenced by hormonal overexpression such as breast cancer, hormone status is also considered in staging (see Chapter 23 regarding genetic mutations and genomics). For the clinician, awareness and knowledge of a patient's cancer staging lend to their ability to understand the patient's prognosis and/or the aggressiveness necessary for the treatment.

The TNM system leads to grouping from 0 to IV where stage 0 represents in situ disease, stages I and II represent local disease, stage III represents regional spread of disease, and stage IV represents distant spread of disease. Typical solid tumors are staged from I to IV, with terminal, or incurable, cancer considered the end stage of any tumor type, generally stages III to IV. Several aggressive forms of cancer are more likely to be diagnosed at, or progress to, later stages of disease as evidenced by their poorer five-year survival rates. Specifically, patients with gastric, lung, or malignant brain cancers are often targeted for early PC due to their tendency to progress rapidly. For those individuals, clinicians must work to palliate the symptoms of their disease that often lead to limitations in their functional mobility.

The mainstays of oncologic medical management in most countries includes *surgical oncology*, for the removal of tumors, *medical oncology*, the treatment of cancer with medicine, and *radiation oncology*, the treatment of cancer with radioactive sources. Access to these treatment modalities varies widely across the globe, and is heavily influenced by the availability of the practitioners, medications and equipment, proximity to cancer centers, and socioeconomic status and insurance status. Depending on the diagnosis, some individuals will receive all three treatment modalities, and may receive medical oncology and radiation oncology interventions simultaneously or *concurrently*. Some treatments occur pre-operatively, or *neoadjuvantly*, or postoperatively, or *adjuvantly*.

For individuals in the postoperative phase of cancer care, postsurgical management involves care initially for the surgical incision, followed by subsequent management of scar tissue, and recovery of incised tissues in the surgical region. For individuals receiving medical oncology interventions, managing medication side effects is most critical for maintaining quality of life and functional mobility. Certain classes of chemotherapeutics are known to cause chemotherapy-induced peripheral neuropathy, such as the Taxanes and Vinca alkaloids, and others are known to be cardiotoxic, such as doxorubicin (Adriamycin) and trastuzumab (Herceptin). Endocrine therapy, also known as hormone therapy, includes the use of medications such as aromatase inhibitors for hormonally driven tumors such as breast cancer. These medications can potentially cause myalgias, arthralgias, and bone loss. For individuals in treatment for radiation therapy, monitoring for radiation dermatitis in the treatment field, or skin irritation to the dermal level commonly seen from external beam radiation therapy, is an important role for treating clinicians. It is critical for any practitioner rehabilitating cancer survivors to be aware of the cancer treatment history, especially treatments in combination which can compound risks for side effects. For example, lymph node status, as well as lymphatic system surgical and radiation therapy history is not only indicative of a patient's cancer stage but also the risk of lymphedema (see lymphedema addressed in Chapter 17).

Globally, as well as in the United States, the most frequent cause of death from cancer for both men and women is primary lung cancer (see Table 9.1).[2,3] Following lung carcinoma, prostate and breast cancers are second in mortality rates for men and women, respectively, in the United States, followed by colorectal as the third, and pancreatic cancers the fourth leading causes of death for both sexes.[2]

The International Agency for Research on Cancer (IARC) estimates the burden of cancer worldwide in countries by the Human Development Index (HDI).[3] The HDI considers such factors as health, education, and standard of living, and is therefore indicative of access to early detection and quality medical treatment. Additionally, the age distribution of a particular geographical population, as well as the prevalence of specific risk factors, alter the prevalence of cancers in particular regions of the world. In countries with a low HDI, the rate of cancers associated with infections demonstrates the greatest disease burden compared to countries with higher HDI.[3] For example, cancers caused by helicobacter pylori (H. pylori) infection, such as gastric cancer, are three times more likely in low HDI countries. Environmental factors suspected to be associated with H. pylori infection include water sources contaminated with human waste.[3]

While focusing on the cancer and cancer treatment-related sequelae is important, considering any and all medical comorbidities and coexisting conditions is also important when treating patients with early stage and advanced cancer. In addition to the metastatic spread of existing primary cancers, cancer survivors may also experience new types of primary cancers, as well as secondary cancers associated with the treatment of their original primary cancer. Non-cancer related diagnoses, such as heart attack, stroke, and diabetes, may also be life-threatening or fatal for cancer survivors. In a population-based study with Surveillance, Epidemiology, and End Results (SEER) Program data from 1992 to 2015, Zaorsky et al.[4] analyzed fatal stroke risk among cancer survivors with the goal of identifying those at highest risk. They determined survivors of gastrointestinal and brain cancers to be at the highest risk level for fatal stroke. Maintaining an awareness of all systems of the body when treating cancer survivors can help the clinician keep an individual's overall health and risk profile in mind.

Monitoring for symptoms, and managing them when identified, is essential for quality cancer survivorship care for individuals with all stages of cancer. For postoperative patients, care should be taken to follow postsurgical protocols from the attending surgeon. Special attention should be paid to devices such as Jackson-Pratt (JP) drains from the surgical region, and/or devices such as urinary catheters, chest tubes, colostomy or urostomy devices, and

Table 9.1 Incidence Rates and Mortality of Cancer in the United States and Worldwide

Type of Cancer	United States (2020)		Worldwide (2018)	
	Estimated New Cancers	Estimated Deaths	Estimated New Cancers	Estimated Deaths
Total: All sites	1,806,590	647,457	17 million	9.5 million
Breast (females)	276,480	42,170	2,088,800	626,700
Prostate (males)	191,930	33,330	1,276,100	359,000
Lung (both sexes)	228,820	135,720	2,093,900	1,761,000
Colorectal (both sexes)	147,950	53,200	1,849,500	880,800
Pancreatic (both sexes)	57,600	47,050	458,918	432,242
Stomach	27,600	11,010	1,033,700	782,700

Sources: American Cancer Society Global Cancer Facts & Figures 4th Edition. *CA Cancer J Clin.* 2020;0:1–24 and *CA Cancer J Clin.* 2018;0:1–31.

intravenous lines. For patients receiving ongoing systemic therapies such as chemotherapy, complete blood count levels should be monitored for immunocompromise, specifically *neutropenia* (low white blood cells) causing risk of infection, *anemia* (low red blood cells) potentially causing fatigue and shortness of breath, and *thrombocytopenia* (low platelets) potentially increasing the risk of bruising and bleeding. Additionally, awareness of venous access devices such as implanted ports, peripherally inserted central catheters (PICC lines), Hickman central catheters, and Ommaya reservoirs (see Figure 9.1) into the ventricles, should be noted with appropriate precautions taken. For patients

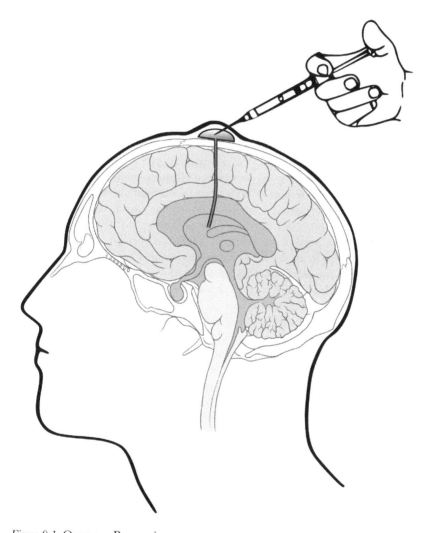

Figure 9.1 Ommaya Reservoir.
Source: https://upload.wikimedia.org/wikipedia/commons/6/63/Ommaya_01.png. Attribution: Patrick L. Lynch / Public domain.

receiving radiation therapy, having sufficient range of motion to achieve the desired positioning during radiation therapy is often an initial goal. Also, routine monitoring of the skin for areas of radiation dermatitis in the treatment field is key.

The symptom burden for patients with advanced cancer can be significant and severe. Ruijs et al.[5] followed 77 palliative care cancer survivors who had a six-month prognosis. The authors found that weakness was the most prevalent unbearable symptom (57%).[5] Decreased functional mobility in advanced cancer survivors, as well as subsequent falls, decubitus ulcers, fatigue, and decreased ability to perform activities of daily living (ADLs), can lead to additional pain and decreased quality of life, increased caregiver demand, and increased costs to the healthcare system. For individuals with metastatic cancer, an awareness of the signs and symptoms of the different types of metastases, as well as necessary precautions is key when treating this patient population.

Skeletal Metastasis

Certain cancers are more likely than others to progress from the primary site to the skeleton, and the lesions can also vary in type (osteoblastic, osteolytic, mixed), size, and location of distribution. Cancer metastasis to the bone can occur in isolated lesions or widespread with multiple lesions. Please see Chapter 17 for a thorough description of bone metastasis principles.

Skeletal-related events (SREs)—defined as pathological fracture, spinal cord compression, the need for surgery or radiation therapy to the skeleton, or hypercalcemia—can be an unfortunate sequela of cancer and cancer treatment for many survivors. SREs associated with bone metastases can include pain, pathological fracture, hypercalcemia, and neurological deficits. A systematic review and meta-analysis by Wang et al.[6] highlighted data from the untreated arms of several clinical trials, which indicated a two-year cumulative incidence of SREs as most prevalent in individuals with skeletal metastasis with primary breast cancer (68%), prostate cancer (49%), and non-small cell lung cancer and other solid tumors (21-month cumulative incidence of 48%). Cancer survivors with skeletal metastases are at risk for SREs, and common treatments include radiation therapy for local pain management and high-dose bisphosphonates for bone strength. Fracture risk in the presence of metastatic cancer to the skeleton deserves keen awareness and strong attention from rehabilitation and fitness practitioners. Please see Chapter 17 for precautions and management principles of pathological fracture risk.

Liver Metastasis

Following tumor-draining lymph nodes, the liver is the second most common organ for the dissemination of metastatic cancer.[7] Individuals with primary or metastatic cancer to major organs can experience progressive loss of organ function, potentially leading to life-threatening organ failure. In spite of the unique capability of the liver to regenerate organ tissue following surgical resection or trauma, liver cancer survivors can experience degrees of reduced liver function which can ultimately lead to symptomatic, or fatal, liver failure. Liver function tests are routinely monitored to assess liver function, but also tolerance for the continuation of chemotherapeutic agents. As systemic chemotherapy must be processed through the liver, reduced liver function limits an individual's ability to continue with these agents for the treatment of advanced cancer.

Progressive liver failure often results in malignant ascites, as well as jaundice. As it progresses due to increased fluid pressure in the liver, ascites distends the peritoneal cavity with an accumulation of fluid which often becomes increasingly uncomfortable for the patient. Shortness of breath can occur due to pressure of ascites on the diaphragm. In advanced cases, fluid can migrate across the diaphragm resulting in pleural effusion. Therapeutic *paracentesis*, when liters of fluid are removed with a large gauge needle, can help to relieve painful pressure. For patients with chronic malignant ascites, paracentesis can be done on a routine basis for palliation or a long-term drain (e.g. PleurX) may be surgically implanted for easier drainage. For refractory cases where surgery is a choice and a viable option, transjugular intrahepatic portosystemic shunts (TIPS) may be considered when severe symptoms are uncontrolled by other interventions.

When treating individuals with ascites, caution should be taken with positioning and activity recommendations. Lying on one's side can be a more comfortable position for many when the abdomen is distended, whereas lying prone may be poorly tolerated. Trunk rotation and side bending may be limited, while excessive trunk and hip flexion should also be avoided. Going through the comfortable, available range of motion and breath work can assist patients in reducing feelings of stiffness and assist in comfort. If ascites is suspected to be impacting breathing, monitoring oxygenation during activity or emphasizing interval exercises or pacing techniques will improve the safety and ability to participate in physical activity.

Central Nervous System Metastases

According to the American Brain Tumor Association, an estimated 200,000–300,000 CNS metastases occur annually in the United States.[8] According to Mehta et al.[9] 80% of brain metastases occur in the cerebral hemispheres, the cerebellum (15%), and the brain stem (5%). Most metastases occur as multiple lesions (>80%), while only an estimated 10–20% present as single lesions.[10] In addition to the number of lesions, the location of lesions will have an impact on clinical presentation. For example, lesions in the occipital lobe may impact visual functioning while frontal lobe lesions may impair executive functioning or motor performance (Figure 9.2).

Rehabilitation approaches with CNS metastases are intended to address and support cancer survivors' impairments. The visual, vestibular, motor,

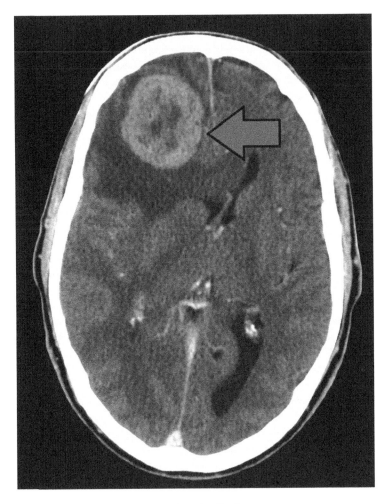

Figure 9.2 Lung Cancer Metastasized to the Brain.
Source: https://upload.wikimedia.org/wikipedia/commons/e/ee/MctstoBrain%28LungPri
%29Mark.png. Attribution: James Heilman, MD / CC BY-SA (https://creativecommons.
org/licenses/by-sa/4.0).

and sensory deficits alone, or in combination, can produce profound balance and functional deficits. This can necessitate interventions to reduce the
risk of falls, and improve function and patient safety. Significant motor deficits
should be assessed with skilled neurological rehabilitation strategies, appropriate bracing, and/or assistive devices for gait training and functional tasks.
Physical activity for individuals with CNS metastases must be tailored to their
disease and clinical presentation. In the presence of balance deficits, caution
should be taken for safety during positional changes. Recommending the use

of various positions, including sitting, supine, and a semi-reclined position (if indicated due to intracranial pressure), can offer improved safety during physical activity and exercise, and reduce fall risk. Clinically, a common medical intervention for brain metastases is high-dose corticosteroids or whole brain radiation. These palliative interventions are not intended to resolve or cure the metastatic disease but to reduce the size or impact of these lesions. These interventions, coupled with aggressive rehabilitative techniques, may result in substantial gains in physical function and mobility and individuals receiving these treatments may benefit from an increased frequency or intensity of rehabilitation to maximize gains for optimization of quality of life.

Pulmonary Metastases

For patients with primary or metastatic lung carcinoma, pulmonary function can become progressively compromised. Individuals with lung metastasis can present with respiratory symptoms more debilitating than the symptoms resulting from their primary cancer. The use of supplemental oxygen can be of assistance for symptom management, including breathlessness and other symptoms of hypoxia, as well as over-the-counter and prescription medications to address throat irritation and cough. Clinicians prescribing physical activity to patients with compromised pulmonary function should be aware of the patient's pulse oxygenation levels, and perceived exertion, to determine the appropriateness of exercise intensity and progression or regression. Please see Chapter 17 for interventions to address breathlessness.

Prior to recommending physical activity to cancer survivors with primary lung carcinoma or pulmonary metastases, a thorough review of their diagnostic imaging is indicated when possible to assess the extent and location of the lesions. Close attention should be paid to large or extensive numbers of metastases in the upper lobes secondary to the potential for close proximity to the cardiac circulation, as well as lesions in the mediastinal region, which may compromise the bronchi and/or the heart. Much like head and neck cancer survivors, these individuals are at risk for conditions such as superior vena cava syndrome where blockages to circulation cause cancer-related emergencies (see Cancer-related Emergencies section), and in advanced cancers, terminal hemorrhage resulting in rapid death.

Prior to initiating physical activity, monitoring of vitals at rest and with activity should include blood pressure, respiratory rate, oxygen saturation levels, and heart rate. During initial attempts at physical activity, cancer survivors with inoperable primary lung carcinoma or metastatic pulmonary lesions should be monitored for their current fatigue, activity tolerance, and levels of dyspnea. For survivors on supplemental oxygen, a physician order should be obtained to increase the liters/minute delivered in the event that their oxygen saturation level drops below 90% on pulse oximetry during physical activity. Patient education on diaphragmatic and pursed-lip breathing techniques incorporated into physical activity may assist survivors in controlling their respiratory rate. Performing exercises while sitting can help to conserve energy in survivors who easily become dyspneic while standing or walking. Instructing cancer survivors to lean forward in the sitting position while resting their hands on their knees can help to reduce symptoms of breathlessness for some (however, this position may exacerbate breathlessness in those with abdominal distension and ascites). Adjusting exercise intensity based on RPE, such as ratings on the Borg scale, can improve exercise tolerance and improve accuracy of exercise prescription.

Widespread Metastases

In cancer survivors with evidence of widely disseminated metastatic disease, clinicians should be aware of both the location, and extent, of all known metastases. These individuals often present with a multitude of symptoms; each additional lesion can present with additional complications, and metastases in one area can compound the symptoms resulting from metastasis elsewhere. The cumulative effects of disease-related symptoms, multiple medications, and degrees of organ system failures can cause varying presentations over time and from day to day. Cancer survivors should be educated on maximizing their abilities on days and times of day (e.g. mid-morning) that permit, while allowing for rest on days when they are more symptomatic. These individuals require close monitoring for new symptom presentation or existing symptom progression; therefore, the skill of an oncology-trained physical or occupational therapist is recommended to prescribe physical activity for these individuals with complex, advanced cancer diagnoses.

For survivors with limited performance status, a homecare therapist can provide several options. Survivors with limited ambulatory endurance can be prescribed an interval walking program of short distances on level surfaces with or without an assistive device multiple times per day. Individuals with limited ambulatory tolerance can be prescribed standing exercises, while holding onto a secure surface for safety, in order to maintain functional lower extremity muscle strength. Advanced cancer survivors spending the majority of time either in a chair or bed should be prescribed exercises in sitting and/ or supine for both range of motion and isometric strengthening. With multiple options, survivors still can maintain some degree of physical activity regardless of their capabilities on any given day. Meeting them where they are, and emphasizing and encouraging cancer survivors' abilities in their current state while keeping safety in mind, will provide empowerment to the individual and yield the best outcomes.

Cancer-related Emergencies

Therapists providing care for individuals with advanced cancer must be familiar with the potential risk for rare metabolic, cardiovascular, neurologic, infectious, hematologic, and respiratory emergencies in the cancer survivors under their care (see Table 9.2). Oncologic emergencies are potentially life-threatening medical events which can occur when the cancer causes either: (1) a serious secretory/metabolic malfunction or (2) an obstruction of a vital structure. Lewis, Hendrickson, and Moynihan[11] eloquently and thoroughly described the pathophysiology, presentation, diagnosis, and treatment of oncologic emergencies, and provided a comprehensive summary of their incidence and management. As individual descriptions of these oncologic emergencies would consume a large portion of this text, the authors recommend accessing appropriate resources to further their knowledge about these important potential conditions in survivors with advanced cancer.

When supervising patients receiving physical activity or skilled rehabilitation as part of their cancer treatment plan, the clinician should be aware of the typical signs and symptoms of oncologic emergencies, and know when to refer cancer survivors for further evaluation and intervention. Clinical examples of diagnoses with an emergent response would be observing and recognizing the signs and symptoms of venous thromboembolism (VTE) and pulmonary embolism (PE), as well as evidence of sepsis or septic shock, and referring the patient for appropriate diagnostics in an immediate response (unless their wishes are for no further medical intervention). Cancer survivors and caregivers should also be educated about the signs and symptoms of the emergencies for which they are at greatest risk, as well as the proper steps to take, who to contact, and where to go if symptoms arise. Basic safety precautions during physical activity such as keeping a phone nearby, staying adequately nourished and hydrated, and avoiding overexertion are always helpful reminders for those at risk.

Early versus Late-stage Disease

In a 1981 text, Dietz[12] articulated the model for the role of oncology rehabilitation throughout the continuum of cancer care that still holds

Table 9.2 Cancer Related Emergencies

Type	Emergency Diagnosis
Metabolic	Hypercalcemia, Hyponatremia, Syndrome of Inappropriate Antidiuretic Hormone Secretion (SIADH), Hypoglycemia, Tumor Lysis Syndrome
Cardiovascular	Superior Vena Cava Syndrome (SVC), Pericardial Effusion/ Cardiac Tamponade
Neurologic	Spinal Cord Compression (SCC), Seizures, Increased Intracranial Pressure (IICP)
Infectious	Neutropenic Fever/ Sepsis
Hematologic	Hyperviscosity Syndrome, Disseminated Intravascular Coagulation (DIC), Leukostasis
Chemotherapeutic	Hypersensitivity Reactions (Anaphylaxis), Extravasation of chemotherapy
Structural	Malignant Airway Obstruction, Small Bowel Obstruction (SBO)

relevant today. This model ranges in scope and intensity of intervention, from the preventative phase for predictable conditions, through the palliative phase for irreversible conditions (see Figure 9.3). The overarching goals across the continuum of cancer survivorship are to have an awareness for identifying and addressing what issues arise, when and how they present. Throughout the phases, patient education and empowerment are key themes.

The continuum of cancer survivorship extends from prevention and pre-treatment to palliation (see Figure 9.4).[13] As with many health conditions, early intervention is key to reducing the risk of future complications after the initial diagnosis of cancer. The pretreatment phase, sometimes referred to as *pre-rehabilitation* (or prehabilitation), can be effective for patients of all stages of disease undergoing aggressive surgical interventions. A systematic review of prehabilitation interventions for cancer survivors found improvements in function and physical capacity within 18 studies of 966 patients.[14] For individuals with early stage cancers, lifestyle modification to reduce the risk for metastasis, secondary cancers, or new primary cancers is appropriate. For individuals in active cancer treatment, oncology rehabilitation and physical activity to address cancer treatment-related side effects are key. Nutrition consultations for weight management are also key in cancer risk reduction in long-term survivorship. Comprehensive survivorship programming for all stages of disease is the ideal format for monitoring cancer survivors for treatment-related sequela including cardiomyopathy from cardiotoxic chemotherapy or immunotherapy, late effects from radiation such as plexopathies and radiation fibrosis, and signs and symptoms of disease progression (Figure 9.4).

For individuals with advanced cancer, life expectancy varies widely based on the type, location, and extent of metastatic disease. For many, such as individuals with metastatic prostate cancer isolated to the skeleton, this can mean a prognosis of several years of survival. For others, such as those with metastatic spread to the liver, life expectancy often shortens to months. For these

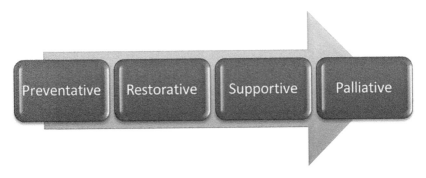

Figure 9.3 Phases of Oncology Rehabilitation. Dietz (1981).

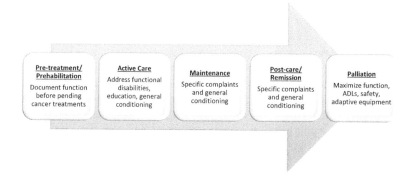

Figure 9.4 The Cancer Survivorship Continuum.
Source: Adapted from Fitzpatrick T. Principles of physical and occupational therapy in cancer. In: Stubblefield MD, O'Dell MW, eds. *Cancer Rehabilitation: Principles and Practice.* New York, NY: Demos Medical Publishing; 2009:785–796.

individuals, quality of life and maintaining functional mobility are key for the longest duration of time possible. Cachexia, or in the oncology setting *cancer cachexia*, is an unfortunate wasting condition that can occur with advanced disease. Please see Chapter 17 for information on cachexia.

Maintaining physical activity levels and ADL performance is best assisted with referral to a rehabilitation professional either on an outpatient basis, in a homecare setting, or through a palliative and hospice care service. As fatigue is the most common symptom in cancer survivorship, physical activity is recommended for individuals with all stages of cancer. Guidelines for cancer-related fatigue from associations such as the National Comprehensive Cancer Network® recommend physical activity throughout all phases of cancer survivorship.[15] A systematic review of physical activity in advanced cancer by Dittus, Gramling, and Ades[16] highlighted data from 19 studies which revealed improvements in quality of life (60%) and fatigue (45%).

Home safety modifications and/or the acquisition of necessary equipment is critical to improve patient safety and reduce fall risk. If the patient is eligible for end-of-life/hospice care based on the prognosis and has not yet been referred, the therapist should initiate a referral or discuss with the interdisciplinary care team as the situation warrants. Additionally, providers of integrative medicine services for symptom management and quality of life become critical team members in the patient's care (see Chapter 6). Caregiver education is also a key component to support individuals facing advanced cancer.

Summary

Advanced cancer is a complex and debilitating progressive disorder, but patients would benefit from physical activity and rehabilitation interventions across the entire continuum of cancer survivorship. As cancer progresses for individuals with advanced disease, the need for our interventions increases rather than lessens but becomes more complex as medical conditions evolve. Being an advocate for movement and functional mobility for cancer survivors at all stages is a vital role to fill, but even more so over the trajectory of progressive disease.

In the United States, oncology is a recognized area of specialty practice for physical therapists by the American Board of Physical Therapy Specialties. It was approved by a unanimous vote at the American Physical Therapy Association's 2016 House of Delegates.[17] This advancement of physical therapist practice will further enhance the standards of care established for the rehabilitation of all cancer survivors, but also certainly those individuals with terminal cancer.

References

1 Louis DN, Perry A, Reifenberger G, et al. The 2016 World Health Organization classification of tumors of the central nervous system: A summary. *Acta Neuropathol.* 2016;131(6):803–820. doi:10.1007/s00401-016-1545-1.
2 American Cancer Society Facts and Figures, 2020. *CA Cancer J Clin.* 2020;0:1–24.
3 American Cancer Society Global Cancer Facts & Figures 4th Edition. *CA Cancer J Clin.* 2018;0:1–31.
4 Zaorsky NG, Churilla T, Egleston BL, et al. Causes of death among cancer patients as a function of calendar year, age, and time after diagnosis. *Ann Oncol.* 2016;27:vi476. doi:10.1093/annonc/mdw387.10.
5 Ruijs CD, Kerkhof AJ, van der Wal G, Onwuteaka-Philipsen BD. Symptoms, unbearability and the nature of suffering in terminal cancer patients dying at home: A prospective primary care study. *BMC Fam Pract.* 2013;14:201. doi:10.1186/1471-2296-14-201.
6 Wang Z, Qiao D, Lu Y, et al. Systematic literature review and network meta-analysis comparing bone-targeted agents for the prevention of skeletal-related events in cancer patients with bone metastasis. *Oncologist.* 2015;20(4):440–449. doi:10.1634/theoncologist.2014-0328.
7 Rafaeva M, Erler JT. Framing cancer progression: Influence of the organ- and tumour-specific matrisome. *FEBS J.* 2020. doi:10.1111/febs.15223.
8 American Brain Tumor Association. Metastatic brain tumors. https://www.abta.org/wp-content/uploads/2018/03/metastatic-brain-tumor-1.pdf. Published 2017. Accessed March 1, 2020.
9 Mehta M, Vogelbaum MA, Chang S, Patel N. Neoplasm of the central nervous system. In: DeVita VT Jr, Lawrence TS, Rosenberg SA, eds. *Cancer: Principles and Practice of Oncology.* 9th ed. Philadelphia, PA: Lippincott Williams & Wilkins; 2011:1700–1749.
10 Lipton A, Theriault RL, Hortobagyi GN, et al. Pamidronate prevents skeletal complications and is effective palliative treatment in women with breast carcinoma and osteolytic bone metastases: Long-term follow-up of two randomized, placebo-controlled trials. *Cancer.* 2000;88:1082–1090.
11 Lewis MA, Hendrickson AW, Moynihan TJ. Oncologic emergencies: Pathophysiology, presentation, diagnosis, and treatment. *CA Cancer J Clin.* 2011;61:287–314. doi:10.3322/caac.20124.
12 Dietz, J. *Rehabilitation Oncology.* New York, NY: John Wiley and Sons; 1981.

13 Fitzpatrick T. Principles of physical and occupational therapy in cancer. In: Stubblefield MD, O'Dell MW, eds. *Cancer Rehabilitation: Principles and Practice.* New York, NY: Demos Medical Publishing; 2009:785–796.

14 Singh F, Newton RU, Galvão DA, Spry N, Baker MK. A systematic review of pre-surgical exercise intervention studies with cancer patients. *Surg Oncol.* 2013;22(2):92–104. doi:10.1016/j.suronc.2013.01.004.

15 National Comprehensive Cancer Network. *Clinical practice guidelines in oncology: Cancer-related fatigue.* https://www.nccn.org/professionals/physician_gls/pdf/fatigue.pdf. Published 2020. Accessed March 20, 2020.

16 Dittus KL, Gramling RE, Ades PA. Exercise interventions for individuals with advanced cancer: A systematic review. *Prev Med.* 2017;104:124–132. doi:10.1016/j.ypmed.2017.07.015.

17 American Board of Physical Therapy Specialties. Specialist certification: Oncology. http://www.abpts.org/Certification/Oncology/. Published 2016. Accessed March, 2020.

10 Accidents and Unintentional Injuries

Amy J. Litterini and Christopher M. Wilson

Introduction

Accidents are an unfortunate cause of unintentional injuries that can result in both short- and long-term disability, and death.[1] The most common causes of unintentional injuries include motor vehicle accidents (MVA), falls, and workplace accidents. Occupational accidents alone result in an annual estimated 340 million injuries globally and pose a major health concern.[2] The subsequent needs of individuals following accident-related injuries are as varied as the possible accidents causing the injuries, and rehabilitation and physical activity play a vital role in restoration of function and quality of life into recovery (Table 10.1).

Motor Vehicle Accidents

MVA, or road traffic accidents, are the leading cause of accidental death globally for pedestrians, cyclists, motorcyclists, and vehicle drivers.[3] According to the World Health Organization (WHO), most traffic accidents occur in developing countries with the highest risks for younger age groups (5–29 years), male gender, and those with low-middle socioeconomic status.[3] Additional risk factors for traffic accidents include: speeding; driving under the influence; nonuse of helmets and seatbelts; distracted driving; unsafe road infrastructure; unsafe vehicles; inadequate post-crash care; and inadequate enforcement of traffic laws.[3] In 2017, the WHO launched the *Save LIVES* campaign, an initiative including the following evidence-based priorities: **S**peed management; **L**eadership; **I**nfrastructure design and improvement; **V**ehicle

Table 10.1 Incidence and Mortality Rates by Type of Accidental Injuries Globally

Type of Accident	Incidence	Mortality
Motor vehicle accidents[3]	20–50 million	1.35 million
Falls[5]	37.3 million	646,000
Work-related Injuries[2]	340 million	11,000

safety standards; **E**nforcement of traffic laws; and post-crash **S**urvival. The goals are to, literally, save lives and reduce the risks of traffic accidents globally with proven strategies.[4]

Falls

Falls are the second leading cause of accidental death worldwide and pose a major public health concern.[5] Although most falls are non-fatal, medical attention is required annually for an estimated 37.3 million individuals post-fall globally, with considerable costs and morbidity.[5] Greater than 80% of fall-related mortality occurs in low to middle-income countries with the majority of deaths occurring in the regions of the Western Pacific and Southeast Asia.[5]

The largest age group impacted by falls are individuals over age 65, with the highest incidence of death also occurring in individuals 60 years of age or older.[5] In this age population, the subsequent need for hospitalization and or long-term institutionalization post-injurious fall increases secondary to complications such as hip fracture and/or head trauma. Contributing factors for falls include sensory (including vestibular), physical, and cognitive deficits, as well as unsafe home environments and public settings not appropriately adapted for aging in place. Therefore, the growing population sector of elderly individuals worldwide poses a greater concern for skilled intervention for both fall risk reduction and post-fall clinical management.

Comprehensive skilled management for an individual with a fall history ideally includes a formal evaluation for the source of the fall, including screening for medical differential diagnoses and contributing factors such as medication side effects. When possible, a home safety assessment of the living environment, with necessary modifications such as addressing low light areas, would occur if suspected to be a contributing factor. The interventions prescribed in the plan of care should address known factors, such as hip and ankle weakness and range of motion restrictions, and/or vestibular hypofunction, for example. Addressing the direct fall-related injuries, as well as education and mitigation of the contributing factors simultaneously provides the greatest likelihood of success for an individualized program.

In addition to traditional rehabilitation, integrative modalities such as tai chi have demonstrated potential effectiveness in fall risk reduction for older individuals. A systematic review and meta-analysis of the effectiveness of tai chi on falls in older and at-risk adults found a short-term medium protective effect for fall incidence (IRR = 0.57; 95% CI = 0.46, 0.70) and a long-term small protective effect (IRR = 0.87; 95% CI = 0.77, 0.98).[6]

Following the geriatric population, children are also at risk for falls at a higher rate than other age ranges due to their inherent stage of development, desire to explore their environment, and risky behaviors associated with younger age.[5] Public health initiatives aimed at reducing fall risk are key to reducing the overall morbidity and mortality attributed to falls globally for all age groups. Assisting individuals to regain their maximum functional mobility and independence post-fall is an integral role for both rehabilitation and fitness professionals.

Workplace Injuries

According to the International Labour Organization, annual workplace accidents account for an estimated 340 million injuries globally and an estimated 11,000 deaths, which are believed to be grossly under-reported.[2] Aside from accidents, poor workplace conditions often associated with exposure to hazardous substances contribute to an additional 160 million illnesses, and subsequent deaths, annually.[2] Addressing poor work conditions remains a major public health concern globally.

Managing the Effects of Accidental Injuries

For the individuals who survive accidents with unintentional injuries, they are often left with permanent, debilitating consequences and may ultimately succumb to those injuries. Subsequent trauma from unintentional injuries often results in orthopedic, neurologic, and/or organ-related deficits that can persist into survival post-accident. Psychosocial and emotional issues may also arise secondary to fear of recurrence of the original accident. Many individuals will present with traumatic deficits in multiple body regions simultaneously following a traumatic injury, and therefore, the treating clinicians should be cognizant of the need to manage issues in different systems simultaneously, as well as refer to the appropriate interdisciplinary professionals. As clinicians, we ideally assist individuals in overcoming the deficits caused by injuries, and/ or allow them to live to the fullest for the remainder of their lives.

For individuals of working age, return to work is a key goal for most following an injurious accident of any kind. When possible and feasible, workplace assessments with recommendations for appropriate modifications and accommodations are ideal. Where available, seeking guidance from an interdisciplinary occupational health team in a specialized work conditioning center is the gold standard of care. Functional capacity evaluations can provide an objective view of an individual's tolerance for a particular physical demand level. Where mandated by law, advocating for the necessary accommodations legally permitted and expected such as part-time employment, adaptive equipment, modified workstations, improved access, and work status such as light duty are warranted.

Cultural Influences

Following an accident-related injury or illness, the challenges of lost functional mobility can be exacerbated by cultural stigmas associated with disability; these stigmas vary widely by nation or region. Some cultures attribute disease and medical conditions to lack of attention to the spiritual domain, curses on individuals or families through witchcraft or possession by evil spirits, or due to supernatural causes (e.g. epilepsy, cerebral palsy).[7–10] Therefore, seeking medical care to address needs may be limited due to a lack of expectation or hope for improvement due to the inherent consideration of a predetermined destiny. Other influences on medical decision-making include religious and spiritual beliefs, limitations on available accommodations within communities, costs and access to care, and varied terrain to navigate within a community in many geographical regions. Additionally, in many African, Asian, and Latin American countries, care is often provided locally by Traditional Medicine (TM) practitioners such as spiritual healers, bone setters, and herbalists within individual communities and tribes, and hospitalizations and/or more aggressive care occurs only in severe medical conditions or life-threatening traumatic injuries.[11] TM includes various health practices and beliefs, medicines from animal, plant and mineral sources, spiritual therapies, and other techniques.[11] The lack of formal research evidence for some TM interventions may result in unclear efficacy and utility for these treatments; however, respecting cultural tradition and having cultural awareness and humility is the role of the treating clinician.[12]

Box 10.1 Kleinman's Questions[13]

Begin with finding a common term for the problem or illness:
 What do you call your illness or problem? What name does it have?

1 What do you think caused this problem?
2 Why do you think this problem started and when did it start?
3 What do you think this problem does inside your body? How does it work?
4 How severe is this problem? Will it have a short or long course?
5 What kind of treatment do you think you should receive?
6 What are the most important results you hope to receive from this treatment?
7 What are the chief problems this illness has caused?
8 What do you fear most about the illness/problem?

Several models have been developed to assist in effective communication with individuals of different cultures regarding their perspectives on the causes of their injuries and/or illnesses and to improve cultural awareness and humility. Kleinman's Questions (see Box 10.1), mnemonics such as LEARN (see Box 10.2), and Campinha-Bacote's Process of Cultural Competence Model using the mnemonic ASKED (**A**wareness, **S**kills, **K**nowledge, **E**ncounters, and **D**esire), are examples of useful strategies to bridge potential cultural divides and improve the effectiveness of the clinician for rehabilitation for an individual of any culture.[13–15] Having a clear understanding of an individual's opinion on their condition, as well as their wishes for the direction of their treatment, creates a solid foundation for a therapeutic alliance.

Box 10.2 LEARN Model for Cultural Competency[13]

L: Listen with empathy and understanding to the person's perception of the situation

E: Elicit culturally relevant information and Explain your perception of the situation

A: Acknowledge the other person's strengths rather than pointing out their deficits

R: Recommend options/alternatives and Respect the person and their choices

N: Negotiate agreement

Summary

In conclusion, unintentional injuries have multiple causes and result in various levels of morbidity and mortality risk. Assisting individuals who survive these injuries to maximize their functional mobility is a critical aspect of rehabilitation, and a potential benefit of physical activity targeted to the individual deficits to enhance quality of life.

References

1 Dobkowski D, Becker R. CDC: Heart disease, cancer leading causes of death in 2017. *Cardiol. Today.* 2019;22(2):1–5. https://search.proquest.com/docview/2225755106.

2 International Labour Organization. World statistic. https://www.ilo.org/moscow/areas-of-work/occupational-safety-and-health/WCMS_249278/lang--en/index.htm. Published 1996–2020. Accessed April 1, 2020.

3 World Health Organization. Road traffic injuries. https://www.who.int/news-room/fact-sheets/detail/road-traffic-injuries. Published 2020. Accessed February 7, 2020.

4 World Health Organization. Save lives: A road safety technical package. World Health Organization. https://apps.who.int/iris/handle/10665/255199. License: CC BY-NC-SA 3.0 IGO. Published 2017. Accessed February 1, 2020.

5 World Health Organization. Falls. https://www.who.int/news-room/fact-sheets/detail/falls Published 2020. Accessed February 7, 2020.

6 Lomas-Vega R, Obrero-Gaitán E, Molina-Ortega F, Del-Pino-Casado R. Tai chi for risk of falls. A meta-analysis. *J Am Geriatr Soc.* 2017;65(9):2037–2043. doi:10.1111/jgs.15008.

7 Mohammed IN, Babikir HE. Traditional and spiritual medicine among Sudanese children with epilepsy. *Sudan J Paediatr.* 2013;13(1):31–37.

8 Nakken KO, Brodtkorb E. Epilepsy and religion. *Tidsskr Nor Laegeforen.* 2011;131:1294–1297.

9   Sidig A, Ibrahim G, Hussein A, et al. Study of knowledge, attitude, and practice towards epilepsy among relative of epileptic patients in Khartoum State. *Sudan J Public Health*. 2009;4:393–399.

10 Adib SM. From the biomedical model to the Islamic alternative: A brief overview of medical practices in the contemporary Arab world. *Soc Sci Med*. 2004;58(4):697–702. doi:10.1016/s0277–9536(03)00221-1.

11 World Health Organization. Traditional Medicine Growing Needs and Potential - WHO Policy Perspectives on Medicines, No. 002. https://apps. who.int/medicinedocs/en/d/Js2293e/. Published May, 2002. Accessed February 7, 2020.

12 Barnes C, Mueller K, Fawcett L, Wagner B. Living and dying in a disparate health care system: Rationale and strategies for cultural humility in palliative and hospice care physical therapy. *Rehabil Oncol*. 2020 January;38(1):30–38.

13 Berlin E, Fowkes W. A teaching framework for cross-cultural health care. *Western J Med*. 1983;139:934–938.

14 London F. Meeting the challenge: Patient education in a diverse America. *J Nurses Staff Dev*. 2008;24(6):283–285. doi:10.1097/01.NND.0000342240.50989.59.

15 Ingram R. Using Campinha-Bacote's process of cultural competence model to examine the relationship between health literacy and cultural competence. *J Adv Nurs*. 2012;68(3):695–704. doi:10.1111/j.1365–2648.2011.05822.x.

11 Respiratory Diseases

Amy J. Litterini and Christopher M. Wilson

Introduction

As introduced in Chapter 8, *Diseases of the Heart*, the function of the cardio-pulmonary system is a strong indication of health. In the presence of disease or dysfunction, it is also indicative of the overall prognosis. The respiratory system is associated with many diagnoses, several of which can prove to be life-limiting. This chapter will discuss the characteristics of several of these diagnoses, as well as the unique role of rehabilitation and physical activity in the management of symptoms and improvement of quality of remaining life.

Respiratory Diseases

Respiratory diseases, including diagnoses arising within the pulmonary system, occur from different causative sources, across the lifespan, and around the globe (see Figure 11.1). Certain non-communicable respiratory diseases, such as cystic fibrosis, have inherited genetic components while others occur primarily due to acquired genetic mutations, such as lung carcinoma. Respiratory infections, such as seasonal influenza and the novel coronavirus COVID-19, are considered communicable diseases transmitted from person to person via droplets and airborne particles, respectively. Progressive, irreversible tissue damage is implicated in diagnoses such as chronic obstructive pulmonary disease (COPD) and pulmonary fibrosis.

The major contributing factors to respiratory diseases include genetic mutations, exposure to environmental and occupational carcinogens, and tobacco use disorder. Ambient air pollution alone is considered a major public health concern globally and is thought to contribute to a mortality rate of 8.8 million per year through non-communicable diseases including cardiovascular and respiratory diagnoses (see Table 11.1).[1] Air pollution, primarily associated with fossil fuel use, is estimated to cause a loss of life expectancy of 2.9 (2.3–3.5) years, which exceeds the effects of smoking and consequences of violence.[1] Certain geographical and lower-income regions, such as Sub-Saharan Africa, experience lower life expectancy as well as higher than average air pollution-induced infant mortality rates, secondary to the additional risk factor of high household air pollution associated with indoor use of solid biofuels.[1]

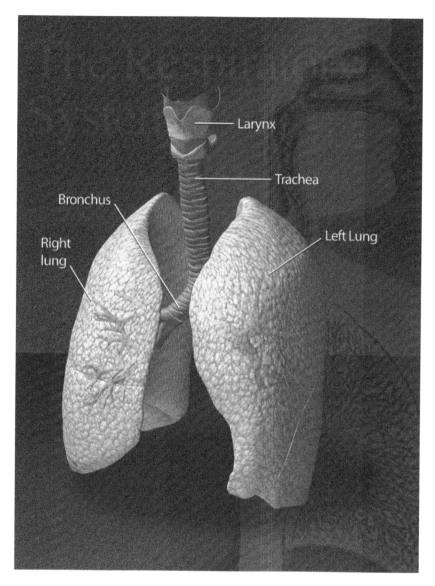

Figure 11.1 The Respiratory System. Nucleus Medical Media. Respiratory System. Smart Imagebase. March 5 2020 10:32 EST. https:// ebsco-smartimagebase-com.une.idm.oclc.org/respiratory-system/ view-item?ItemID=18332. Accessed April 10, 2020.

Table 11.1 Incidence Rates and Mortality in Respiratory Disease in the United States and Globally

Type of Respiratory Disease	United States		Globally	
	Incidence	Mortality	Incidence	Mortality
Chronic obstructive pulmonary disease	12.8 million	160,201	251 million	3.1 million
Chronic bronchitis	9 million			
Emphysema	3.8 million			
Influenza	9–45 million	12,000– 61,000	3–5 million	650,000
Coronavirus (COVID-19) (January, 2021)	20,470,169	348,962	84,474,195	1,848,704

Sources: Center for Disease Control and World Health Organization.
World Health Organization. Burden of COPD. https://www.who.int/respiratory/copd/burden/en/. Published 2020. Accessed April 10, 2020.
World Health Organization. Up to 650,000 people die of respiratory diseases linked to seasonal flu each year. https://www.who.int/mediacentre/news/statements/2017/flu/en/. Published December 17, 2017. Accessed April 7, 2020.
Centers for Disease Control and Prevention. Disease burden of influenza. https://www.cdc.gov/flu/about/burden/index.html. Published January 10, 2020. Accessed April 10, 2020.
World Health Organization. Coronavirus pandemic (COVID-19). https://www.who.int/emergencies/diseases/novel-coronavirus-2019. Published 2021. Accessed January 5, 2021.
National Heart, Lung and Blood Institute. Cystic fibrosis. https://www.nhlbi.nih.gov/health-topics/cystic-fibrosis. Published date unknown. Accessed April 7, 2020.

Chronic Obstructive Pulmonary Disease

COPD, previously known as emphysema, is a life-threatening respiratory diagnosis characterized by chronic inflammation and obstruction of the alveoli, or air sacs, of the lungs. COPD is considered a combination of those diagnosed with *emphysema*, an abnormal accumulation of air secondary to damaged and scarred alveoli, and *chronic bronchitis*, or inflammation of the mucous membranes of the bronchial tubes. For individuals presenting with symptoms such as cough, sputum production, dyspnea, and/or exposure to known risk factors, a formal diagnosis of COPD is made via spirometry. Confirmatory results of spirometry include measurements of forced vital capacity (FVC), the total volume during exhalation, as well as the volume of air exhaled in the first second, known as the forced expiratory volume in one second (FEV1). COPD is then staged from 1 (mild) to 4 (severe), where results of spirometry are compared to normative values to distinguish staging and monitor the status of disease.

Risk factors for COPD include tobacco use, exposure to second-hand smoke, air pollution, and occupational dust and chemicals, and recurrent lower respiratory infections in childhood.[2] The use, particularly by women, of biomass fuels for cooking contribute to the higher rates of COPD among non-smoking women in regions of the Middle East, Africa, and Asia.[2] The global burden of COPD is estimated to affect 65 million individuals, with a disproportionate number of cases diagnosed in low-middle socioeconomic status countries. Due to the excessive disease burden, public health strategies to address issues such as air pollution and smoking cessation are critical in order to slow the projected growth of COPD in the coming decades, as it is projected to be the third leading cause of death worldwide by 2030.[3]

The World Health Organization recommends four critical components of the comprehensive management of COPD: (1) assessment and monitoring of disease; (2) reduction of risk factors; (3) management of stable COPD; and (4) management of exacerbations.[4] Goals for comprehensive management of COPD should ideally include: prevention of disease progression; symptom management; improvement of exercise tolerance; improvement of health status; prevention and treatment of complications; prevention and treatment of exacerbations; and reduction of mortality.[4]

Pulmonary rehabilitation is considered the gold standard for the management of patients with COPD at any stage (see Box 11.1), as well as other

Box 11.1 Pulmonary Rehabilitation Components

Exercise training	Supervised, individualized endurance training (including a walking program), interval training, resistance/strength training, postural exercises, flexibility, and inspiratory muscle training. May also include neuromuscular electrical stimulation and biofeedback from a wearable device.
Patient education	Provides information, offers advice, encourages the acquisition of knowledge for behavioral change
Self-management	Personalized intervention with the goal of motivating and training in healthy behaviors and skills to better manage disease. May also include a negotiated, written action plan for worsening symptoms
Breathing strategies	Education and training on techniques such as pursed lip breathing, diaphragmatic breathing, and positioning to enhance respiratory function and control breathlessness and dyspnea
Nutritional counseling	Components include nutritional supplements to maintain ideal body weight and reduce the risk of malnutrition or low body mass index. Nutritional antioxidant supplementation may be recommended.
Energy conservation techniques	Components include training in the use of adaptive equipment, efficient techniques for the performance of activities of daily living, and pacing strategies.
Counseling	Psychosocial and emotional support to manage transition to illness, as well as teaching coping strategies with ongoing needs for disease management.
Peer support	Learning from and supporting others with shared experiences
Mind-body strategies	Integrative medicine techniques can be helpful to address symptoms such as dyspnea, fatigue, anxiety, insomnia, and stress.

respiratory diseases. Strong evidence supports the use of comprehensive pulmonary rehabilitation programming for improving dyspnea, health status, and exercise tolerance, and it has been shown to reduce hospitalizations in patients with a recent exacerbation (within the previous month).[5] Programs consisting of individualized exercise programming with hybrid types of exercise for durations of six to eight weeks, with supervision provided, are considered the most effective.[5]

Infection: Pneumonia, Influenza, and COVID-19

Respiratory infections are a major public health concern globally. Pneumonia, a viral, bacterial, or fungal infection of the alveoli, can occur in one or both lungs. Most frequently diagnosed on a chest radiograph, pneumonia is usually defined as community-acquired or hospital-acquired. The most common form of bacterial pneumonia is associated with streptococcus (pneumococcus), while many types of viral pneumonia are associated with pathogens such as influenza and coronavirus. Those at a higher risk for acquiring bacterial pneumonia include older individuals, those recovering from injury, illness, or surgery, those with concurrent medical conditions, and/or individuals with tobacco use disorder. Those with viral pneumonia are at risk of developing bacterial pneumonia. A rarer form of pneumonia, *chemical pneumonia*, is associated with lung inflammation caused by exposure to liquids, gases, or small particles.

Seasonal influenza, an acute viral infection transmitted via droplets, causes an estimated 650,000 deaths worldwide annually.[6] In the United States, the disease burden of influenza is estimated to result in 9–45 million illnesses, 140,000–810,000 hospitalizations, and 12,000–61,000 deaths annually.[7] The types of viruses associated with seasonal influenza include A, B, C, and D, with only type A associated with epidemics and pandemics, and B associated with epidemics. The greatest mortality rates secondary to influenza are seen among individuals over the age of 75 and occur in regions with low socioeconomic status.[6] The world's greatest flu mortality risk is in Sub-Saharan Africa, followed by the Eastern Mediterranean, and Southeast Asia.[6] The ideal prevention strategy for seasonal flu is routine vaccination of populations across the globe, and most specifically those individuals at high risk including pregnant women, children, the elderly, individuals with chronic medical conditions, and healthcare workers. As influenza viruses mutate, new forms of the vaccine are needed to effectively treat them.

The diagnosis of influenza is typically made clinically, however, laboratory confirmation is possible where testing is readily available. Typical symptoms of influenza include rapid onset of fever, cough, body aches, headache, malaise, sore throat, and runny nose. Front-line management ideally includes isolation to protect others from the spread of the virus; however, achieving this in households with many people or in communities with tight living quarters is quite challenging. Routine treatment is generally focused on symptom

management and use of antiviral medication such as neuraminidase inhibitors, with corticosteroids used only when indicated for the management of
concurrent diagnoses such as asthma and bronchitis. Although most individuals with influenza recover within approximately one week, conditions
associated with fatal cases are often attributed to concurrent pneumonia and
bronchitis, advanced age, or concurrent health conditions.[8]

The novel COVID-19, or coronavirus, viral pandemic, which swept the
globe in 2019–2021, caused record setting incidence and death rates. At the
time of print, 220 countries had cases with a total of 84,474,195 diagnosed,
and 1,848,704 deaths globally.[9] Initially identified in Wuhan, China, the virus rapidly spread to countries such as South Korea, Italy, Spain, France,
Germany, the United Kingdom, the United States, and many other regions
around the world. As of 2021, the highest death toll was ultimately seen in
the United States.[9] Initially considered a viral pathogen with droplet transmission, the ease of coronavirus transmission by even asymptomatic infected
people and the apparent need for and significant use of N-95 particulate
masks indicated the potential concern for both airborne and droplet transmission. Ultimately, airborne transmission was cautioned by several national
health authorities several months into the pandemic. Additionally, the high
utilization of intensive care unit beds and the need for mechanical ventilators
set this pandemic apart from other viral epidemics and pandemics experienced previously. The exhausted systems resources, including staff fatigue
and facilities at full capacity and beyond, as well as rapidly dwindling stock-
piles of personal protective equipment (PPE), became readily apparent as
the pandemic progressed globally. Techniques such as *proning*, or placing the
patient in prone for extended periods of time, were applied with acute coronavirus to improve air exchange to healthier, less damaged alveoli as it was
hypothesized that the posterior lung tissues were more damaged, restricting
air exchange in supine. In institutions where a substantial number of individuals with COVID-19 were cared for, physical therapists and occupational
therapists were included as key members of proning teams to assist in rolling
orally intubated patients from prone to supine. Some practice guidelines recommended patients lying prone for 12–18 of 24 hours daily during their stay
in intensive care unit.

The need for social distancing, mandatory quarantines, and isolation
during stay-at-home orders, placed severe restrictions not only on socialization within societies and economies of the world but also on traditional rehabilitation and physical activity practices. In order to protect public health
and prevent gatherings of more than ten individuals, fitness gyms were shut-
tered, and public parks and recreational areas were closed. Often deemed
"non-essential" within the healthcare system, most outpatient therapy clinics
closed, and inpatient rehabilitation occurred only in the most extreme cases,
and often via telehealth methods (see Chapter 23). Schools, colleges, and uni-
versities were closed, and therefore, school-based rehabilitation and physical
activity did not occur formally during the pandemic. Home care and hospice

care services were seriously limited, and rehab care in long-term facilities was virtually halted.

Although the volume of deaths was high, with over 1,848,704 succumbing to the virus, millions of people were infected and survived (as of January, 2021). Nonetheless, many continued to be physically and emotionally affected after initial recovery. Issues such as ongoing respiratory dysfunction, critical illness myopathy, and associated functional limitations and participation restrictions occurred. As this specific virus is so novel to humans, there is certainly a role for therapists in the rehabilitation of survivors. However, due to the limited (though rapidly growing) body of knowledge, a therapist may need to employ the concept of disease/symptom triangulation in establishing a patient-centered treatment plan as described in Chapter 22 until there are sufficient studies to establish a valid, reliable clinical pathway.

Many individuals succumbing to symptoms of COVID-19, as well as those who died from other diagnoses during the pandemic, passed away in isolation and without the full support of a traditional interdisciplinary hospice team, or support of loving families. Circumstances required some families to say goodbye to loved ones in a hospital or nursing home via telecommunications because of visitor restrictions aimed at curtailing the rapid spread of COVID-19. Funerals and traditional burial services were not possible, and therefore the normal grieving process for many individuals was seriously disrupted. Support groups and traditional bereavement counseling was also interrupted, not allowing time for the appropriate support for grieving loved ones.

The coronavirus pandemic resulted in unprecedented lapses in care for individuals in need of customary traditional medical care, wellness services, and rehabilitation around the world for extended periods of time. The full effects of this lapse in care, specifically for physical activity and skilled rehabilitation for the public health of populations globally, will need close, thoughtful analysis for years to come. The gravity and sheer magnitude of this pandemic demonstrated an obvious lack of preparedness globally for such a significant outbreak. One can only hope that when faced with inevitable future outbreaks, our countries and healthcare systems will be far more efficiently and effectively prepared to prevent epidemics from progressing to worldwide pandemics, and/or respond swiftly and efficiently to control a pandemic should the world be faced with a similar unfortunate situation in the future.

Cystic Fibrosis

Cystic fibrosis, an inherited genetic disease associated with mutations in copies of the cystic fibrosis transmembrane conductance regulator (CFTR) gene, is passed on from both parents.[10] Individuals inheriting only one copy of the CFTR gene mutation do not develop cystic fibrosis but are asymptomatic carriers of the gene mutation for the disease. The CFTR protein is responsible for the normal production of mucus as a protective lubricant throughout the body. Subsequent dysfunction in the CFTR protein results in excessive mucus production in the lungs and the digestive tract. Risk factors for cystic fibrosis include a family history of the CFTR gene mutation, as well as northern European ancestry. Asian Americans also present with an above-average prevalence. The diagnosis is made based on symptoms and genetic testing, as well as sweat chloride measurement, or sweat test. Screening for the CFTR genetic mutation is now standard of care for newborns in the United States, and allows for early diagnosis and intervention.[10]

As cystic fibrosis most frequently affects the lungs, the most common symptom is a wheezing cough. Potential complications associated with cystic fibrosis include pulmonary exacerbations, hemoptysis, and pneumothorax.[10] Other complications may be associated directly with other involved organs such as pancreatitis and diabetes associated with damage to the pancreas, heart, liver, and kidney disease, as well as osteoporosis, malnutrition, and/ or cancers of the digestive tract. Although the median survival has steadily increased over time, it is presently only 45 years of age in the United States.[11]

There is no definitive cure for cystic fibrosis, and therefore, treatment primarily centers around symptom management. Pharmacological interventions as well as airway clearance techniques are the mainstays of care; however, lifestyle and behavioral choices including a healthy diet, physical activity, and avoiding tobacco use are recommended to improve health outcomes. Supplemental oxygen is recommended when indicated, and lung transplant is a consideration for some with advanced disease.[11]

Pulmonary rehabilitation should be considered at any stage of disease, but most certainly in the recovery of individuals post lung transplantation (see Box 11.1). A systematic review of physical activity with the diagnosis of cystic fibrosis was unable, based on the limited number of small studies with low-to-moderate methodological quality, to strongly advocate for physical activity as a standard of care.[12] However, since there were minimal risks and potential benefits identified with no evidence to discourage physical activity in this instance, the authors advise thoughtful consideration of integration of physical activity and also recommend further investigation with large-scale randomized control trials. An interdisciplinary team centered around pulmonary rehabilitation and respiratory therapy is recommended, as is a center specializing in care for individuals with cystic fibrosis.

Pulmonary Fibrosis

Defined by chronic, progressive, fibrosing interstitial pneumonia, idiopathic pulmonary fibrosis (IPF) is seen primarily in older adults and has no known cause. Diagnosis is one of exclusion, confirmed by high-resolution computed tomography (HRCT) and histopathological features, and is improved in accuracy by consultation with a multidisciplinary team.[12] IPF has a poor prognosis and although it has an unpredictable course, it is considered a fatal condition due to the symptoms of progressive fibrosis and worsening of dyspnea, diminishing lung function, and acute respiratory decline.[13] Although the cause of IPF is unknown, risk factors including tobacco use, environmental exposures, microbial agents including chronic viral infections, gastroesophageal reflux disease, and genetic factors have been suspected.[13]

In an international consensus statement published by the American Thoracic Society and European Respiratory Society (ATS/ERS), in collaboration with the American College of Chest Physicians (ACCP), management recommendations were presented for IPF. Despite insufficient evidence for specific pharmacological intervention recommendations, the authors strongly recommend the consideration for lung transplantation and supplemental oxygen use in patients with IPF.[13] The use of mechanical ventilation was not recommended for the majority of the patients; however, it was recommended for consideration for some selected patient populations. The evidence for the treatment of comorbidities such as pulmonary hypertension and gastroesophageal reflux disease was weak, as was the recommendation for pulmonary rehabilitation.[13] Pertaining specifically to pulmonary rehabilitation (see Box 11.1), the authors state that although it is recommended for the majority of patients with IPF, it would also be a reasonable decision to not use pulmonary rehabilitation for the minority of patients.[13]

Although it could be considered intuitive that early palliative care should be the standard for individuals diagnosed with IPF due to the heavy symptom burden and ultimate fatality rate, the utilization data does not support this notion. According to a retrospective study of 404 decedents by Lindell et al.,[14] individuals with IPF had a median survival of three years from the time of diagnosis, with most dying in the hospital (>50%), and 13.7% of individuals dying without the benefit of a referral for palliative care or hospice. For those receiving a referral for palliative care, the referral occurred within one month of death (71.7%).[14] In a qualitative study by Samson et al.[15] key care concepts were identified in interviews with patients (n = 27) and paired carers/caregivers (n = 21). These authors identified: (1) focus of clinical encounters; (2) timely identification of changes in health status and functional activity; (3) understanding of symptoms and medical interventions; and (4) coping strategies and carer roles, to be key elements of focused support provided to individuals and families with IPF.[15]

Early versus Late-stage Pulmonary Disease

At the time of original diagnosis of respiratory disease, treatment modalities are generally focused on acute and immediate symptom management. Following the acute phase of initial diagnosis, rehabilitation interventions and prescriptions for physical activity are generally targeted at the return of functional capacity from periods of prolonged immobility during recovery, in not only the respiratory system but also the cardiovascular and musculoskeletal systems. Most individuals with a diagnosis of a respiratory disease would benefit from referral for services such as respiratory therapy, pulmonary rehabilitation, physical therapy (PT) and occupational therapy (OT), and exercise prescription from a fitness professional. Co-treatment of PT or OT with speech therapy has shown benefits of the dual task of coordinating physical activities with speech and singing. Caution should be taken for appropriate monitoring of exercise tolerance as well as oxygen saturation levels during physical activity and with changes in the intensity level of physical activity (see Chapter 17 for management of breathlessness).

Strategies to address overall physical capacity, including functional mobility and activity of daily living performance, should be considered for patients at the later stages of disease. Adaptive equipment, activity modification, and energy conservation techniques should be employed to preserve capacity during waking hours. Time spent out of bed, as well as regular position changes, should be encouraged and scheduled when possible to promote proper organ function, maintain skin integrity, and reduce the risk of infection.

For individuals at the end of life secondary to respiratory disease, the symptom burden is often greatest and in need of close attention and intervention. The course of illness is frequently unpredictable and presents with exacerbations, hospitalizations, and periods of decline. Pharmacological interventions, particularly opioid-based regimens, can be effective for both dyspnea and pain management.[16] Higher levels of oxygen may be required to address symptoms of respiratory panic and/or unresolved breathlessness (see Chapter 17). Fatigue should be addressed with pulmonary rehabilitation and education on self-management techniques (see Box 11.1). Nutritional support, including the consideration for antioxidant supplementation, can be valuable for individuals presenting with malnourishment to assist with weight gain, improvements in respiratory muscle strength, and overall health-related quality of life.[16] Symptoms of anxiety, respiratory panic, and/or depression should be monitored and addressed with appropriate medications, cognitive behavioral therapy and/or mind-body therapies.[16] As with all terminal illnesses, discussions regarding end-of-life decisions and advanced care planning are critical as early on in the disease process as possible.

Summary

Respiratory diseases vary widely in origin, risk factors, and disease trajectory. Global public health concerns, such as air pollution and widespread viral transmission, remain contributing factors to the prevalence of these life-limiting diseases. Early detection, and thoughtful intervention including pulmonary rehabilitation strategies, can result in the best outcomes and highest quality of life for those diagnosed.

References

1 Lelieveld J, Pozzer A, Pöschl U, Fnais M, Haines A, Münzel T. Loss of life expectancy from air pollution compared to other risk factors: A worldwide perspective. *Cardiovasc Res.* 2020;116(11):1910–1917. doi:10.1093/cvr/cvaa025.

2 World Health Organization. Causes of COPD. https://www.who.int/respiratory/copd/causes/en/. Published 2020. Accessed April 10, 2020.

3 World Health Organization. Burden of COPD. https://www.who.int/respiratory/copd/burden/en/. Published 2020. Accessed April 10, 2020.

4 World Health Organization. COPD management. https://www.who.int/respiratory/copd/management/en/. Published 2020. Accessed April 10, 2020.

5 2020 Global Strategy for Prevention, Diagnosis and Management of COPD. https://goldcopd.org/wp-content/uploads/2019/12/GOLD-2020-FINAL-ver1.2-03Dec19_WMV.pdf. Pg. 56, Published 2020. Accessed April 10, 2020.

6 World Health Organization. Up to 650,000 people die of respiratory diseases linked to seasonal flu each year. https://www.who.int/mediacentre/news/statements/2017/flu/en/. Published December 17, 2017. Accessed April 7, 2020.

7 Centers for Disease Control and Prevention. Disease burden of influenza. https://www.cdc.gov/flu/about/burden/index.html. Published January 10, 2020. Accessed April 10, 2020.

8 World Health Organization. Influenza (seasonal). https://www.who.int/en/news-room/fact-sheets/detail/influenza-(seasonal). Published December 17, 2017. Accessed April 7, 2020.

9 World Health Organization. Coronavirus pandemic (COVID-19). https://www.who.int/emergencies/diseases/novel-coronavirus-2019. Published 2021. Accessed January 5, 2021.

10 National Heart, Lung and Blood Institute. Cystic fibrosis. https://www.nhlbi.nih.gov/health-topics/cystic-fibrosis. Published date unknown. Accessed April 7, 2020.

11 Sockrider MM, Ferkol TW. Twenty facts about cystic fibrosis. *Am J Respir Crit Care Med*. 2017;196:23–24. doi:10.1164/rccm.19612P23.

12 Radtke T, Nevitt SJ, Hebestreit H, Kriemler S. Physical exercise training for cystic fibrosis. *Cochrane Database Syst Rev*. 2017;11(11):CD002768. Published November 1, 2017. doi:10.1002/14651858.CD002768.pub4.

13 Raghu G, Collard HR, Egan JJ, et al. An official ATS/ERS/JRS/ALAT statement: Idiopathic pulmonary fibrosis: Evidence-based guidelines for diagnosis and management. *Am J Respir Crit Care Med*. 2011;183(6):788–824. doi:10.1164/rccm.2009-040GL.

14 Lindell KO, Liang Z, Hoffman LA, et al. Palliative care and location of death in decedents with idiopathic pulmonary fibrosis. *Chest*. 2015;147(2):423–429. doi:10.1378/chest.14-1127.

15 Sampson C, Gill BH, Harrison NK, Nelson A, Byrne A. The care needs of patients with idiopathic pulmonary fibrosis and their carers (CaNoPy): Results of a qualitative study. *BMC Pulm Med*. 2015;15:155. Published December 4, 2015. doi:10.1186/s12890-015-0145-5.

16 2020 Global Strategy for Prevention, Diagnosis and Management of COPD. https://goldcopd.org/wp-content/uploads/2019/12/GOLD-2020-FINAL-ver1.2-03Dec19_WMV.pdf. Pg. 59, Published 2020. Accessed April 10, 2020.

12 Cerebrovascular Diseases

Acute and Chronic Stroke

Amy J. Litterini and Christopher M. Wilson

Introduction

Cerebrovascular diseases include diagnoses in which the blood vessels to the brain are deformed or damaged, affecting cerebral circulation. Cerebrovascular accidents (CVA), also commonly referred to as *strokes*, are life-threatening diagnoses affecting arteries that lead to the brain causing them to rupture or occlude (see Figure 12.1).[1]

Each year in the United States, 800,000 people experience a new or recurrent stroke; strokes are the leading cause of adult disability and the fifth leading cause of death.[2] Globally, strokes pose a major public health concern

Hemorrhagic Stroke   Ischemic Stroke

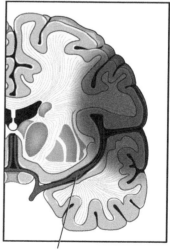

Hemorrhage / blood leaks   Clot stops blood supply
into brain tissue   to an area of the brain

Figure 12.1 Hemorrhagic versus Ischemic Stroke.

Source: Nucleus Medical Media. Hemorrhagic versus Ischemic Stroke. Smart Imagebase. https://ebsco-smartimagebase-com.une.idm.oclc.org/hemorrhagic-vs.-ischemic-stroke/view-item?ItemID=37065. Published January 20, 2019 4:22 EST. Accessed April, 14 2020.

(see Table 12.1). The strongest predictors of stroke survival are severity of the stroke, including neurologic impairment, and age.[3]

There are several risk factors for stroke, many being associated with health factors and lifestyle choices. According to the American Heart Association, atrial fibrillation, tobacco use disorder, physical inactivity, poor diet, overweight /obesity, high cholesterol, diabetes, and hypertension are commonly associated with the incidence of stroke.[1] Worldwide, individuals from the regions of Eastern Europe, Africa, and Central Asia have the highest rates of stroke mortality, with most attributable to ischemic stroke.[1]

Signs and symptoms of stroke include: a sudden onset of numbness in the face or extremities, particularly on one side of the body; sudden confusion; difficulty in speaking and/or understanding speech; altered gait pattern; reduced vision in one or both eyes; and/or sudden onset of severe headache with no known origin. The formal diagnosis of stroke is made through a medical examination including: neurologic testing and blood pressure assessment; laboratory assessments to analyze the clotting cascade; a CT of the head and/or MRI of the brain; and in some cases, a cerebral angiogram to assess the blood flow of the brain and neck. Differential diagnosis of stroke includes seizures, hypoglycemia, migraine headaches, systemic infection, encephalitis, toxic metabolic syndromes, dementia, and other neurological disorders.[4] Carotid ultrasound and echocardiogram are confirmatory tests also used to reveal underlying causes for stroke, such as blockages elsewhere, causing blood clots to travel into the bloodstream.

Medical management following stroke is acutely focused on addressing issues associated with the specific type of stroke. During an *ischemic stroke*, when a blocked artery reduces circulation to a portion of the brain, the immediate concern is restoration of blood flow. Most often when a thrombotic event is causing ischemia, this is achieved with emergency intravenous medications. Given ideally within three hours of the onset of symptoms to relieve clotting, the medication considered the gold standard is recombinant tissue

Table 12.1 Incidence Rates and Mortality in Cerebrovascular Disease in the United States and Worldwide

Type of Cerebrovascular Disease	United States		Worldwide	
	Incidence	Mortality	Incidence	Mortality
Total: Cerebrovascular Diseases	795,000	146,383		5.5 million
Ischemic Stroke	691,650		9.5 million	2.7 million
Hemorrhagic Stroke	103,350		4.1 million	2.8 million

Sources: Centers for Disease Control and Prevention. Stroke facts. https://www.cdc.gov/stroke/facts.htm and World Stroke Organization. Global stroke fact sheet. https://www.world-stroke.org/assets/downloads/WSO_Global_Stroke_Fact_Sheet.pdf.

plasminogen activator (tPA). Other strategies utilized may include emergency endovascular surgical procedures to address blockages directly.[5]

With a *hemorrhagic stroke*, most frequently caused by a ruptured blood vessel, the initial goal is to stop the bleeding and reduce pressure within the brain. Often this involves surgical intervention to repair any blood vessel deficits which led to the stroke initially, including aneurysms and arteriovenous malformations, or procedures intended to remove blood and reduce pressure. Surgical clamps can be used to stop bleeding from occurring or progressing, and stereotactic radiosurgery can be used to repair blood vessel malformations.[5] Considered a third type of stroke, *transient ischemic attacks* (TIA) are similar to ischemic strokes in that they are also generally caused by blood clots. TIAs are typically short in duration, with symptoms often resolving within minutes. Ideally, the cause of a TIA should be formally diagnosed in the hope of preventing future ischemic strokes that might result in persistent, residual deficits.

Assessments of function and performance status of individuals post-stroke in the inpatient setting vary depending on institution. The National Institute of Health Stroke Scale (NIHSS), the Postural Assessment Scale for Stroke (PASS), and the Functional Independence Measure (FIM) are often the standard of care in some US facilities.[6–8] Additionally, depending on level of consciousness, a full systems review including cardiopulmonary, musculoskeletal, neuromuscular, and integumentary assessments are generally completed by physical therapists and/or occupational therapists, while a full communication assessment is performed by speech-language pathologists. Residual stroke symptoms may include *expressive aphasia*, the inability to speak, *receptive aphasia*, the inability to understand spoken words, or *global aphasia*, which presents with symptoms of both receptive and expressive aphasia. For individuals with aphasia, alternative means of communication should be provided for effective medical management and rehabilitation. These may include communication boards, text-to-talk apps using technology on devices such as cellular phones or computer tablets, or writing surfaces such as whiteboards or paper tablets. For individuals experiencing *dysphagia*, or difficulty swallowing, speech-language pathologists and dietitians can work to address issues to reduce the risk of death from choking and/or aspiration pneumonia. Nasogastric (NG) tubes or percutaneous endoscopic gastrostomy (PEG) tubes are often used as temporary nutrition sources for patients with dysphagia.

Rehabilitation tests and measures are applied on a case-by-case basis and are dependent on the amount of time since the initial onset of symptoms, current functional mobility tolerance of the individual, level of alertness and cognition, and ability to communicate sufficiently to complete the testing. A systematic review by Moore, Potter, Blankshain, Kaplan, O'Dwyer, and Sullivan[9] led to a clinical practice guideline on outcome measures for adults with neurologic conditions in rehabilitation. The Berg Balance Scale was recommended for the assessment of static and dynamic sitting and standing balance, and the Activities-specific Balance Confidence Scale was recommended for assessing confidence in balance, based on the strength of the evidence. The Functional Gait Assessment was recommended for determining changes in dynamic balance during ambulation. The six-minute walk test and the 10-meter walk test were also recommended for determining changes in ambulation.[9]

Impairments associated with strokes are numerous, and can persist from acute to chronic functional deficits. The specific neurological deficits are indicative of the portion of the brain affected by the stroke, and the extent of the tissue damage. The most frequently experienced impairments include hemiparesis, loss of sensation in the face or extremities, and/or difficulties with speech, vision, and gait.[5] *Hemiparesis*, significant weakness on one side of the body, often poses the greatest challenges to functional mobility post-stroke, and dictates a high demand for intensive multidisciplinary rehabilitation. Hemiparesis may present as *hypotonicity*, or low resting muscular tone, which may clinically present as weakness or flaccidity (no muscular activity). Conversely, some individuals with stroke may present with *hypertonicity*, a high resting muscle tone, that impairs movement. With hypertonicity or hypotonicity, if range of motion (ROM) activities are not performed regularly, joint or soft tissue stiffness may present, which may result in contracture or permanent deformity. Some individuals may have mixed hypertonicity/hypotonicity and symptoms may be highly variable based on internal and external stimuli. There is a subset of stroke that affects the cerebellum which often presents quite differently from cerebral strokes, having symptoms more often related to balance and coordination. Other commonly encountered symptoms include *neglect*, where the individual appears to be "ignoring" things on the affected side of their body. This often occurs in response to neurological damage of the sensory or processing systems in the damaged part of the brain. In individuals presenting with neglect, rehabilitative efforts should be focused on engaging the patient in stimulating activities on the affected side.

Standard of care in recovery from stroke includes comprehensive multidisciplinary rehabilitation including PT, OT, and speech-language pathology (SLP) to address impairments, in collaboration with medical doctors, nurses, counselors, dietitians, and clergy members. When possible, individuals should be cared for in a facility designated as a stroke center of excellence or an equivalent designation. Depending on the severity of deficits and overall prognosis, care of the individual after a stroke often begins at the intensive care or acute care level, possibly followed by acute rehabilitation at an inpatient rehab facility (IRF), or sub-acute rehab within a skilled nursing facility. The general progression, when feasible, based on recovery and prognosis, is to home care rehabilitation, and ultimately the outpatient setting for extended care. Comprehensive rehabilitation is best initiated immediately, as restoration of functional gains and mobility are more likely to occur early, rather than late, in the recovery process.

Many interventions are utilized for individuals following stroke to address gait and balance deficits. A systematic review by Hornby, Reisman, and Ward,[10] which led to a clinical practice guideline on the management of patients with chronic stroke, summarized the available evidence from 1995 to 2016. Strong evidence was identified for the use of moderate-to-high intensity task-oriented locomotor therapy, augmented by virtual reality methods to increase patient engagement. The recommended goals of therapy, specifically for gait training, are to address the parameters of gait speed and distance through rehabilitation.[10]

Body weight support treadmill training (BWSTT), in combination with functional electrical stimulation (FES), may improve gait mechanics, and balance training may reduce fall risk.[11–13] Gait training can also be performed using FES to the anterior tibialis to facilitate dorsiflexion during ambulation. Early FES on a paretic lower extremity (LE) has been shown to improve walking ability and performance of activities of daily living (ADLs) in patients following strokes.[13] Devices such as ankle-foot orthoses (AFO) can be used to assist with dorsiflexion during ambulation. AFOs have demonstrated an improvement in weight-bearing through affected LE's along with an improvement in gait pattern.[14,15] These skilled interventions can improve safety, balance, gait mechanics, and cadence, thus promoting overall functional independence. Procedural interventions are often focused on task-oriented training for bed mobility, transfers, and ambulation. Research regarding task-oriented training approaches has found that it may improve functional mobility, ADL performance, balance, and self-efficacy in patients with stroke.[16,17] Interventions also routinely include therapeutic exercise, therapeutic activities, neuromuscular re-education, balance training, stair training, and community re-integration. Therapeutic exercises are often utilized for upper and lower extremity strengthening, ROM exercises, and pre-gait activities to increase strength and control of the trunk and extremities. Resistance training has been shown to be an effective intervention to improve strength for patients with hemiparesis in order to enhance performance of functional activities.[18] Neuromuscular re-education, tone normalization, and pre-gait exercises such as weight-shifting exercises and stepping strategies, are frequently incorporated into rehab programs to improve the patient's body awareness and positional stability. Previous studies have shown that weight-shift training can improve overall gait pattern and speed.[19] Tactile facilitation, including stroking and tapping the involved musculature, and pre-gait exercises can help facilitate movement of hemiparetic extremities. Repetitive facilitation exercises (RFE) have demonstrated improvements in LE motor performance and functional ambulation.[20]

Early versus Late-stage Disease

For individuals with an acute onset of stroke, the immediate concerns are for medical management and the early initiation of rehabilitation. Attention should be paid to reducing the number, and extent, of known risk factors (e.g. smoking cessation) that may have contributed to the onset of stroke, to reduce the risk of recurrent strokes. For those surviving acute stroke with persistent symptoms of chronic stroke, the goals shift to maximizing functional mobility and performance of ADLs. Custom devices such as AFOs and equipment for independence in daily activities become critical for long-term survivors with symptoms of chronic stroke. For individuals maintaining the ability to operate a motor vehicle, modifications to steering and pedal operations for individuals with right-sided hemiparesis of the lower extremity can be instrumental in maintaining one's independence with transportation. Driver retraining, often provided by occupational therapists, can assist in gaining independence in driving.

For individuals in the later stages of stroke and near the end of life, the goals of therapy include symptom management, comfort, care coordination, and caregiver training. Due to the multiple impairments associated with stroke, especially for patients in a persistent vegetative state, attention is required for maintenance of skin integrity, prevention of contractures affecting personal care, and position changes for comfort and proper organ function to reduce the risk for infection of the lungs and/or bladder. For those experiencing progressive decline following a stroke, or the inability to achieve successful medical management of the progression of stroke symptoms, hospice care is recommended. In a study of 2,446 patients following acute ischemic stroke, the factors associated with discharge from a hospital setting to home hospice care include older age, high NIHSS score, and altered mental status.[21] Adequate training for caregivers of individuals with terminal stroke symptoms in proper bed care and appropriate devices to assist with the mechanical lifting of dependent patients if needed are critical for injury prevention (see Chapter 5).

Summary

Stroke is one of the leading causes of morbidity and mortality globally. The key to survival and symptom mitigation remains early intervention with appropriate medical management. This intervention includes early rehabilitation to optimize long-term outcomes; individuals with residual stroke symptoms that have been present for years can also experience improvements in adapted function with comprehensive rehabilitation and physical activity strategies. End-of-life care for patients with terminal stroke is best delivered with an interdisciplinary hospice team, which includes care both for the stroke survivor as well as the caregivers.

References

1 American Heart Association. 2020 Heart disease and stroke statistical update fact sheet at-a-glance. https://professional.heart.org/idc/groups/ahamah-public/@wcm/@sop/@smd/documents/downloadable/ucm_505473.pdf. Accessed March 19, 2020.

2 Winstein CJ, Stein J, Arena R, et al. Guidelines for adult stroke rehabilitation and recovery: A guideline for healthcare professionals from the American

Heart Association/American Stroke Association. *Stroke.* 2016;47(6):e98–e169. doi:10.1161/STR.0000000000000098.

3 Edwardson MA, Dromerick AW. Ischemic stroke prognosis in adults. *UpToDate.* 2017;14086(16). http://www.uptodate.com/contents/ischemic-stroke-prognosis-in-adults. Accessed June 20, 2017.

4 Yew KS, Cheng EM. Diagnosis of acute stroke. *Am Fam Physician.* 2015;91(8):528–536.

5 The Mayo Clinic. Stroke: Diagnosis. https://www.mayoclinic.org/diseases-conditions/stroke/diagnosis-treatment/drc-20350119.Published2020.Accessed April 17, 2020.

6 Kwah LK, Diong J. National Institutes of Health Stroke Scale (NIHSS). *J Physiother.* 2014;60(1):61. doi:10.1016/j.jphys.2013.12.012.

7 Huang YC, Wang WT, Liou TH, Liao CD, Lin LF, Huang SW. Postural Assessment Scale for Stroke Patients Scores as a predictor of stroke patient ambulation at discharge from the rehabilitation ward. *J Rehabil Med.* 2016;48(3):259–264. doi:10.2340/16501977-2046.

8 Glenny C, Stolee P. Comparing the Functional Independence Measure and the interRAI/MDS for use in the functional assessment of older adults: A review of the literature. *BMC Geriatr.* 2009;9:52. doi:10.1186/1471-2318-9-52.

9 Moore JL, Potter K, Blankshain K, Kaplan SL, O'Dwyer LC, Sullivan JE. A core set of outcome measures for adults with neurologic conditions undergoing rehabilitation: A clinical practice guideline. *J Neurol Phys Ther.* 2018;42(3):174–220. doi:10.1097/NPT.0000000000000229.

10 Hornby TG, Reisman DS, Ward IG, et al. Clinical practice guideline to improve locomotor function following chronic stroke, incomplete spinal cord injury, and brain injury. *J Neurol Phys Ther.* 2020;44(1):49–100. doi:10.1097/NPT.0000000000000303.

11 Mulroy S, Klassen T, Gronley J, Eberly V, Brown D, Sullivan K. Gait parameters associated with responsiveness to treadmill training with body-weight support after stroke: An exploratory study. *Phys Ther.* 2010;90(2):209–223. doi:10.2522/ptj.20090141.

12 Mehrholz J, Thomas S, Elsner B. Treadmill training and body weight support for walking after stroke. *Cochrane Database Syst Rev.* 2017;8(8):CD002840. Published August 17, 2017. doi:10.1002/14651858.CD002840.pub4.

13 You G, Liang H, Yan T. Functional electrical stimulation early after stroke improves lower limb motor function and ability in activities of daily living. *Neurorehabilitation.* 2014;35(3):381–389. doi:10.3233/NRE-141129.

14 Kim K. Effect of ankle-foot orthosis on weight bearing of chronic stroke patients performing various functional standing tasks. *J Phys Ther Sci.* 2015;27(4):1059–1061. doi:10.1589/jpts.27.1059.

15 Nikamp CD, Hobbelink MS, van der Palen J, Hermens HJ, Rietman JS, Buurke JH. A randomized controlled trial on providing ankle-foot orthoses in patients with (sub-)acute stroke: Short-term kinematic and spatiotemporal effects and effects of timing. *Gait Posture.* 2017;55:15–22. doi:10.1016/j.gaitpost.2017.03.028.

16 Kim K, Jung SI, Lee DK. Effects of task-oriented circuit training on balance and gait ability in subacute stroke patients: a randomized control trial. *J Phys Ther Sci.* 2017;29(6):989–992. doi:10.1589/jpts.29.989.

17 Choi JU, Kang SH. The effects of patient-centered task-oriented training on balance activities of daily living and self-efficacy following stroke. *J Phys Ther Sci.* 2015;27(9):2985–2988. doi:10.1589/jpts.27.2985.

18 Wist S, Clivaz J, Sattelmayer M. Muscle strengthening for hemiparesis after stroke: A meta-analysis. *Ann Phy Rehabil Med.* 2016;59(2):114–124. doi:10.1016/j.rehab.2016.02.001.

19 Nam SH, Son SM, Kim K. Changes of gait parameters following constrained-weight shift training in patients with stroke. *J Phys Ther Sci.* 2017;29(4):673–676. doi:10.1589/jpts.29.673.

20 Tomioka K, Matsumoto S, Ikeda K, et al. Short-term effects of physiotherapy combining repetitive facilitation exercises and orthotic treatment in chronic post-stroke patients. *J Phys Ther Sci.* 2017;29(2):212–215. doi:10.1589/jpts.29.212.

21 Chauhan N, Ali SF, Hannawi Y, Hinduja A. Utilization of hospice care in patients with acute ischemic stroke. *Am J Hosp Palliat Care.* 2019;36(1):28–32. doi:10.1177/1049909118796796.

13 Progressive Neurological Diseases

Amy J. Litterini and Christopher M. Wilson

Introduction

Neurodegenerative disorders, conditions characterized by progressive decline with accentuated symptoms occurring over time, pose substantial functional limitations for the individuals diagnosed. Many of these conditions are associated with both significant morbidity and mortality, such as Alzheimer's disease (AD) and amyotrophic lateral sclerosis (ALS), or *Lou Gehrig's disease* (see Table 13.1), due to their terminal prognosis. Other diagnoses such as Parkinson's disease (PD) and multiple sclerosis (MS) often have varied disease courses which are not always immediately correlated with mortality, though with differing severity levels and morbidity, which make them more individualized and unpredictable regarding disease trajectory.

According to the World Health Organization (WHO), the burden of neurological disorders not only results in morbidity and mortality but also substantial healthcare expenditures. Globally, the spectrum of these disorders includes conditions within the neuropsychiatric category (epilepsy, AD and other dementias, PD, MS, and migraine), cerebrovascular disease (see earlier in Chapter 12), neuroinfections and neurological sequelae of infections (poliomyelitis, tetanus, meningitis, Japanese encephalitis, syphilis, pertussis, diphtheria, malaria), neurological sequelae secondary to nutritional deficiencies and neuropathies (protein/energy malnutrition, iodine deficiency, leprosy, and diabetes mellitus), and neurological sequelae associated with injuries (road traffic accidents, poisonings, falls, fires, drownings, other unintentional injuries, self-inflicted injuries, violence, war, and other intentional injuries).[1] When estimating and projecting the burden of healthcare conditions, the metric often applied considers both (1) premature mortality (years of life lost because of premature mortality [YLL]), and (2) disability (years of healthy life lost as a result of disability [YLD]).[1] The two components, YLL + YLD, equal disability-adjusted life years (DALYs), which equates to the number of healthy years of life lost due to a condition. The top five neurological conditions contributing to the greatest number of DALY's globally include cardiovascular disease (53,815), AD and other dementias (13,540), migraine (7,736), epilepsy (7,419), and tetanus (4,871).[1] In order to address those conditions requiring the greatest demand for rehabilitative interventions and palliative care, dementia, PD, and ALS will be described in this chapter.

Table 13.1 Progressive Neurological Disease Statistics in the United States and Worldwide[2-7]

Type of Neurologic Disease	United States		Worldwide	
	Incidence	Mortality	Incidence	Mortality
Dementia[2,3]	5.8 million	121,404	10 million	unknown
	Incidence	Death rate	Incidence	Mortality
Parkinson's disease[4,5]	60,000	8.7/100,000	10 million	211,296
	Prevalence		Prevalence (median)	
Amyotrophic lateral sclerosis[6,7]	5.2 per 100,000		5.4 per 100,000	

Sources:
[2] Centers for Disease Control and Prevention. Alzheimer's facts and figures 2019. https://www.alz.org/media/documents/alzheimers-facts-and-figures-2019-r.pdf.
[3] World Health Organization. Dementia. https://www.who.int/news-room/fact-sheets/detail/dementia.
[4] Centers for Disease Control and Prevention. Parkinson's disease mortality by state. https://www.cdc.gov/nchs/pressroom/sosmap/parkinsons_disease_mortality/parkinsons_disease.htm.
[5] GBD 2016 Parkinson's Disease Collaborators. Global, regional, and national burden of Parkinson's disease, 1990–2016: A systematic analysis for the Global Burden of Disease Study 2016. *Lancet Neurol.* 2018;17(11):939–953. doi:10.1016/S1474-4422(18)30295-3.
[6] Centers for Disease Control and Prevention. Prevalence of amyotrophic lateral sclerosis — United States, 2015. https://www.cdc.gov/mmwr/volumes/67/wr/pdfs/mm6746a1-H.pdf. https://www.cdc.gov/mmwr/pdf/ss/ss6307.pdf.
[7] Chiò A, Logroscino G, Traynor BJ, et al. Global epidemiology of amyotrophic lateral sclerosis: A systematic review of the published literature. *Neuroepidemiology.* 2013;41(2):118–130. doi:10.1159/000351153.

Dementia

Dementia is a medical syndrome characterized by a cluster of symptoms which includes the deterioration of memory, cognitive function, and the ability to successfully perform usual activities of daily living secondary to damage or loss of nerve cells within the brain. There are several different types of dementia based on the pathological features and presenting symptoms of an individual (see Table 13.2). As dementia is a fatal disease with no known cure, it has recently begun to be referred to as *brain failure* to emphasize the severity of the condition, and to equate its seriousness with other potentially fatal organ diseases such as heart failure and kidney failure. The diagnosis of dementia is made by obtaining a personal and family history, including psychiatric history, as well as evident changes in behavior or cognition. Cognitive testing, as well as physical and neurological exams, aid in the diagnosis. Brain imaging such as CT, MRI, and PET scans may also be used in the diagnostic workup, while lab work can rule out other causes of such changes.

Table 13.2 Types of Dementia[2]

Alzheimer's disease	Most common form of dementia (60–80% of cases)
Vascular dementia	Estimated 10% of cases; most often from blood vessel blockage or damage associated with cerebrovascular disease
DLB	Associated with hallucinations and Parkinsonian-type movement features. May occur in the absence of significant memory losses
Mixed dementia	More than one cause (e.g. Alzheimer's + vascular dementia, Alzheimer's + DLB)
FTD	Frontal and temporal lobe degeneration. Early symptoms include marked changes in personality and behavior (versus memory lapses)

Dementia with Lewy bodies, DLB; Frontotemporal dementia, FTD.

As of 2019 in the United States, an estimated 5.8 million Americans have been diagnosed with AD.[2] Of these individuals, the majority, or 5.6 million people, were aged 65 and older, with 81% aged 75 or older.[2] An estimated 200,000 individuals younger than 65 years have early onset AD. Globally, an estimated 50 million individuals currently have a diagnosis of dementia, with the numbers expected to rise to 152 million by the year 2050.[3]

The hallmark in the diagnosis of AD is the accumulation of amyloid protein plaque formation outside neurons in the brain, and twisted tau protein strands (aka neurofibrillary tangles) inside neurons, with damage and subsequent death of brain neurons. The pathological changes are thought to begin many years before symptoms become evident or obvious. Three stages of AD have been identified as follows: (1) preclinical AD; (2) mild cognitive impairment (MCI) due to AD; and (3) dementia due to AD. In stages two and three, symptoms are observable but vary in severity from individual to individual. There are several modifiable and non-modifiable risk factors for dementia (see Table 13.3).[2]

As a diagnosis, dementia has a high level of both morbidity and mortality. AD is one of the leading causes of disability in the United States resulting in: immobility; swallowing disorders and malnutrition; pneumonia; a high rate of nursing home admissions; utilization of the emergency department; and hospital admissions.[2] Individuals with dementia also contribute to substantial utilization of hospice and palliative care, estimated at 15.6% of total individuals enrolled in hospice in the United States.[8] Dementia places a heavy burden on society for caregiver needs, both in intensity level and duration. The average survival for patients with dementia is four to eight years, with 40% of time with the diagnosis spent in the most advanced stage.[2] AD is the sixth leading cause of death in the United States and the fifth cause of death in individuals aged 65 and older. The diagnosis of dementia is often underreported as cause of death (e.g. *from* versus *with* dementia).[2] As death certificates routinely list pneumonia or other medical conditions as the primary cause of death rather than dementia, the WHO emphasizes the diagnosis of dementia

Table 13.3 Modifiable and Non-modifiable Risk Factors for Dementia[2]

Type of Risk Factor		
Non-modifiable risk factors	Single gene mutations	• FAD; familial vascular dementia; and familial frontotemporal dementia • 50% chance of inheriting from a parent with the mutation • APOE allele on chromosome 19: Inherit one gene from each parent (ε2, ε3, ε4) Two copies of APOE-4 = 8–12-fold risk of AD • Tend to develop early onset (30s–50s)
	Multi-gene variants	More frequently associated with dementia
	Age	Dementia risk increases dramatically with age
	Other conditions	• Down's Syndrome • Huntington's Disease • MCI
Modifiable risk factors	Lifestyle	High cholesterol, hypertension, type 2 diabetes, and a personal or family history of stroke or heart disease increases the chances of developing vascular dementia
	Education level	More years of formal education thought to build "cognitive reserve"
	Social and cognitive engagement	Thought to build cognitive reserve
	Traumatic brain injury (moderate-severe)	Falls, motor vehicle accidents, boxing, football, combat veterans
	CTE	Same tangles of tau protein similar to those seen in dementia are observed in CTE

Familial Alzheimer's disease (FAD); Apolipoprotein (APOE); Mild Cognitive Impairment (MCI); Chronic Traumatic Encephalopathy (CTE)

as "the disease or injury which initiated the train of events leading directly to death."[2(pg25),9]

There are several common behaviors manifested by individuals with dementia. Many behaviors often start as mild on the spectrum, and can progress in severity over time. Some examples include: aggression; anxiety; agitation; confusion; repetition (e.g. activities and comments); suspicion/paranoia; sleep disturbances; and wandering/getting lost.[10] Symptoms with greater severity are referred to as *behavioral and psychological symptoms of dementia* (BPSD). BPSD often lead to institutionalization due to manifestations such as: delusions/hallucinations; depression/apathy; inappropriate sexual behavior; aggressiveness; criminal behavior; aberrant motor behaviors; disinhibition; and abnormal eating behaviors.[11]

Managing symptoms for an individual with a diagnosis of dementia often includes addressing contributing factors and underlying symptoms. Scenarios such as physical discomfort, overstimulation, unfamiliar surroundings, complicated tasks, and frustrating interactions can and should be minimized to reduce their influence on symptoms of dementia. During a new onset or worsening of existing confusion, other medical diagnoses such as delirium, urinary tract or other infection, medication interactions, dehydration, low blood sugar, and substance use disorder should be investigated for a differential diagnosis.

Dementia severely affects the level of one's home safety. According to the Alzheimer's Association, reduced home safety is associated with cognitive decline in individuals with dementia, including changes in judgment, awareness of time and place, behaviors, physical abilities, and alterations to vision, hearing, and proprioception.[12] In order to maintain independence and the potential to remain in one's home, a multidisciplinary team approach to home safety assessment and safety modifications are necessary. Depending on the needs of the individual, safety strategies for patient location and identification may include the use of medical alert bracelets and GPS tracking capabilities. High deadbolts and/or painted doorknobs, as well as Velcro stop sign banners across door frames, can prevent unsupervised access to off-limits or potentially unsafe environments. Unintentional injuries and fire hazards can be minimized by securing car keys to prevent driving, locking or removing firearms, securing lighters and/or combustible materials, and removing knobs from stoves.[12]

The issue of wandering by individuals with dementia is one of grave concern for both loved ones and healthcare professionals. According to the Alzheimer's Association, six out of ten individuals with dementia are estimated to wander.[2] *Purposeful wandering,* or deliberately trying to go somewhere such as a childhood home or former place of employment, is also a common occurrence. The risks associated with wandering are numerous, and include dehydration/malnutrition, cold weather exposure, premature permanent placement, resident-to-resident violence, and even death. A study by Kikuchi et al.[13] examined the concept of fatality associated with wandering. Information provided by families of 388 deceased patients with dementia from missing persons reports revealed three identified causes/patterns: (1) traumatic injury or drowning (on the day of wandering); (2) hypothermia (within days of wandering); and (3) other causes of death.[13] In addition to wandering, *boundary transgressions* (BT) are also observed in individuals particularly with severe dementia. BT is considered wandering-related locomotion that takes a person with dementia into hazardous or out-of-bounds areas (such as busy streets, industrial areas, or construction zones).[14] Associated outcomes for long-term care residents secondary to BT include: injury from resident-to-resident altercation; becoming lost or trapped; and accidental exit from a safe environment without being able to return safely unassisted.[14] In addition to dedicated memory care units and facilities, the creation of "dementia friendly" communities and businesses like the *Dementia Village* in Denmark, are being designed to promote the comfort, support, and safety needed for the growing number of individuals living with dementia across the globe.

The availability of outcome measures specifically for individuals with a diagnosis of dementia is limited. However, there is available evidence for the application for certain outcome measures to be valid for the dementia patient population (see Table 13.4).

Traditional treatment for individuals with dementia includes both pharmacological and non-pharmacological interventions. Historically speaking, pharmacological interventions for dementia have proven to be a disappointment in both short and long-term outcomes, as there is no cure and no medication presently able to effectively slow the progression of the disease. Research

Table 13.4 Outcome Measures Research: Dementia[15–17]

Study	Authors	Design	Results/Conclusions
Test-retest reliability and minimal detectable change scores for the Timed "Up & Go" Test, the Six-Minute Walk Test, and gait speed in people with Alzheimer disease	Ries et al. (2016)[15]	Prospective, non-experimental, descriptive methodological study, n = 51	"The TUG, the 6MWT, and gait speed are reliable outcome measures for use with people with AD, recognizing that individual variability of performance is high. Minimal detectable change scores at the 90% confidence interval can be used to assess change in performance over time and the impact of treatment."[p569]
The Groningen Meander Walking Test (GMWT): A dynamic walking test for older adults with dementia	Bossers et al. (2013)[16]	Repeated-measures design, n = 42	"The GMWT is a feasible test for people with dementia. With the GMWT time score, a reliable and sensitive field test to measure walking abilities in older adults with dementia is available. The GMWT overstep score can be used to give information about the execution according to protocol and should be emphasized during the instructions. Future studies need to investigate the validity of the GMWT."[p262]
Reliability of six physical performance tests in older people with dementia	Blankevoort, van Heuvelen, and Scherder (2012)[17]	Prospective, nonexperimental study, n = 58	"The relative reliability of the F8W, TUG, and Jamar dynamometer was excellent (ICC = 0.90–0.95) and good for the 6-m walk test, FICSIT-4, and CRT (ICC = 0.79–0.86). The SEMs and MDCs were large for all tests. The absolute reliability of the TUG and CRT was significantly influenced by the level of cognitive functioning (as assessed with the Mini-Mental State Examination [MMSE])."[p69]

GMWT, The Groningen Meander Walking Test; F8W, Figure-of-Eight Walk Test; TUG, Timed "Up Go" Test; FICSIT-4, Frailty and Injuries: Cooperative Studies of Intervention Techniques–4 (FICSIT-CRT, Chair Rise Test is under way to improve options for patients and families with the hope for more effective medication options.

Non-pharmacological interventions include recommendations for formal skilled rehabilitation, as well as computerized memory training, music therapy, physical activity, and Cognitive Stimulation Therapy (CST). The goals of non-pharmacological therapy include: maintaining or improving cognitive function and the ability to perform activities of daily living (ADLs); and maintain a quality of life while reducing behavioral symptoms of depression/apathy, wandering/sleep disturbances, and agitation/aggression. Additional goals should include reducing the burden on caregivers, which is inordinately high for individuals caring for loved ones with dementia, often elderly spouses (see Chapter 5).

The evidence supporting the role of physical activity for individuals with dementia has become more robust in recent years. A systematic review and meta-analysis by Farina, Rusted, and Tabet[18] found physical activity to have a positive effect on cognitive decline as well as a positive effect on global cognitive function for exercising individuals (0.75 [95% CI = 0.32–1.17]). A meta-analysis by Lee et al.[19] determined that physical activity for patients with dementia demonstrated an improvement in physical capacity, and the most effective physical activity was combined exercise. In a meta-analysis by Groot et al.,[20] physical activity interventions were found to be equally beneficial for individuals with AD as well as individuals with non-Alzheimer's related diagnoses of dementia. They found both combined and aerobic-only exercise to have a positive effect on cognition.[20]

Appropriate communication strategies are necessary to be effective in caring for individuals with dementia (see Chapter 7). Ideally, a calming voice, soft facial expressions, and a kind presence can portray a non-threatening verbal and non-verbal level of messaging. Therapists should strive to avoid confrontation and instead attempt gentle redirection, which can help prevent situations from escalating to aggression or an argument. Opportunities to orient the individual to name, day, place, and time such as use of whiteboards and items to creatively decorate an individual's door to ease in recognition, can improve awareness. Remembering that if a person with dementia is engaged in an activity that will not hurt them or others, and they are pleasantly occupied with the activity (e.g. packing a suitcase, folding and refolding clothes, playing with a doll), then there is minimal risk or harm in allowing the activity to persist or be performed on a repeated basis. Activities to keep individuals participating in meaningful tasks, such as those proposed by a recreational therapist or an activities coordinator, can provide purpose and maintain a level of engagement in daily tasks and recreation.

Due to the fatal nature of dementia, documentation of an advance directive is a key step and completion is encouraged early upon the diagnosis. Due to the inevitable loss of competence and the ability to make one's own medical decisions at some point in the disease trajectory, documentation of the individual's wishes and preferences is important to individuals and their families. Please see Appendix 1 for more information regarding dementia-specific advance directives.

Parkinson's Disease

PD, a complex condition associated with loss of dopaminergic neurons in the substantia nigra, is estimated to affect 60,000 newly diagnosed individuals in the United States annually and 10 million individuals globally.[4,5] The diagnosis of PD is often made as one of exclusion, as there are limited definitive diagnostic tests available. Patient history, neurological exam, and response to Parkinson's medications are generally used in the diagnosis process.

Based on work by Hoehn and Yahr,[21] PD is staged on a 1 to 5 scale representing the severity of the condition and movement deficits, with Stage 1 being early disease with unilateral involvement, and Stage 5 representing advanced disease.[22] The Unified Parkinson's Disease Rating Scale (UPDRS) also grades the severity of PD symptoms, but takes the following into consideration: mentation, behavior, and mood, as well as performance of ADLs; motor examination results; and complications of therapy to provide a more comprehensive perspective on a patient's presentation.[23]

The most common signs and symptoms associated with PD include tremors, rigidity (stiffness), bradykinesia (slow movements), balance and coordination impairments, and fall risk often associated with a shuffling gait pattern.[24] Additional symptoms may include: depression and other emotional changes; dysphagia, difficulty chewing, and/or speaking; incontinence and/or constipation; and sleep disturbances. Advanced Parkinson's can also be associated with hallucination-type symptoms, confusion, and/or delusions. The cause of PD remains unknown, but it is thought to be attributed to a combination of both environmental and genetic factors. Contributing factors for the development of PD may include increasing age (60 and older), male gender, and pesticide exposure. *Early onset* PD is considered in those with an onset at 50 or younger years of age.[24]

Outcome measure application is an important component to rehabilitation for initial assessment, and monitoring for progress or decline, in individuals with PD. A study by Steffen and Seney[25] identified the Berg Balance Scale (BBS), the Activities-specific Balance Confidence (ABC) Scale, Sharpened Romberg Test (SRT) with eyes closed, the six-minute walk test (6MWT), and the assessment of gait speed to have high test-retest reliability for individuals with PD. The recommended measures for assessment of quality of life and disease severity were the SF-36 and the UPDRS.[25]

The prognosis of PD, and the progression of the condition, varies from individual to individual. Treatment is heavily dependent on pharmaceuticals, and successful treatment is generally considered to be a result of improvements in physical function and symptoms resulting from a positive response to the prescribed medications. For rehabilitation clinicians and physical activity professionals, the goals are to assist with symptoms of rigidity through regular range of motion activities, use of gait training strategies to address gait deviations and reduce fall risk, and prescribed exercise to maintain strength and cardiovascular endurance. Due to symptoms of bradykinesia and lost automaticity for individuals with PD, repetitive, reciprocal activities such as cycling, boxing, and treadmill training have been incorporated into exercise prescription with growing popularity. However, evidence of efficacy for these interventions is still needed in well-designed, large-scale, randomized trials.[26–28]

Amyotrophic Lateral Sclerosis
(Lou Gehrig's Disease)

ALS, also known as *Lou Gehrig's disease*, is a progressive neurodegenerative disease that involves the motor neurons within the corticospinal tract, brain stem, spinal cord, and primary motor cortex.[29] ALS may begin with an initial *bulbar* or *limb* onset. Limb onset shows signs of weakness, spasticity, paralysis, and abnormal reflexes, presenting with either upper or lower motor neuron dysfunction.[29] *Bulbar* onset refers to the involvement of the medulla oblongata and pons, which control the bulbar muscles of the face, jaw, soft palate, larynx, pharynx, and tongue.[30] With a bulbar onset, oral motor dysfunction including dysarthria, dysphagia, and sialorrhea (drooling or excessive salivation) are observed.[29] In *limb* onset, muscle atrophy as well as muscle fasciculation are common, and diagnosis occurs at approximately 60 years of age.[29] As the course of ALS progresses, it often leads to pulmonary complications.[29] ALS progresses in stages based on symptom presentation, muscle function, and physical effects of the disease from Stage 1, or *early stage*, to Stage 4, or *end-stage*.

ALS is initially a diagnosis of exclusion, where other possible neurological causes of symptomatology are ruled out by the absence of electromyographic and neuroimaging proof of other diagnoses. According to the El Escorial criteria, after ruling out other neurologic conditions, the specific diagnosis is made with evidence of: lower motor neuron degeneration by clinical, electrophysiological, and or neuropathological examination; evidence of upper motor neuron degeneration by clinical examination; and progressive spread of signs and symptoms within a region, or throughout another region of the body, by history and examination.[31]

As the presentation and progression of ALS varies from person to person, an additional classification of ALS phenotypes has been suggested by Al-Chalabi et al.[32] These authors propose an enhanced classification system which incorporates the following components: (1) stage of disease; (2) phenotype; (3) diagnosis; and (4) El Escorial category, including other diagnostic modifiers (e.g. family history) and optional terms.[32]

The typical presentation of ALS symptoms includes persistent weakness and/or spasticity in one or more extremities, with initial presentation often unilateral. Difficulty with swallowing and/or speech may accompany the extremity symptoms. Bowel and bladder dysfunction may also be noted by individuals with ALS, and chronic constipation leads to increased risk for bowel obstruction. Prolonged immobility can also contribute to symptoms of pain for these individuals. Fasciculations are also seen, as well as cognitive and behavioral issues for some people. Risk factors for ALS which are consistently reported include older age, male gender, and tobacco use disorder.[33]

In addition to the outcome measures for assessing balance and functional mobility recommended earlier (see Chapter 12 on cerebrovascular disease), the Assessment of Activities of Daily Living in Patients with Amyotrophic Lateral Sclerosis (ALSFRS) is also considered a valuable tool for individuals with ALS. In a study of 75 patients with ALS, internal consistency and test-retest reliability for the ALSFRS were found to be high, and the assessment demonstrated good construct validity. The ALSFRS also showed close agreement with muscle strength and pulmonary function.[34]

The management of ALS requires a complex and comprehensive approach by a multidisciplinary team. Based on a systematic review, an expert panel developed consensus recommendations which indicate the best practices from diagnosis throughout the disease course (see Table 13.5).[35]

The literature on the benefits of skilled rehabilitation for ALS continues to be limited. Regarding physical rehabilitation and physical activity for individuals with ALS, Bello-Haas[36] summarized the role of rehabilitation in addressing symptoms. Despite the progressive nature of the disease, having a multidisciplinary team available for issues such as cognitive, behavioral, and psychological impairments, pain, fall risk, appropriate exercise prescription, and respiratory impairments, promotes maximization of functional mobility and participation in ADLs for the greatest duration possible. According to Macpherson and Bassile,[37] pulmonary physical therapy interventions such as inspiratory muscle training (IMT), lung volume recruitment training (LVRT), and manually assisted cough (MAC), have shown effectiveness in improving respiratory outcome measures and increasing survival for individuals with ALS.

Respiratory failure is the most frequent cause of death for individuals with ALS. Other less frequent causes of death include malnutrition,

Table 13.5 European Federation of Neurological Societies' Guidelines on the Clinical Management of Amyotrophic Lateral Sclerosis[35]

Diagnosis	Early identification of disease, by an experienced neurologist, including neurophysiological testing
Education	Patient and family education regarding the disease state and expected progression
Medical management	Initiation of the medication riluzole Control of symptoms including pain, spasticity, cramps, excessive mucus and sialorrhea
Supportive care	Skilled rehabilitation to maintain functional mobility and patient autonomy Speech and language pathology to assist in communication strategies Dietary consultation and potential for peg tube placement to maintain nutrition Counseling on development of advanced directives Early initiation of multidisciplinary palliative care

pulmonary embolism, cardiac arrhythmias, and aspiration pneumonia.[38] Most individuals diagnosed with ALS survive for an average of three years from diagnosis, with poorer outcomes seen with either an older age of onset or bulbar type ALS.[39]

Other Neurodegenerative Disorders

There are several additional neurodegenerative conditions that have progressive symptom presentations, high care demand components, and feature gradual declines, such as MS, spinal muscular atrophy, and Huntington's disease. Other conditions causing chronic, recurrent neurologic symptoms include those with diagnoses such as epilepsy and/or migraines. Regardless of the particular diagnosis, many of the same outcome measures, principles of maintenance of functional mobility with interventions, caregiver training, patient education, symptom management and palliation, similarly apply. In addition, respiratory failure and associated infections are often the ultimate cause of death for many of these neurological conditions. Maintaining functional mobility, and retaining physical capabilities for both occupation and recreation, while enhancing quality of life, remain the overarching goals regardless of the primary diagnosis. As discussed in Chapter 4, the concept of *Rehabilitation in Reverse* is most applicable to the care of people with neurodegenerative disorders experiencing the sequential loss of function over time.

Early versus Late-stage Disease

In the early stages of many neurodegenerative conditions, individuals may be able to compensate quite well for minor neurologic deficits. Some individuals may have a delayed diagnosis due to minimizing or dismissing their symptoms, while assuming they are unrelated to a potential neurologic diagnosis (e.g. chronic memory loss attributed to 'senior moments'). Once diagnosed, individuals could ideally function successfully with the appropriate rehabilitative strategies and maintenance of physical activity levels during their early stages. As with many diagnoses, early identification and referral to rehabilitation offer the highest likelihood of prolonged functional mobility, participation in ADLs, and quality of life. For diagnoses such as ALS, the early acquisition of appropriate durable medical equipment, and patient and caregiver training, helps to maintain independence for the greatest duration possible.

In the later stages of neurodegenerative diseases, there are often multiple levels of support required for the individual to maintain a degree of functional mobility and quality of life. Caregivers and loved ones carry a higher burden of the demand for care as the diseases progress. It is imperative for appropriate screening and referral for the necessary rehabilitative and higher capability durable medical equipment options for patients at each stage of decline during disease progression. For example, in individuals who were initially able to transfer independently, or with the assistance of a caregiver, transfer devices such as transfer boards and mechanical lifts can ultimately maintain the individual's ability to regularly assume the sitting position while protecting the caregiver in the circumstance of an increasingly physically demanding transfer. Hospital beds, and equipment for the bathroom such as tub seats and elevated toilet seats, become necessary to allow an individual to remain within a home setting. If or when ambulatory capabilities are lost, wheelchair fitting becomes necessary. If unable to self-propel in a manual wheelchair, individuals may benefit from a transport chair. If an individual's cognitive status allows for safe operation, a power chair rental or purchase could be considered as equipment if resources allow. In instances where an individual can no longer be cared for in the home, placement in a facility where higher intensity care is available is often the next step. Comprehensive management from an interprofessional hospice team provides the best option for symptom management and quality of life. Referring the patient and family for psychosocial and/or spiritual counseling can assist them as they transition towards the end of life. Admission to an inpatient hospice unit might be considered for those with a prognosis of fewer than two weeks or whose quality of care would not be sufficient in a home environment.

Summary

Due to the progressive cognitive and neuromuscular impairments, physical activity plays a key role throughout the neurological disease process. This presentation requires the therapist to tailor their care to the patient presentation, and meet the individual where they are in their disease journey, as keys to success in managing these difficult neurodegenerative conditions. Preparing the patient and caregivers for the potential and anticipated future physical and functional losses with resultant decline, and how to best manage it, is a responsibility of the treating clinician team members. Staying present throughout the process assures the patient-family unit they are not alone in their time of need, and that they will receive the support necessary when the time comes for enhanced levels of care.

References

1 World Health Organization. Global Burden of neurological disorders estimates and projections. In: Neurological Disorders: Public Health Challenges.   https://www.who.int/mental_health/neurology/chapter_2_neuro_disorders_public_h_challenges.pdf?ua=1. Published date unknown. Accessed April 23, 2020.
2 Centers for Disease Control and Prevention. Alzheimer's facts and figures 2019. https://www.alz.org/media/documents/alzheimers-facts-and-figures-2019-r.pdf. Published 2019. Accessed March 1, 2020.
3 World Health Organization. Dementia. https://www.who.int/news-room/fact-sheets/detail/dementia. Published 2020. Accessed March 1, 2020.
4 Centers for Disease Control and Prevention. Parkinson's disease mortality by state. https://www.cdc.gov/nchs/pressroom/sosmap/parkinsons_disease_mortality/parkinsons_disease.htm. Published 2020. Accessed March 1, 2020.

5 GBD 2016 Parkinson's Disease Collaborators. Global, regional, and national burden of Parkinson's disease, 1990–2016: A systematic analysis for the Global Burden of Disease Study 2016. *Lancet Neurol.* 2018;17(11):939–953. doi:10.1016/S1474-4422(18)30295-3.

6 Centers for Disease Control and Prevention. Prevalence of Amyotrophic Lateral Sclerosis — United States, 2015 https://www.cdc.gov/mmwr/volumes/67/wr/pdfs/mm6746a1-H.pdf. Published 2018. Accessed March 1, 2020.

7 Chiò A, Logroscino G, Traynor BJ, et al. Global epidemiology of amyotrophic lateral sclerosis: A systematic review of the published literature. *Neuroepidemiology.* 2013;41(2):118–130. doi:10.1159/000351153.

8 National Hospice and Palliative Care Association. Facts and figures 2018 edition. https://www.nhpco.org/wp-content/uploads/2019/07/2018_NHPCO_Facts_Figures.pdf. Published 2019. Accessed April 20, 2020.

9 World Health Organization. *International Statistical Classification of Diseases and Related Health Problems.* 10th revision, 2nd ed. Geneva, Switzerland: WHO Press; 2004.

10 Alzheimer's Association. Behaviors. https://www.alz.org/national/documents/brochure_behaviors.pdf. Published 2020. Accessed April 21, 2020.

11 Torrisi M, Cacciola A, Marra A, De Luca R, Bramanti P, Calabrò RS. Inappropriate behaviors and hypersexuality in individuals with dementia: An overview of a neglected issue. *Geriatr Gerontol Int.* 2017;17(6):865–874. doi:10.1111/ggi.12854.

12 Alzheimer's Association. Home safety. https://www.alz.org/help-support/caregiving/safety/home-safety#safetytips. Published 2020. Accessed April 21, 2020.

13 Kikuchi K, Ijuin M, Awata S, Suzuki T. A study on the mortality patterns of missing and deceased persons with dementia who died due to wandering. *Nihon Ronen Igakkai Zasshi.* 2016;53(4):363–373. doi:10.3143/geriatrics.53.363.

14 MacAndrew M, Fielding E, Kolanowski A, O'Reilly M, Beattie E. Observing wandering-related boundary transgression in people with severe dementia. *Aging Ment Health.* 2017;21(11):1197–1205. doi:10.1080/13607863.2016.1211620.

15 Ries J, Echternach J, Nof L, Gagnon Blodgett M. Test-retest reliability and minimal detectable change scores for the Timed "Up & Go" Test, the Six-Minute Walk Test, and gait speed in people with Alzheimer disease. *Phys Ther.* 2009;89(6):569–579. doi:10.2522/ptj.20080258.

16 Bossers W, van der Woude L, Boersma F, Scherder E, van Heuvelen M. The Groningen Meander Walking Test: A dynamic walking test for older adults with dementia. *Phys Ther.* 2014;94(2):262–272. doi:10.2522/ptj.20130077.

17 Blankevoort C, van Heuvelen M, Scherder E. Reliability of six physical performance tests in older people with dementia. *Phys Ther.* 2013;93(1):69–78. doi:10.2522/ptj.20110164.

18 Farina N, Rusted J, Tabet N. The effect of exercise interventions on cognitive outcome in Alzheimer's disease: A systematic review. *Int Psychogeriatr.* 2014;26(1):9–18. doi:10.1017/S1041610213001385.

19 Lee HS, Park SW, Park YJ. Effects of physical activity programs on the improvement of dementia symptom: A meta-analysis. *BioMed Res Int.* 2016; 2920146. doi:10.1155/2016/2920146.

20 Groot C, Hooghiemstra AM, Raijmakers PG, van Berckel BN, Scheltens P, Scherder E, et al. The effect of physical activity on cognitive function in patients with dementia: A meta-analysis of randomized control trials. *Ageing Res Rev.* 2016;25:13–23.

21 Hoehn M, Yahr M. Parkinsonism: onset, progression and mortality. *Neurology.* 1967(17)5;427–442.

22 Parkinson's Resource Organization. The five stages of Parkinson's. https://parkinsonsresource.org/news/articles/five-stages-of-parkinsons/. Published 2020. Accessed March 5, 2020.

23 Unified Parkinson's Disease Rating Scale. https://www.etas.ee/wp-content/uploads/2013/10/updrs.pdf. Published date unknown. Accessed March 20, 2020.

24 Kalia L, Lang A. Parkinson's disease. *Lancet.* 2015;386:896–912.

25 Steffen T, Seney M. Test-retest reliability and minimal detectable change on balance and ambulation tests, the 36-Item Short-Form Health Survey, and the Unified Parkinson Disease Rating Scale in people with Parkinsonism. *Phys Ther.* 2008;88(6):733–746. doi:10.2522/ptj.20070214.

26 Morris ME, Ellis TD, Jazayeri D, et al. Boxing for Parkinson's disease: Has implementation accelerated beyond current evidence? *Front Neurol.* 2019;10:1222. Published December 4, 2019. doi:10.3389/fneur.2019.01222.

27 Wu T, Hallett M, Chan P. Motor automaticity in Parkinson's disease. *Neurobiol Dis.* 2015;82:226–234. doi:10.1016/j.nbd.2015.06.014.

28 Schenkman M, Moore CG, Kohrt WM, et al. Effect of high-intensity treadmill exercise on motor symptoms in patients with de novo Parkinson Disease: A phase 2 randomized clinical trial. *JAMA Neurol.* 2018;75(2):219–226. doi:10.1001/jamaneurol.2017.3517.

29 Wijesekera L, Leigh PN. Amyotrophic lateral sclerosis. *Orphanet J Rare Dis.* 2009;4:3. doi:10.1186/1750-1172-4-3.

30 Diagnosis and treatment of bulbar symptoms in amyotrophic lateral sclerosis. Medscape Web site. https://www.medscape.org/viewarticle/575966_2. Accessed March 20, 2020.

31 Brooks BR, Miller RG, Swash M, Munsat TL, World Federation of Neurology Research Group on Motor Neuron Diseases. El Escorial revisited: Revised criteria for the diagnosis of amyotrophic lateral sclerosis. *Amyotroph Lateral Scler Other Motor Neuron Disord.* 2000;1(5):293–299. doi:10.1080/146608200300079536.

32 Al-Chalabi A, Hardiman O, Kiernan MC, Chiò A, Rix-Brooks B, van den Berg LH. Amyotrophic lateral sclerosis: Moving towards a new classification system. *Lancet Neurol.* 2016;15(11):1182–1194.

33 Ingre C, Roos PM, Piehl F, Kamel F, Fang F. Risk factors for amyotrophic lateral sclerosis. *Clin Epidemiol.* 2015;7:181–193.

34 The Amyotrophic Lateral Sclerosis Functional Rating Scale. Assessment of activities of daily living in patients with amyotrophic lateral sclerosis. The ALS CNTF treatment study (ACTS) phase I-II Study Group. *Arch Neurol.* 1996;53(2):141–147.

35 EFNS Task Force on Diagnosis and Management of Amyotrophic Lateral Sclerosis: Andersen PM, Abrahams S, et al. EFNS guidelines on the clinical management of amyotrophic lateral sclerosis (MALS)-revised report of an EFNS task force. *Eur J Neurol.* 2012;19(3):360–375. doi:10.1111/j.1468-1331.2011.03501.x.

36 Bello-Haas VD. Physical therapy for individuals with amyotrophic lateral sclerosis: Current insights. *Degener Neurol Neuromuscul Dis.* 2018;8:45–54. Published July, 16 2018. doi:10.2147/DNND.S146949.

37 Macpherson CE, Bassile CC. Pulmonary physical therapy techniques to enhance survival in amyotrophic lateral sclerosis: A systematic review. *J Neurol Phys Ther.* 2016;40(3):165–175. doi:10.1097/NPT.0000000000000136.

38 Muscular Dystrophy Association. Stages of ALS. https://www.mda.org/disease/amyotrophic-lateral-sclerosis/signs-and-symptoms/stages-of-als. Published 2020. Accessed April 20, 2020.

39 Couratier P, Corcia P, Lautrette G, Nicol M, Preux PM, Marin B. Epidemiology of amyotrophic lateral sclerosis: A review of literature. *Rev Neurol (Paris).* 2016;172(1):37–45. doi:10.1016/j.neurol.2015.11.002.

14 Diabetes

Amy J. Litterini and Christopher M. Wilson

Introduction

Blood sugar, or blood *glucose*, is a simple carbohydrate which is a critical fuel source for energy and basic metabolic functions to occur properly in the body. The stomach converts the foods and liquids one consumes into blood glucose, with the normal ranges being <100 mg/dL after fasting, to <140 mg/dL two hours after a meal. In response to fluctuating levels of blood glucose, the pancreas secretes insulin to maintain proper levels of blood glucose in the bloodstream. The diagnosis of *diabetes mellitus* is made when elevated blood glucose levels (hyperglycemia) occur and persist due to (1) the body's inability to produce sufficient amounts of the hormone insulin, or (2) the body cannot effectively use, or is resistant to, the insulin it is capable of producing. There are several types of diabetes with the primary categories including type I, type II, hyperglycemia in pregnancy (HIP), and other types of diabetes (see Table 14.1).

Type I diabetes, or *insulin-dependent diabetes*, occurs when the body does not sufficiently produce insulin. Type I diabetes is associated with autoimmune β-cell destruction, which usually leads to absolute insulin deficiency. Type II diabetes, or *non-insulin-dependent diabetes*, occurs when the body does not properly utilize insulin. Type II diabetes is characterized by a progressive loss of β-cell insulin secretion associated with insulin resistance. Whereas type II diabetes had historically been referred to as *adult-onset diabetes*, both type I and II diabetes are now observed in both adults and children. Impaired glucose tolerance (IGT), and impaired fasting glucose (IFG), indicate the presence of elevated blood glucose levels above normal values but below the diagnostic threshold for diabetes. Labels such as *prediabetes, non-diabetic hyperglycemia,* and *intermediate hyperglycemia* are also used to classify these conditions.[1]

HIP includes the conditions of gestational diabetes mellitus (GDM), as well as diabetes in pregnancy (DIP). GDM occurs for the first time at any point of gestation during pregnancy while DIP occurs in women with either a past history of diabetes, or hyperglycemia that meets the criteria for a diagnosis of diabetes in a non-pregnant state. Screening for HIP is an important aspect of prenatal care, particularly for those women at high-risk.

Symptoms of type I diabetes include *polydipsia* (excessive thirst), bedwetting, *polyuria* (excessive urination), lack of energy, fatigue, constant hunger, and/or sudden weight loss. *Diabetic ketoacidosis*, a serious complication of diabetes that

Table 14.1 Other Causes of Diabetes

Diseases of the pancreas	Pancreatitis, trauma, infection, pancreatic cancer, cystic fibrosis and pancreatectomy
Endocrine disorders	Excess secretion of hormones which antagonize insulin
Drug and chemical-induced	Medications which alter or disrupt insulin secretion or action (e.g. glucocorticoid use, HIV/AIDS treatment, post-organ transplantation)
Infection-related	Viral infection resulting in destruction of beta cells
Immune-mediated	Immunological disorders
Genetic syndromes	Prader-Willi syndrome, Down syndrome, Friedreich's Ataxia
Monogenic diabetes syndromes	Neonatal diabetes and maturity-onset diabetes of the young (MODY)

Sources: International Diabetes Federation. IDF Atlas 9th Edition: 2019. https://www.diabetesatlas.org/upload/resources/material/20200302_133351_IDFATLAS9e-final-web.pdf#page=38&zoom=auto. Published 2019. Accessed April 27, 2020.
Centers for Disease Control and Prevention. National diabetes statistics report, 2017. Atlanta, GA: Centers for Disease Control and Prevention, U.S. Department of Health and Human Services; 2017.
Centers for Disease Control and Prevention. Gestational diabetes. https://www.cdc.gov/diabetes/basics/gestational.html. Published 2019. Accessed August 27, 2020.

occurs when the body produces high levels of blood acids called ketones, is seen in approximately one-third of individuals with type I diabetes. Symptoms of type II diabetes can have some similarities with those of type I diabetes; however, individuals with type II diabetes may also be completely asymptomatic.

The formal diagnosis of diabetes is made via testing of plasma glucose levels. The types of testing include fasting glucose testing (FGT), the 2-hour plasma glucose (2-h PG) test with a 75g oral glucose tolerance test (OGTT), and/or hemoglobin A1c testing (the average blood glucose level over the previous three months).[2] See Table 14.2 for tests and blood glucose values indicating a diabetes diagnosis. Diabetes is formally staged based on phenotypic characteristics, diagnostic criteria, and the clinical presentation of symptoms, but is clinically staged from *pre-diabetes* to *diabetes with complications*. There are several modifiable risk factors for diabetes (see Table 14.3).

The incidence of diabetes has increased precipitously over the last several decades, with the rates of type II diabetes coinciding directly with the obesity epidemic. Globally, an estimated 463 million people are living with a diagnosis of diabetes in 2019, with the number projected to climb to 700 million by 2045.[1] According to the Centers for Disease Control and Prevention's National Diabetes Statistics Report, 30.3 million children and adults had the diagnosis of diabetes in the United States in 2015, representing 9.4% of the population.[4] Also in the year 2015, close to 80,000 deaths occurred in the United States as a result of diabetes, with over 250,000 having the diagnosis of diabetes listed as an underlying or contributing cause of death.[4]

Table 14.2 American Diabetes Association: Diagnostic Criteria[2]

Fasting Plasma Glucose (FPG)	FPG ≥ 126 mg/dL (7.0 mmol/L). Fasting is defined as no caloric intake for at least eight hours

OR

Two-hour Plasma Glucose (2-h PG)	2-h PG ≥ 200 mg/dL (11.1 mmol/L) during OGTT. The test should be performed as described by the WHO, using a glucose load containing the equivalent of 75-g anhydrous glucose dissolved in water

OR

A1C	A1C ≥ 6.5% (48 mmol/mol). The test should be performed in a laboratory using a method that is NGSP certified and standardized to the DCCT assay

OR

Random Plasma Glucose Test	In a patient with classic symptoms of hyperglycemia or hyperglycemic crisis, a random plasma glucose ≥200 mg/dL (11.1 mmol/L)

Source: American Diabetes Association. 2. Classification and diagnosis of diabetes: *Standards of Medical Care in Diabetes-2018. Diabetes Care.* 2018;41(Supplement 1):S13–S27. doi:10.2337/dc18-S002.

OGTT, oral glucose tolerance test; NGSP National Glycohemoglobin Standardization Program; DCCT, Diabetes Complication and Control Trial.

Table 14.3 Modifiable and Non-modifiable Risk Factors for Diabetes[3]

Non-modifiable Risk Factor

Age	Age 45 or older
Race/ethnicity	Black, Hispanic/Latino, American Indian, Asian American, or Pacific Islander
Family history	First-degree relative with a diagnosis of diabetes
Past medical history	History of diabetes during pregnancy; diagnosis of Polycystic Ovary Syndrome

Modifiable Risk Factor

Weight	Overweight or obese
Activity level	Inactive
Co-existing conditions	Hypertension; low HDL cholesterol and/or high triglycerides

Source: American Diabetes Association. Diabetes risk. https://www.diabetes.org/diabetes-risk. Published 2020. Accessed April 27, 2020.

The prevalence of diabetes increases with age, with the youngest category having the lowest percentage of diabetes in the age range of 20–24 years (1.4%), while it is highest for those aged 75–79 (19.9%).[1] Adult men (age 20–79) are also more likely to be diagnosed with diabetes globally, with a prevalence rate of 9.6% versus adult women at 9.0%.[1] Geographically, the countries with the highest prevalence rates of diabetes include China, India, and the United States.[1] Urban areas have higher rates of diabetes (10.8%) compared to rural areas (7.2%), with this percentage expected to rise in the upcoming years due to global urbanization.[1]

Many individuals with a diagnosis of diabetes are undiagnosed. According to the International Diabetes Federation, 50.1% of the estimated 463 million individuals worldwide with diabetes are undiagnosed. Due to limited access to healthcare, low-income countries have the highest percentage of undiagnosed residents (66.8%). However, even in high-income countries, it is estimated that 38.3% of citizens are also undiagnosed.[1]

The late effects of chronic diabetes are associated with several negative medical consequences, including increased mortality rates (see Table 14.4). These consequences include, but are not limited to: retinopathy often associated with blindness; peripheral neuropathy, which can progress to limb amputation; kidney failure; and major cardiovascular events including cerebrovascular accidents and myocardial infarction (see Figure 14.1). Due to the high rate of complications from diabetes, the diagnosis is a frequent cause of both emergency room visits and hospitalizations.[3]

Intervention for Diabetes

Many individuals with diabetes will require a prescription of an insulin-related medication, delivered either by mouth in pill form, or by injection.

Table 14.4 Incidence Rates and Mortality in Diabetes in the United States and Worldwide[1]

Type of Diabetes	United States (2017)		Worldwide	
	Incidence	Mortality	Incidence (2019)	Mortality (2019)
Total: All types	30.3 million	83,564	463 million	4.2 million
Incidence				
Type I (0–19 years)	17,900	nk	128,900	nk
Type II	2.87 million	nk		nk
Hyperglycemia in pregnancy	Occurs in 2–10% of pregnancies	nk	20.4 million	nk
Impaired glucose tolerance	84.1 million	nk	373.9 million	nk

nk: not known.
Source: International Diabetes Federation. IDF Atlas 9th Edition: 2019. https://www.diabetesatlas.org/upload/resources/material/20200302_133351_IDFATLAS9e-final-web.pdf#page=38&zoom=auto.

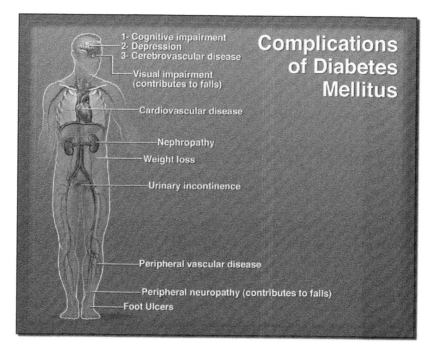

Figure 14.1 Complications of Diabetes.
Source: Nucleus Medical Media. Diabetes, complications and symptoms. Smart Imagebase. https://ebsco-smartimagebase-com.une.idm.oclc.org/diabetes-complications-and-symptoms/view-item?ItemID=14604. Published March 5, 2020 10:32 EST. Accessed April 30, 2020.

According to the American Diabetes Association (ADA), a comprehensive care plan should include lifestyle management strategies as standard recommendations for individuals with diabetes. The components of the ADA recommendations include: (1) diabetes self-management education and support (DSMES); (2) medical nutrition therapy (MNT); (3) physical activity; (4) smoking cessation counseling; and (5) psychosocial care.[5] An interprofessional care team representing these areas of care, including a diabetes educator with the direction and collaboration of primary care and/or endocrinology, is the ideal standard.

Physical Activity

A comprehensive physical activity prescription is a key component of diabetes management. According to the International Diabetes Federation *Clinical Practice Recommendations for managing Type 2 Diabetes in Primary Care*, physical activity is one of the lifestyle modifications beneficial to individuals with diabetes. Their recommendations for individuals with type II diabetes include: (1) increased physical activity; (2) start walking for at least 150 minutes per week with intervals less than 48 hours; and (3) if overweight, a more intensive physical activity program to facilitate weight loss and avoid regain may be indicated.[6] The precise parameters of *increased physical activity* are subject to some debate. According to a meta-analysis by Nery et al.,[7] the existing evidence comparing the effects of resistance exercise with aerobic activity in individuals with type II diabetes not receiving insulin therapy is limited.

Early versus Late-stage Disease

Risk reduction is a vital component of public health, and millions of people worldwide are either at risk for, or are undiagnosed, when it comes to diabetes. Considering the dramatic rise in projected numbers of individuals to be diagnosed with diabetes in the next several decades, risk reduction will be even more critical to mitigate the disease burden of diabetes globally. A Cochrane Review of 12 randomized controlled trials with 5,238 people concluded that diet combined with physical activity reduces or delays the onset of type II diabetes in individuals with impaired glucose tolerance.[8]

As with other disease processes that are often associated with lifestyle choices, early stage diabetes should be addressed with lifestyle and behavioral modification strategies. Many individuals have the option to reverse the state of their disease, particularly type II diabetes, by appropriate lifestyle modifications such as dietary changes and weight management. With a known correlation of diabetes with heart disease, kidney disease, and certain types of cancer, reversing the early presentation of type II diabetes can help to reduce the risk of the diagnosis of comorbidities. Additionally, the risk of pancreatic cancer increases significantly for those individuals with alterations in fasting blood glucose levels. A meta-analysis of nine studies with 2,408 patients demonstrated that a 0.56 mmol/L increase in fasting blood glucose was associated with an increased risk in the rate of pancreatic cancer by 14%.[9]

It is incumbent upon the therapist to be aware of the associated risk factors coexisting with a diagnosis of diabetes, and appropriately counsel their patients on preventative measures in the presence of progressive disease. Secondary to the associated elevated cardiovascular risk factors, monitoring of vital signs is a critical component to routine medical care and rehabilitation. Encouraging and maintaining a level of physical fitness to assist with the regulation of blood glucose levels is recommended, with the incorporation of techniques such as motivational interviewing (see Chapter 7). Ensuring that the individual is regularly monitoring their blood glucose levels, maintaining adherence with their prescriptions, and monitoring their intake of carbohydrates, are key components of care. Maintaining range of motion and performing regular movement of the extremities can assist with maintenance of functional mobility, tissue integrity, and oxygenation. Continuing with the highest performance level of activities of daily living can also contribute to the maintenance of activity tolerance and encourage independence for a patient with progressive disease. Interprofessional collaboration with a dietitian is indicated to assist in education on proper diet and fluid intake, and education on regular skin checks secondary for risks of wounds. Occupational therapy for adaptive equipment and adaptations for limited visual acuity or peripheral neuropathy can improve independence for the greatest duration of time possible. Collaboration with speech language pathologists can also provide alternatives for means of communication in the presence of the diagnosis of blindness.

Side effects of diabetes such as peripheral neuropathy and diabetic retinopathy are diagnoses important for targeted screening both at the time of diabetes diagnosis and through all stages of diabetes. Diabetic neuropathy (DN) is the most frequently diagnosed complication, which results in a high disease burden and a significant economic burden on health systems. DN is a common cause of non-traumatic amputations and is associated with increased balance and fall risk, as well as the onset of wounds.[10] When compared to gender and age-matched controls, individuals with type I diabetes (n = 36,872) were 40 times more likely to experience amputation.[11]

For individuals with advanced-stage disease, greater deficits associated with the integumentary and cardiovascular systems place them at significant risk for morbidity and mortality. Repeated amputations of ascending portions of diseased extremities secondary to non-healing wounds, severe limb ischemia, and chronic infection pose risks for sepsis. Advanced cardiac and kidney disease, associated with the primary diagnosis of diabetes, become challenging to the overall disease burden as diabetes progresses. Diabetes is associated with an increased risk of both sudden cardiac death as well as non-sudden cardiac-related deaths when compared to controls.[12]

Death as a result of diabetes can occur due to both hypoglycemia and hyperglycemia. Additionally, sudden death is often attributed to myocardial infarction and/or cerebrovascular accidents. Patients with chronic ulcers associated with diabetic neuropathy and limb ischemia can present with recurrent infections, which may in some instances result in sepsis and/or death. The World Health Organization estimates diabetes and diabetes-related complications to contribute to 11.3% of deaths globally with 46.2% occurring in individuals of working-age, or 60 years of age or less.[13]

Summary

Reduced activity tolerance and functional mobility, accompanied by the need to address several comorbidities, makes end-of-life care in diabetes complex. Managing these comorbidities becomes a focus in both a medical and a supportive capacity. Maintaining appropriate levels of physical activity and functional mobility are key as with any other advanced disease. Specific to signs and symptoms of diabetes, screening for conditions such as peripheral neuropathy, which increases the risk for falls, and the integumentary system, which increases the risk for wound development, become hallmarks of comprehensive management.

References

1 International Diabetes Federation. IDF Atlas 9th Edition: 2019. https://www.diabetesatlas.org/upload/resources/material/20200302_133351_IDFATLAS9e-final-web.pdf#page=38&zoom=auto. Published 2019. Accessed April 27, 2020.
2 American Diabetes Association. 2. Classification and diagnosis of diabetes: *Standards of Medical Care in Diabetes-2018. Diabetes Care.* 2018;41(Supplement 1):S13–S27. doi:10.2337/dc18-S002.
3 American Diabetes Association. Diabetes risk. https://www.diabetes.org/diabetes-risk. Published 2020. Accessed April 27, 2020.
4 Centers for Disease Control and Prevention. National diabetes statistics report https://www.cdc.gov/diabetes/pdfs/data/statistics/national-diabetes-statistics-report.pdf. Published 2020. Accessed April 27, 2020.
5 American Diabetes Association. 4. Lifestyle management: *Standards of Medical Care in Diabetes-2018. Diabetes Care.* 2018;41(Supplement 1):S38–S50. doi:10.2337/dc18-S004.
6 International Diabetes Federation. Clinical practice recommendations for managing type 2 diabetes in primary care. https://idf.org/e-library/guidelines/128-idf-clinical-practice-recommendations-for-managing-type-2-diabetes-in-primary-care.html. Published 2017. Access April 27, 2020.
7 Nery C, Moraes SRA, Novaes KA, Bezerra MA, Silveira PVC, Lemos A. Effectiveness of resistance exercise compared to aerobic exercise without insulin therapy in patients with type 2 diabetes mellitus: a meta-analysis. *Braz J Phys Ther.* 2017;21(6):400–415. doi:10.1016/j.bjpt.2017.06.004.
8 Hemmingsen B, Gimenez-Perez G, Mauricio D, Roqué I Figuls M, Metzendorf MI, Richter B. Diet, physical activity or both for prevention or delay of type 2 diabetes mellitus and its associated complications in people at increased risk of developing type 2 diabetes mellitus. *Cochrane Database Syst Rev.* 2017;12(12):CD003054. Published December 4, 2017. doi:10.1002/14651858.CD003054.pub4.
9 Liao WC, Tu YK, Wu MS, Lin JT, Wang HP, Chien KL. Blood glucose concentration and risk of pancreatic cancer: systematic review and dose-response meta-analysis. *BMJ.* 2015;350:g7371. Published January 2, 2015. doi:10.1136/bmj.g7371.
10 Vinik AI, Nevoret ML, Casellini C, Parson H. Diabetic neuropathy. *Endocrinol Metab Clin North Am.* 2013;42(4):747–787. doi:10.1016/j.ecl.2013.06.001.
11 Ólafsdóttir AF, Svensson AM, Pivodic A, et al. Excess risk of lower extremity amputations in people with type 1 diabetes compared with the general population: amputations and type 1 diabetes. *BMJ Open Diabetes Res Care.* 2019;7(1):e000602. Published April 14, 2019. doi:10.1136/bmjdrc-2018-000602.
12 Eranti A, Kerola T, Aro AL, et al. Diabetes, glucose tolerance, and the risk of sudden cardiac death. *BMC Cardiovasc Disord.* 2016;16:51. Published February 24, 2016. doi:10.1186/s12872-016-0231-5.
13 Saeedi P, Salpea P, Karuranga S, et al. Mortality attributable to diabetes in 20–79 years old adults, 2019 estimates: Results from the International Diabetes Federation Diabetes Atlas, 9th edition. *Diabetes Res Clin Pract.* 2020;162:108086. doi:10.1016/j.diabres.2020.108086.

15 Kidney Disease

Amy J. Litterini and Christopher M. Wilson

Introduction

The kidneys are small, symmetrical organs, situated bilaterally adjacent to the spine in the retroperitoneum of the lower abdominal cavity (Figure 15.1). Their purpose is to filter the blood, via *nephrons*, the structural and functional units within the kidney. Reabsorbed fluids are returned to the bloodstream, while waste products are secreted, then excreted from the renal pelvis through the ureter into the bladder to be removed from the body during urination. A process of filtration, reabsorption, secretion, and excretion occurs several times daily in order to remove waste products from the blood and maintain appropriate fluid balance and electrolyte levels within the body.

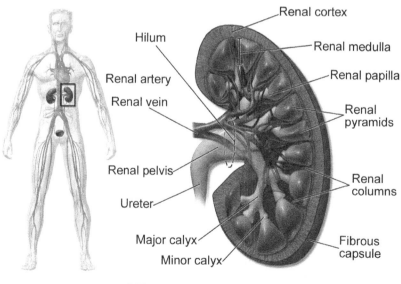

Kidney Anatomy

Figure 15.1 Kidney Anatomy.

Source: Blausen.com staff. Medical gallery of Blausen Medical 2014. *Wiki J Med.* 2014;1(2). doi:10.15347/wjm/2014.010. ISSN 2002-4436.

Chronic kidney disease (CKD) results from conditions which either damage or reduce the function of one or both kidneys. *Nephritis* refers to inflammation of the kidneys, while *nephrosis* refers to non-inflammatory kidney disease associated with damage or degeneration. *Nephrotic syndrome* refers to small vessel damage within the kidneys causing excess protein to be released into the urine.

The incidence of CKD causes significant disease burden worldwide (see Table 15.1). In the United States, CKD occurs most often in older adults, with the highest rates for individuals 65 years of age or older.[1] The rates are higher in women (15%) than in men (12%) while end-stage kidney disease (ESKD) is more likely in men; with regard to race, CKD is more common in non-Hispanic blacks (16%), followed by Hispanics (14%), while the highest rates of ESKD occur in African Americans.[1] Geographically, the location of residence for one-third of the total individuals with CKD globally was China and India.[2] Limited access to care, including dialysis, poses health disparities for countries with low socioeconomic profiles and results in higher mortality rates.[2]

There are several medical conditions associated with CKD including diabetes, hypertension, polycystic kidney disease, interstitial nephritis, recurrent kidney infections, chronic obstruction of the urinary tract, *glomerulonephritis* (inflammation of the glomeruli), and *vesicoureteral reflux* (backup of urine into the kidneys). According to the Mayo Clinic (Rochester, Minnesota, United States), several potential symptoms arise from kidney disease (see Table 15.2), although many individuals with reduced kidney function are actually asymptomatic.[3] Several conditions such as fluid retention, particularly in the extremities, is frequently experienced by individuals with CKD. Hypertension and pulmonary edema can also be diagnosed, as can cardiovascular disease and *pericarditis* (inflammation of the lining of the heart). *Hyperkalemia* (elevated potassium in the blood), *uremia* (elevated levels of urea/waste products in the blood), *proteinuria* (elevated levels of protein in the urine), and *anemia* (low red blood cells) can be found on laboratory analysis. CKD is also associated with *immunocompromise* (reduced immune response causing increased risk for

Table 15.1 Kidney Disease in the United States and Worldwide[1,2]

Type of Kidney Disease	United States		Worldwide	
	Incidence	Mortality	Incidence	Mortality
Chronic kidney disease	37 million	50,633	697 million	1–2 million

Sources: 1. Centers for Disease Control and Prevention. Chronic kidney disease in the United States, 2019. https://www.cdc.gov/kidneydisease/pdf/2019_National-Chronic-Kidney-Disease-Fact-Sheet.pdf. Published 2019. Accessed April 30, 2020.
2. GBD Chronic Kidney Disease Collaboration Global, regional, and national burden of chronic kidney disease, 1990–2017: A systematic analysis for the Global Burden of Disease Study 2017. *Lancet*. 2020;395(10225):709–733. doi:10.1016/S0140-6736(20)30045-3.

infection), as well as increased likelihood of bone fragility. Mineral and bone disorders are observed secondary to alterations in vitamin D utilization in CKD, as well as high levels of phosphorus, causing excess production of parathyroid hormone (PTH). PTH in high concentrations causes calcium to leach from the bone into the bloodstream (*hypercalcemia*), potentially resulting in lowered bone mineral density.

The diagnosis of kidney disease is made with imaging studies such as renal ultrasound and CT scanning. Renal biopsy can also confirm the diagnosis through pathological assessment of gross tissue specimens.[4] Kidney function is assessed through lab analysis of both blood and urine.[5] Urine tests include: urinalysis to assess for *hematuria* (blood in the urine), *proteinuria* (protein in the urine), and *cystitis* (bacteria indicative of infection); creatinine clearance, which compares a 24-hour urine sample to the creatinine level in blood; and dipstick urine testing for *microalbuminuria* (albumin level in the urine). Blood tests include: serum creatinine (normal = <1.2 for women; <1.4 for men); glomerular filtration rate (GFR [normal = >90]); and blood urea nitrogen (BUN [normal = 7–20]). CKD is staged by GFR, with stage 1 (>90; kidney damage with normal GFR) to stage 5 (<15; end-stage renal disease [ESRD]/kidney failure).[5] Routine assessment of kidney function is necessary to monitor the stability or the progression of CKD. There are several risk factors for the development of kidney disease (Table 15.3).

Table 15.2 Signs and Symptoms of Chronic Kidney Disease by System[3]

System	Symptoms
Gastrointestinal	Nausea, vomiting, loss of appetite
Musculoskeletal	Weakness, muscle cramps, muscle twitching, low bone density, sarcopenia
Integumentary	Pruritis, fluid retention
Cardiopulmonary	Hypertension, angina
Pulmonary	Dyspnea
Genitourinary	Urinary changes
Cognitive/ psychosocial	Depression, altered mental acuity
General	Fatigue, sleep disorders

Source: Mayo Clinic. Chronic kidney disease. https://www.mayoclinic.org/diseases-conditions/chronic-kidney-disease/symptoms-causes/syc-20354521. Published 2020. Accessed April 30, 2020.

Table 15.3 Risk Factors for Kidney Disease

Comorbidities/ conditions	Diabetes, hypertension, abnormal kidney structure, heart and blood vessel (cardiovascular) disease
Modifiable risk factors	Obesity, smoking
Non-modifiable risk factors	Older age; race: African-American, Native American or Asian-American; family history of kidney disease
Globally[2]	Diarrheal diseases, HIV infection, low birth weight, malaria, preterm birth

Rehabilitation Considerations

Regarding physical activity and rehabilitation, there are several musculoskel-etal considerations for treating clinicians. As CKD is associated with impaired muscle mitochondrial metabolism and mitochondrial oxidative stress, *sarcope-nia* (loss of muscle mass), *dynopenia* (muscle weakness), and frailty (see Chap-ter 17) are frequently observed in these individuals.[6] Monitoring functional mobility through objective assessments such as gait speed, the Timed Up and Go Test, the Six-minute walk test, and the Short Physical Performance Bat-tery (SPPB) can play a key role in determining risk for morbidity and mortal-ity, frailty status, and the need for referral to skilled rehabilitation.[6] According to Hernandez, Obamwonyi, and Harris-Love,[7] areas of focused attention for individuals with CKD should include screening for sarcopenia and fall risk, as well as an increased awareness of bone mineral density. Regarding out-come measures to address these key areas, the authors suggest: grip strength assessment via dynamometry; the SPPB for assessment of functional mobility, balance, and fall risk; dual energy X-ray absorptiometry (DEXA) for bone mineral density; and DEXA or bioelectrical impedance analysis (BIA) for as-sessing muscle mass. They conclude that incorporating strength training to address these musculoskeletal concerns, in combination with aerobic training for cardiovascular health, may produce the most broad spectrum results for individuals with CKD.[7] One key consideration in the presence of kidney dis-ease is avoiding excessive or aggressive exercise, or traumatic muscle damage via contact sports, as these may elicit *rhabdomyolysis*. This occurs after muscle damage from a variety of causes including substance misuse, medications, trauma, prolonged immobilization, or exercise.[8] Muscle damage releases the protein myoglobin which is too large for the nephrons to filter, thereby causing acute kidney injury and fluid retention. Myoglobin-induced rhabdomyolysis is characterized by tea-colored urine and an increase in creatinine phosphoki-nase.[8] Rhabdomyolysis has the potential to be life-threatening, especially in the context of underlying CKD; a slow, graded introduction of exercise with individuals having CKD or a history of rhabdomyolysis is warranted when starting a new exercise regimen.

Early versus Late-stage Disease

The medical management of individuals with chronic kidney disease present-ing with early kidney failure includes treatment of the underlying disease and comorbidities, as well as education on lifestyle and behavioral management to address comorbid conditions. For individuals with advanced kidney failure, hemodialysis (dialysis) should be considered. *Hemodialysis* is a process where the blood, and toxins within the blood, normally filtered by the kidneys, are perfused mechanically and filtered by a dialyzer (see Figure 15.2). The filtered blood, after toxins are removed, is then returned to the body. Venous access is required for hemodialysis by either an atrial venous (AV) fistula, AV graft,

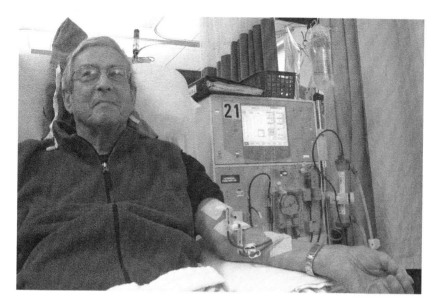

Figure 15.2 Patient Receiving Hemodialysis.
Source: https://commons.wikimedia.org/wiki/File:Patient_receiving_dialysis_03.jpg#/
media/File:Patient_receiving_dialysis_03.jpg.

or central venous catheter. For individuals choosing to forego hemodialysis, maximum medical management and pharmacological interventions should be targeted towards aggressive control of underlying conditions per the individual's wishes.

For individuals with ESRD secondary to severe kidney damage and/or very low kidney function, consideration for dialysis and/or kidney transplantation comes into play to improve chances of survival. Once an individual becomes dialysis-dependent, they often experience high rates of hospitalization, including intensive care unit admission, and declining functional mobility. For example, conditions such as infections, potentially leading to sepsis, can acutely exacerbate kidney failure. Additionally, the high intensity of care required for dialysis can become excessive for some and may result in further reductions in quality of life. For both medical providers and patients, the conversation to begin dialysis is much easier than the conversation about when to end it. Declining the initiation of dialysis may generate a hospice referral, although some marginal kidney function may sustain life. Similarly, discontinuing dialysis after prolonged use would warrant a similar referral, though again, life expectancy might vary from days to weeks or months, depending on remaining kidney function. The uncertainty in predicting prognosis also adds additional barriers to serious illness conversations, but broaching the topic of patient goals is a critical aspect of comprehensive patient care for individuals with ESRD.[9]

For patients not receiving adequate success from medical management, including ongoing dialysis, and for those who are not appropriate candidates for kidney transplantation, palliative care or hospice admission is an appropriate consideration secondary to the poor prognosis with ESRD. The goals of palliative care and hospice for individuals with ESRD include management of symptoms including pain, stiffness, fatigue, anorexia, nausea, pruritus, dyspnea, insomnia, anxiety, and depression. Functional mobility training for the patient, and caregiver training for the caregivers, can provide the longest period of independence possible with a patient/family-centered approach.

Summary

Overall, CKD and ESRD pose a substantial symptom burden for both the individuals diagnosed and health systems globally. Early identification of the disease, as well as education to empower the patient to experience the optimum medical management for their condition, are the ideal standards of care. For individuals with end-stage disease, a comprehensive interdisciplinary team approach offers the best quality of life possible, with maximal functional mobility for the duration of life that remains.

References

1 Centers for Disease Control and Prevention. Chronic kidney disease in the United States, 2019. https://www.cdc.gov/kidneydisease/pdf/2019_National-Chronic-Kidney-Disease-Fact-Sheet.pdf. Published 2019. Accessed April 30, 2020.
2 Global Burden of Disease Chronic Kidney Disease Collaboration. Global, regional, and national burden of chronic kidney disease, 1990–2017: A systematic analysis for the Global Burden of Disease Study 2017. *Lancet.* 2020;395(10225):709–733. doi:10.1016/S0140-6736(20)30045-3.
3 Mayo Clinic. Chronic kidney disease: Symptoms and causes. https://www.mayoclinic.org/diseases-conditions/chronic-kidney-disease/symptoms-causes/syc-20354521. Published 2020. Accessed April 30, 2020.
4 Mayo Clinic. Chronic kidney disease. Diagnosis and treatment. https://www.mayoclinic.org/diseases-conditions/chronic-kidney-disease/diagnosis-treatment/drc-20354527. Published 2020. Accessed April 30, 2020.
5 National Kidney Foundation. Tests to measure kidney function, damage and detect abnormalities. https://www.kidney.org/atoz/content/kidneytests. Published 2020. Accessed April 30, 2020.
6 Roshanravan B, Gamboa J, Wilund K. Exercise and CKD: Skeletal muscle dysfunction and practical application of exercise to prevent and treat physical impairments in CKD. *Am J Kidney Dis.* 2017;69(6):837–852. doi:10.1053/j.ajkd.2017.01.051.
7 Hernandez HJ, Obamwonyi G, Harris-Love MO. Physical therapy considerations for chronic kidney disease and secondary sarcopenia. *J Funct Morphol Kinesiol.* 2018;3(1):5. doi:10.3390/jfmk3010005.
8 Zutt R, Van Der Kooi AJ, Linthorst GE, Wanders RJ, De Visser M. Rhabdomyolysis: Review of the literature. *Neuromuscul Disord.* 2014 August 1;24(8):651–659.
9 Mandel EI, Bernacki RE, Block SD. Serious illness conversations in ESRD. *Clin J Am Soc Nephrol.* 2017;12(5):854–863. doi:10.2215/CJN.05760516.

16 Substance Use Disorder, Intentional Self-Harm, Gun Violence, and HIV/AIDS

Amy J. Litterini and Christopher M. Wilson

Introduction

Rehab clinicians and fitness professionals routinely encounter individuals with common diagnoses associated with major organs and diseases (see Chapters 8–15), and likely feel comfortable and competent with their basic management strategies. Other conditions may be experienced much less frequently, leading to limited awareness and perhaps a reduced comfort level in patient-client management. Certain clinical scenarios, such as drug misuse, gun violence, and suicidal ideation, may be associated with personal, cultural, religious, and/or political biases. The process of gaining knowledge where needed, and setting aside biases, is key to success in helping people in these instances. The ability to recognize important signs and symptoms may lead to accurate identification of a problem and the appropriate next steps. This chapter will outline the important diagnoses of substance misuse and human immunodeficiency virus (HIV), and the clinical and societal challenges of intentional self-harm and gun violence.

Substance Use Disorder

Substance use disorder (SUD), a chronically relapsing brain disease characterized by the compulsive misuse of alcohol, nicotine, and/or illicit drugs despite negative consequences, is a major societal and economic public health concern globally. *Illicit drug use* includes the misuse of illegal substances such as cocaine and methamphetamine, and/or the misuse of prescription drugs and household substances. In 2017, an estimated 7.5 million people in the United States had SUD involving illicit drug use (4.1 million: marijuana use; 2.1 million: opioid use; 1.7 million: prescription pain relievers;.7 million: heroin use).[1] Of the 70,237 drug overdose deaths in the United States in the year 2017, 68% of them involved an opioid (see Table 16.1).[2] Globally, estimates of illicit drug use are 27 million people with 450,000 deaths.[11]

SUD first begins by experimentation with substances, which leads to stimulation of the dopamine reward pathway of the brain. Depending on the form of the substance, a stimulant or a depressant, certain physiological effects are experienced by users, with some causing feelings of euphoria through reward

Table 16.1 Substance Use Disorder, Intentional Self-Harm, Gun Violence, and HIV/AIDS in the United States and Globally[1-11]

Pathological Condition	United States		Globally	
	Incidence	Mortality	Incidence	Mortality
Substance use disorder				
Illicit drug misuse[1,2,11]	7.5 million	67,367	27 million	450,000
Alcohol use disorder[1,10]	14.5 million	72,558	nk	3.3 million
Tobacco use disorder[3,4]	48.7 million	480,000	1.1 billion	8 million
Intentional self-harm (suicide)[1,5]	1.4 million attempts	47,173	nk	800,000
Gun violence[6,7]	134,000	39,773	730,000	182,500
HIV/AIDS[8,9]	HIV: 37,832 AIDS: 17,032	16,350	1.7 million	770,000

circuit activation (e.g. cocaine, methamphetamine, and heroin). *Addiction* is subsequently marked by symptoms of craving, followed by increased physiologic tolerance for the substance. *Tolerance* is demonstrated by the need for increased amounts to achieve the desired effect, and markedly diminished effects with continued use of the same amount of the substance. Attempts to reduce, or eliminate use of the substance, are met with withdrawal symptoms, which is indicative of *dependence*.

There is a high prevalence of comorbidity between SUD and mental illness. Mental health disorders include a wide range of diagnoses that affect mood, thinking, and behavior, such as generalized anxiety disorder, panic disorder, and post-traumatic stress disorder (PTSD). Other mental disorders that have been correlated with SUD include depression, psychotic illness, borderline personality disorder, and antisocial personality disorder.[12] Serious mental illnesses (SMI), including major depression, schizophrenia, and bipolar disorder, are also correlated with SUD. In 2017, there were an estimated 46.6 million US adults who suffered from any mental illness (AMI), while 11.2 million had SMI.[1] Adults diagnosed with mental illness disorders are approximately twice as likely to suffer from SUD. Likewise, for adolescents, those with a history of major depressive episodes (MDE) are twice as likely to experience SUD when compared to their age match counterparts.[1]

The effects of SUD with co-occurring conditions can include negative influences on other aspects of one's life. SUD and mental health disorders are a predictor of underachievement and failure at work and school, difficulty with family responsibilities, abuse, violence, non-compliance with treatment, incarceration, poverty, and homelessness.[13] Additionally, individuals within the lesbian, gay, bisexual, transgender, and queer (LGBTQ) community are also at high risk for developing SUD. A survey on SUD in the LGBTQ population from the National Institute on Drug Abuse concluded that individuals in a sexual minority group (i.e. lesbian, gay, or bisexual) were twice as likely as heterosexual counterparts to have used illicit drugs in the previous year.[14]

It is estimated that 8.5 million US adults who had AMI also had at least one SUD.[1] Adverse childhood experiences (ACEs), are correlated with the likelihood of developing AMI and/or SUD in adolescence or adulthood.[15] ACEs are stressful or traumatic aspects of early life associated with abuse (e.g. physical, sexual, verbal), neglect (e.g. emotional, physical), or a disadvantaged home setting with inadequate parenting and/or role models (e.g. parents divorced/separated, SUD, domestic violence, adults who have been incarcerated). Due to the contributing factor of ACE's and the high incidence of co-occurring mental illnesses, the psychosocial and emotional health role of counseling and the co-management of mental health are critical aspects in the recovery for individuals with SUD.[15]

SUD is also associated with the development of several comorbid medical conditions. For example, cerebrovascular accidents, or strokes, occur in individuals with SUD at a rate of 6.5 times that of the general population.[16] The risk of stroke is higher for individuals who misuse drugs and also have known risk factors for stroke such as hypertension, diabetes, heart disease, tobacco use disorder, older age, and male gender.[16] As alcohol and tobacco both contain carcinogenic chemicals, their use is also a risk factor for the development of several forms of cancer, especially head and neck, and gastrointestinal cancers.[17]

Alcohol Use Disorder

According to the National Survey on Drug Use and Health, the most common substance misused in the United States is alcohol.[1] Alcohol is produced by the chemical process of *fermentation*, where grains, fruit, and other sugar sources are broken down into ethyl alcohol. Alcohol is consumed in the form of fermented beverages such as beer and wine, *malt liquor* including beverages made with malt barley with 5% or more alcohol by volume (ABV), or *distilled spirits*, such as whiskey and vodka (40% ABV). Sparkling wines such as French champagne and Italian Prosecco are created through a process of secondary fermentation. Other alcoholic drinks consumed around the world include *cider* (made from fruit juices), *fermented tea* (e.g. kombucha), *mead* (made from honey), *moonshine* (distilled alcohol, often illegally produced), *rice wine* (e.g. saké), and *pulque* (e.g. tequila and mescal made from the Agave Americana plant).[18] Regionally, alcohol consumption is highest in the countries of France and Australia, while the lowest rates of consumption are in Northern Africa in the Middle East, due to the widely held ban on consumption of alcohol in the Muslim culture.[19]

Alcoholism, or *alcohol use disorder* (AUD), is the diagnosis of uncontrolled dependence on alcohol. Morbidity secondary to AUD is associated with alcohol-related diseases such as cardiovascular disease, liver disease, and traumatic injuries, as well as increased needs for emergency medical care and hospitalizations. The increased mortality rate associated with AUD is secondary to cirrhosis, increased incidence of certain cancers, overdoses, and suicides. According to the National Institute on Alcohol Abuse and Alcoholism (NIAAA), death certificates in the United States in 2017 mentioned alcohol as an underlying or contributing cause in the death of 72,558 individuals, although these numbers are suspected to be underreported.[20] Chronic alcohol consumption is also associated with significant neurological sequelae, including brain atrophy with reduced white matter volume, altered gene expression within the brain, and peripheral neuropathies, which can lead to further morbidity secondary to balance issues and increased fall risk. Recent studies have indicated that the health risks associated with AUD are greater for women than men, theorized to be attributed to the differences in how alcohol is metabolized in the body.[21]

Many individuals using alcohol to excess may be unaware of the problem or its consequences. Additionally, most are unaware of what constitutes a single serving of alcohol (e.g. 1.5–2.5 oz of liquor; 5 oz. of table wine; 8 oz. of malt liquor; 12 oz. of beer [variable with craft brews]), and how many alcoholic beverages are recommended daily for moderate consumption (one for women; two for men). For providers, asking about consumption and starting the dialogue is key. Common assessments for AUD are routinely available and easily accessible. The CAGE, MAST, and AUDIT assessments are free to use, easy to complete, and can be administered in a short period of time (see Table 16.2).[22–24]

Table 16.2 Screening Assessments for Substance Use Disorder[22–26]

Test	Substance	Description
CAGE assessment[22]	Alcohol	1 Have you felt the need to **C**ut down on your drinking? 2 Do you feel **A**nnoyed by people complaining about your drinking? 3 Do you ever feel **G**uilty about your drinking? 4 Do you ever drink an **E**ye-opener in the morning to relieve shakes? Two or more affirmative responses suggest that the client is a problem drinker
MAST assessment[23]	Alcohol	The **M**ichigan **A**lcohol **S**creening **T**est is a 24-item questionnaire with yes or no responses weighted from 1 to 5 points depending on the seriousness of the concepts. A total score of 5 or more is indicative of a problem drinker.
AUDIT[24]	Alcohol	The **A**lcohol **U**se **D**isorder **I**dentification **T**est is a 10-question assessment which focuses on drinking patterns and alcohol-related behaviors in adolescents aged 14–18. A score of 3 indicates alcohol abuse or dependence.
ASSIST[25]	All	**A**lcohol, **S**moking, and **S**ubstance **I**nvolvement **S**creening **T**est
DAST[26]	Drugs other than alcohol or tobacco	**D**rug **A**buse **S**creening **T**est (–10, –20, and –28 question versions). Considers illicit drug use, including one's own prescriptions.

Following a formal diagnosis of AUD by a medical professional, the management should be comprehensive and person-centered and include both pharmacological and non-pharmacological interventions. The pharmacological management of SUD and AUD is referred to as *medication-assisted therapy* (MAT). According to the American Psychiatric Association practice guideline, along with management of co-occurring conditions, the recommended first-line medications for individuals of moderate-to-severe AUD include naltrexone or acamprosate.[27] Assessment of the individual's goals for abstinence, moderation, and/or harm reduction, and agreement to and documentation of the goals, allows the care team to produce a person-centered approach in partnership with the individual.

Tobacco Use Disorder

Nicotine, a naturally or synthetically produced stimulant and strong parasympathetic alkaloid, is a highly addictive organic compound found in the leaves of certain plants, most notably the family of tobacco plants within the Nicotiana genus. Nicotine is delivered to the body in various forms including cured tobacco leaves for smoking (e.g. cigarettes, cigars, pipes, and hookahs), smokeless tobacco (e.g. loose-leaf chewing tobacco, loose powder pouches, or grains [snus]), and/or synthetic forms such as transdermal patches, gums, and lozenges. New delivery devices growing in popularity worldwide include heated tobacco products (which produce aerosols containing nicotine), and electronic nicotine delivery systems (e.g. e-cigarettes and vaporizer [vape] pens).

Addiction to nicotine is generally referred to as *tobacco use disorder* (TUD). Each inhaled/direct contact (e.g. chewing) form of tobacco or nicotine poses major health risks for the individual, and serious public health risks globally. Long-term use of tobacco products is associated with both high morbidity and mortality. Diagnoses associated with TUD include diseases such as coronary artery disease, chronic obstructive pulmonary disease, cerebrovascular disease, as well as several forms of cancer, most notably, lung carcinoma. Individuals with TUD are three times more likely to die than their age match counterparts who never used tobacco, with a reduced life expectancy of ten years.[28] In the United States, tobacco use is the leading preventable cause of death annually;[3] second-hand smoke is also associated with numerous deaths each year from both heart disease (33,951) and lung cancer (7,333).[28]

Globally, smoking is second only to hypertension as a risk factor for death, with 15% of all deaths worldwide attributed to tobacco. Most smokers reside in low-to-middle income countries, and subsequently, the economic burden related to the purchase of tobacco products is greater in the context of existing financial demands for food and shelter.[4] Healthcare systems across the globe have initiated smoking cessation programs, including MAT and counseling, often at reduced or no cost to citizens, with the goal of reducing the heavy burdens of TUD at the community and individual level.

Opioid Use Disorder (OUD)

Derived from the opium poppy, *opiates* are natural chemical compounds with psychoactive properties best known for their pain-relieving effects. Opioid drugs are synthetic chemical compounds that produce opiate-type effects, which are physiologically highly addictive. *Semi-synthetic* opioids include oxy-codone, hydrocodone, and oxymorphone, while *synthetic* opioids include meth-adone, tramadol, and fentanyl. The *illegally produced* street drug heroin is a synthesized version of the natural opioid morphine.

Opioids are used in the medical profession for the management of moderate-to-severe acute and chronic pain, including terminal pain in hospice and palliative care settings. However, the over-prescription of opioid medications for pain management, particularly in the United States as a reaction to drug-seeking behaviors by individuals "doctor shopping" from one or multiple doctors, has created an epidemic of misuse which has led to overdoses and skyrocketing deaths nationwide.[2]

In response to this national health crisis in the United States including over-prescription of high dose opioids, the Centers for Disease Control and Prevention (CDC) released a set of new guidelines in 2016. These guidelines advocated for healthcare providers to reduce the use of opioids in favor of safer alternatives like physical therapy (PT).[29,30] The American Physical Therapy Association (APTA) subsequently launched a national public aware-ness campaign about the safety and effectiveness of PT for pain management, #ChoosePT.[31] This campaign has raised awareness about the dangers of pre-scription opioids, and encourages consumers and prescribers to follow guide-lines for conservative pain management best practices by the CDC.

Due to the high level of respiratory depression from opioids, overdoses occur at an alarming rate. The signs and symptoms of an opioid overdose include: low to no respiratory rate; constriction of the pupils; bradycardia; and/or extreme drowsiness or the inability to wake the person from sleep. Injectable naloxone, the medication available to reverse the effects of an overdose, is routinely used by first-line emergency responders and emergency room clinicians.[32] The avail-ability of naloxone in healthcare settings such as PT clinics, other busy public areas, and even in the homes of individuals with SUD, has been advocated for by policy makers as a potentially life-saving strategy for individuals at risk for or experiencing an unintentional or intentional overdose in the presence of an-other person.[33] After naloxone administration following an overdose episode, emergency medical attention is still required to prevent long-term sequelae and/or death. MAT for OUD may include the opiate agonist, methadone, the partial opiate agonist, buprenorphine, or the opiate antagonist, naltrexone.

Early versus Late Disease

Harm reduction is a global public health philosophy designed to reduce the risks associated with SUD such as unwitnessed overdose episodes and deaths, trans-mission of blood-borne pathogens due to shared/used needles for injectable drugs (e.g. HIV, hepatitis), and the incidence of other forms of trauma or violence associated with drug impairment and intoxication (see suicide and gun violence later in this chapter). The goals for clinicians advocating for harm reduction are as follows: (1) create a safer environment for individuals actively using drugs without fear of legal repercussions; (2) offer clean needles to reduce the risk of disease transmission; (3) provide resources and education about help for treating addiction; and (4) have a commitment to social justice to respect the rights of individuals with SUD.[34]

The root cause for the initiation of substance experimentation and use, or the actual progression to SUD, is often multifaceted. Therefore, treatment ideally occurs in an interdisciplinary fashion to address the medical, physical, psychosocial, and emotional needs of the individuals with the disorder, from prevention through treatment. In addition to the risks previously stated, genetic predisposition has been implicated as a risk factor for developing SUD. By addressing the risks for experimentation with substances, especially by children and adolescents, and acknowledging other risk factors such as family history which can contribute to the progression to addiction, clinicians, educators, and policy makers can work collaboratively to intervene for the health and wellness of their communities. Public policy efforts can be focused on counteracting or limiting the often-positive portrayal of substances in music lyrics and advertising/marketing, as well as establishing minimum age restrictions and taxes on items such as cigarettes and alcohol. Through these efforts, parents, community members, and societies can work to combat the early use of substances, which have the potential to become lifelong addictions.

Screening, **B**rief **I**ntervention, and **R**eferral for **T**reatment (SBIRT) is a standard method of care being applied in healthcare to address the crisis of SUD by shifting the focus to earlier detection and an open dialogue between individuals and their healthcare providers. All clinicians treating patients/clients, regardless of the reason for treatment, should screen for the use of substances (*screening*), educate on their levels of consumption and the associated risks (*brief intervention*), and, if necessary, provide opportunities to seek care to address misuse (*referral for treatment*). Early identification through screening (see Table 16.2), and educational resources, can potentially make the difference for individuals struggling with the consequences of SUD. For clinicians, reducing the stigma associated with SUD by engaging in meaningful and supportive conversations can create a dialogue with individuals wishing to break the cycle of addiction and find help.

The recovery from SUD depends on the specific substance(s) being misused, but the processes have the similarities of combining: (1) access to supportive medical care of the appropriate level of intensity; (2) availability of counseling to address co-occurring conditions; and (3) guidance for MAT. The philosophical aspects of SUD recovery generally center on the concepts of *health, home, purpose,* and *community*.[34] *Health* includes management of diseases and symptoms as well as maintaining healthy lifestyle choices. *Home* includes establishing secure shelter and promoting a safe living environment. *Purpose* entails that the person has meaningful daily activity participation in both their personal life and society. Finally, *community* includes that the individual engages in supportive relationships and social networks. In the absence of one of these components, the success of early and long-term recovery is significantly challenged.

Depending on the methodology used in recovery (e.g. harm reduction, moderation [reduce use], abstinence [eliminate use]), and the acuity and severity of the addiction disease, multiple phases or steps are required in the process. *Early recovery* generally includes acute detoxification, which may involve brief inpatient medical care for monitoring and management of acute symptoms, and involves the initiation of MAT to combat the cravings for the addicted substance. Following the acute phase, many individuals will progress to 30, 60, or 90-day residential or community-based outpatient programs. *Long-term recovery* typically includes some form of intensive outpatient care for ongoing peer support, counseling, and medical management for several months to years. Methods for clinicians to address mental health and wellness, and improve resiliency and self-efficacy, include motivational interviewing, cognitive behavioral therapy (CBT), and trauma-informed care. Treatment methods designed to harness individual motivation include motivational enhancement therapy and contingency management. Psychotherapeutic treatment methods include dialectical behavioral therapy, family focused therapy, and 12-step programs.

The available literature on the therapeutic effects of physical exercise (PE) on SUD is somewhat limited. However, some authors have suggested that PE may have positive effects when treating persons with SUD.[35,36] A meta-analysis by Wang et al.[35] concluded there was strong evidence that PE may increase the abstinence rate, reduce withdrawal symptoms, and decrease symptoms of anxiety and depression in persons with SUD. The effects on individuals misusing illicit drugs were significantly greater than on individuals using other substances. The authors concluded that aerobic exercise of moderate and high-intensity, along with mind-body exercises, may be an effective and persistent treatment for persons with SUD.[35] A systematic review of exercise and physical activity interventions in the management of SUD by Zschucke, Heinz, and Strohle[36] found strong evidence for the efficacy of PE in smoking cessation, but weak evidence in alcohol and illicit drug misuse due to poor methodology and insufficient generalizability. The authors did, however, provide several possible mechanisms of potential benefit for patients with SUD including: neurochemical alterations by PE; reduction in acute cravings; endogenous reward mechanisms; mood regulation; reduction of anxiety and depressive symptoms; stress reactivity; benefits of group activity and support; improved coping mechanisms; and improved self-efficacy.[36] A systematic review of physical activity and AUD by Vancampfort et al.[37] found barriers to participation. The authors concluded that TUD, obesity, co-occurring mental illnesses, and a lower self-efficacy may reduce physical activity participation for individuals with AUD.[37] For fitness and rehabilitation professionals treating these individuals, strategies to mitigate these barriers should be incorporated into the plan of care.

For individuals with chronically relapsing disease, the risk for death from overdose increases, as does advanced illness from comorbid conditions such as cirrhosis, chronic obstructive pulmonary disorder, and cancer. Chronic addictive behaviors can lead to physical deterioration without the likelihood of cure. Harm reduction is key to support individuals unsuccessful at, or unable to, gain recovery over SUD. Even for those who eventually do transition into SUD recovery, diagnoses acquired during prior substance use may, in turn, limit their life expectancy.

The literature for palliative care and hospice in SUD is limited, despite the multiple needs of these individuals and its frequency as a secondary diagnosis. As one's personal course of disease progression is an unpredictable entity, the prognosis is also difficult to anticipate. According to Ebenau et al.,[38] challenges to palliative and hospice care access for patients at end of life with SUD include stigmatization of SUD; limited provider training in SUD; altered response to pain medication due to current SUD; risks of patients misusing medication; patients' non-compliance; and non-disclosure of SUD. Effective pain management at the end of life often still requires opioid-based regimens. Additionally, the legalization of cannabis for medical use in several jurisdictions has offered a new treatment option for many individuals on hospice, including those with advanced cancer. Having a skilled medical team to manage medication options is key to successful symptom management at end of life for individuals with a history of SUD.

In conclusion, the incorporation of SBIRT as a routine strategy with all individuals and employing the principles of harm reduction within care systems and local communities are critical components within the role of the rehabilitation and fitness professional. In addition, therapists should advocate for access and availability of naloxone in the event that it is required in an overdose situation. Physical activity and exercise are safe and effective alternatives to opioids and should be considered first-line therapy for individuals in need of chronic pain management. PE should also be incorporated into a comprehensive, interdisciplinary program of recovery from SUD.

Intentional Self-Harm: Suicidal Ideation

Intentional self-harm is a difficult topic for many healthcare providers to understand, with our lens of helping people recover from injury and/or helping people live out their life to the fullest potential possible. *Suicide*, the intentional act of taking one's own life, is unfortunately more common than most can conceptualize. According to the World Health Organization, suicide takes a life every 40 seconds globally.[6] Although it occurs throughout the lifespan, suicide is the second leading cause of death for individuals 15–29 years of age. The societal impacts are greatest for low-to-middle income countries where 79% of all suicides occurred in the year 2016.[6] Men die of suicide three times more often than women, with men using firearms and women using poison as the most common method.[39]

For every suicide, an estimated 20 suicidal attempts (i.e. any non-fatal sui-cidal behavior) occur.[6] In healthcare settings, when a new onset of injurious behavior is determined to be self-inflicted, the identification of whether it was intentional or accidental (e.g. drug or alcohol overdose) should follow. If deemed intentional, follow-up care for suicidal ideation should be initiated. Several ICD-10 codes exist for intentional self-harm (X60–X84).[40] In the ab-sence of a terminal illness with a six month or less prognosis where medical aid in dying (MaiD) may be an appropriate, legal option (see Appendix 2), suicidal ideation is pathological and a medical emergency.

For individuals surviving a suicide attempt, the prior act is the single most important predictor of death by suicide. In addition to prior attempts, there are several other risk factors that increase the risk of suicide.[41] Demographi-cally, individuals between 15–24 years or older than 60 are at the highest risk. In addition, those with a history of suicide attempts, AMD, SUD, or medical illnesses, and/or those with a family history of suicide, physical violence, or sexual violence are also at an increased risk of suicide. An individual is also at an increased risk if they live in an environment with guns or firearms within the home or are incarcerated. Finally, it has been noted that suicide rates increase with increased exposure through others' suicidal behavior, including a family member, peer, or a media personality. Recognizing the risks, under-standing warning signs for suicidal ideology, and making timely referrals for care become pivotal responsibilities for clinicians treating individuals in any setting.

Early versus Late Disease

The warning signs for suicide are complex, and most individuals at risk or displaying signs do not attempt suicide. However, displays of suicidal ideation should be recognized and considered an emergency with immediate medical attention sought for the individuals. Individuals talking about suicide or death often, or expressing extreme feelings of hopelessness, shame, guilt, pain, or being a burden, can be indicative of suicidal intentions. If the person voices that they have a plan for suicide, such as researching a method or obtaining lethal weapons, it should be considered an emergency situation. Actions such as reckless behaviors, or demonstrations of extreme mood swings or changes in sleeping and eating patterns, should not be dismissed. Additionally, activ-ities such as getting affairs in order, giving away possessions, and/or saying goodbye to family and friends should be met with significant concern in the absence of a terminal illness.[41] Asking the person if they are having thoughts of doing harm to themselves or taking their life, though difficult, is the first step to be taken, as well as alerting other appropriate resources and support people. For individuals with a terminal illness, discussing wishes for the end of life should be encouraged (see Chapter 7 and Appendix 1), and patients eligible for MAiD, where legal, should be supported in their decisions (see Appendix 2).

The effects of prior suicide attempts, and ongoing suicidal ideation, can persist and significantly impact quality of life. The residual effects following survival of a severe fall, a gunshot wound, lacerations, or attempted poisoning can have detrimental effects on all the major body systems. Ongoing mental health problems, as well as SUD, can compound suffering for survivors of suicide attempts and limit their motivations about the future. Having an interdisciplinary team involved, specifically with training in surveillance and monitoring of suicide attempts, can help to reduce the risk of suicide and self-harm, or at the very least identify them early to allow for referral for treatment. Broaching the topic of suicidal ideation is the responsibility of the healthcare provider when it is suspected, and asking the question if someone is considering suicide can expedite access to necessary supportive care.[40] Managing co-occurring conditions and making the necessary referrals for patients and clients can help to save a life and reduce the public health burden of this unfortunate scenario.

Gun Violence

Violence is a major global health concern. Lethal violence includes victims in both conflict and non-conflict settings, with two-thirds of deaths occurring as intentional homicides in non-conflict situations. For those societies and cultures most vulnerable to war-related violence, gun violence is prevalent. The countries of Syria, El Salvador, Venezuela, Honduras, and Afghanistan experienced the most violence in the year 2016.[42]

Globally, over 500 people are killed and 2,000 people are injured by gun violence each day.[43] Deaths secondary to gun violence are classified as either suicide or homicide, and an estimated 44% of homicides committed worldwide involve the use of a firearm.

As a result of gun violence, an estimated 2 million people are living with the residual physical and psychological effects of gunshot wounds around the world.[43] The United States is particularly vulnerable to gun violence due to significant access to firearms and loose regulations, with per capita deaths exceeding that of other industrialized countries. Approximately 134,000 Americans were injured, and 39,000 killed, in the year 2017.[43]

Those at greatest risk for gun violence, as a victim or a perpetrator, are men, with 6.1 times greater risk for gun-related mortality than women.[5] Specifically for the United States, non-Hispanic black men and women have higher rates of gun-related mortality than non-Hispanic white men and women, respectively.[5] Women are at greatest risk of gun violence from an intimate partner through domestic violence and during acts of sexual violence.[43,44] A systematic review by Sorenson and Schut[44] of gun violence by intimate partners in the United States revealed that approximately 4.5 million women had been threatened with a gun, and 1 million had been shot, or shot at, by an intimate partner. Other risk factors for perpetrating gun violence include: a personal history of violence; exposure to individuals with violent tendencies; untreated mental health disorders; substance use disorder; and access to weapons.[45]

The economic burden of gun violence is enormous. In the United States alone, the annual costs of firearm injuries and deaths are 3 and 20 billion dollars, respectively, due to medical expenses and lifetime work losses.[45] For survivors of gunshot wounds, the most common locations of injuries involve the extremities, with the majority of wounds seen in soft tissues.[46] Wounds are managed non-surgically when possible, and surgically in the presence of significant soft-tissue or vascular injuries, instances of substantial skin loss, unstable fractures or intra-articular damage, and/or hematomas.[46]

Early versus Late Stages

Additional societal burdens come from individual fears and threats of personal injury and/or the risks to self and loved ones from scenarios receiving media attention such as mass shootings, armed conflicts during wartime, or acts of terrorism. For survivors of gun violence, the psychological and emotional toll as well as the loss of functional mobility and opportunities for employment are substantial. In addition to rehabilitation for recovery of acute injuries, long-term occupational therapy is key for return to work in a modified duty capacity. Routine screening for access to firearms, and for domestic violence at home, is the role of the medical professional for all the new patients seeking care in any setting but is especially relevant in the home health setting. Referring to appropriate resources and care for co-occurring conditions such as mental health disorders and SUD should be standard of care to mitigate the risks of gun violence.

For individuals not expected to survive their injuries, stays in a hospital or intensive care unit setting can be brief during rapid decline or lengthy with progressive organ failures. The integration of palliative care and hospice in surgical and trauma intensive care units is sporadic. Recommendations from the Improving Palliative Care in the Intensive Care Unit (IPAL-ICU) Project Advisory Board call for consultative and integrative models of care that foster a culture for referrals within an institution.[47] Opportunities to bridge gaps between palliative care and surgical/trauma intensive care should be investigated to promote best practices at end of life for individuals experiencing life-limiting trauma.

HIV/AIDS

HIV, a retrovirus which attacks the CD4 (T-cells) of the immune system, was initially identified in humans in the United States in June of 1981 in Los Angeles, California, with the first reported cases in five otherwise healthy gay men presenting with rare lung infections, *pneumocystis carinii pneumonia*.[48] Similar presentations were seen in others at the same time, with concurrent opportunistic infections and cases of *Kaposi's sarcoma*, a rare, aggressive form of cancer. In response, the United States Center for Disease Control convened a *Task*

Force on Kaposi's Sarcoma and Opportunistic Infections to investigate the phenomenon. In September 1982, the term *Acquired Immune Deficiency Syndrome* (AIDS) was used for the first time to describe the condition.[48] In November 1984, the World Health Organization began international surveillance of the diagnosis. Scientists theorized the virus originated from the chimpanzees of Central Africa as early as the 1800s, with transmission to humans through hunting and subsequently butchering of infected meat. Since the formal identification of the disease, significant gains have been made in testing and treatment; however, HIV and AIDS continue to pose a global health concern.

There are two viral subtypes of HIV, HIV1 and HIV2. HIV1 is the most common form of the virus, and is responsible for the majority of infections worldwide.[8] HIV is transmitted person-to-person through blood, pre-ejaculate, semen, vaginal secretions, rectal fluids, and breast milk. Activities that permit the transmission of HIV include sexual contact including unprotected anal or vaginal sex, sharing of contaminated needles and syringes for the injection of drugs, blood transfusions, unsterile procedures (e.g. cutting or piercing), and accidental needle sticks among healthcare workers.[9] Additionally, HIV can pass from mother to child during pregnancy and delivery.[9] HIV is not transmitted through saliva, sweat, or tears; however, universal precautions should be practiced in the same manner for individuals with a known or suspected diagnosis of HIV, as for all individuals.

HIV is initially diagnosed biochemically with serum or plasma specimens by the assessment for HIV1 and HIV2 antibodies to the virus, and the HIV1 p24 antigen, through a reaction to antigens via *enzyme-linked immunosorbent assay* (ELISA) testing.[49] Results should be differentiated for HIV1 versus HIV2, and further evaluated with HIV1-NAAT (nuclear acid amplification test) analysis for reactive or intermediate results. CD4 cell count and percentage are used to determine the risk for HIV-associated complications, including opportunistic infections. Quantitative plasma HIV RNA level, or *viral load*, is used to predict the rapidity of disease progression (e.g. magnitude of viral replication) and is a consideration for the medication regimen to be prescribed. Once diagnosed, testing allows for initial staging, and retesting allows for reclassification of staging with changes in infection status (see Table 16.3). HIV testing is recommended annually for those with risk factors, and more frequently (e.g. every three to six months), for those at high risk.[50]

HIV infection, if left untreated, can progress to AIDS. A clinical syndrome, AIDS is defined: (1) *biochemically* (a drop of CD4 cell count below 200 cells/μL); (2) *clinically* (the emergence of opportunistic infections indicating immune compromise); and/or (3) *historically* (having either biochemical or clinical features of AIDS in the past). Depending on the individual, the time of progression from HIV to AIDS ranges from 2 to 15 years.[9] HIV is staged from 0 to 3 (see Table 16.3).[51,52]

Due to lack of access to testing and treatment, HIV remains a substantial public health concern globally, with 1.7 million new cases and 690,000 deaths in 2019.[9] Of the new cases, 95% have occurred in eastern European, central

Table 16.3 Stages of HIV/AIDS in Adolescents and Adults[51,52]

Stage	Description/Presentation	CD4 Count	CD4 %	Possible Symptoms
Stage 0	Early HIV infection			
Stage 1	Acute HIV infection; flu-like symptoms within two to four weeks of exposure	≥500 cells/mm^3	≥26	• Fever • Chills • Rash • Night sweats • Muscle aches • Sore throat • Fatigue • Swollen lymph nodes • Mouth ulcers • No AIDS-defining condition
Stage 2	Clinical latency	22–499 cells/mm^3	14–25	HIV inactivity or dormancy
Stage 3	Acquired Immune Deficiency Syndrome (AIDS)	<200 cells/mm^3	<14	• Rapid weight loss • Recurring fever or profuse night sweats • Extreme and unexplained tiredness • Prolonged swelling of the lymph glands in the armpits, groin, or neck • Diarrhea that lasts for more than a week • Sores of the mouth, anus, or genitals • Pneumonia • Red, brown, pink, or purplish blotches on or under the skin or inside the mouth, nose, or eyelids • Memory loss, depression, and other neurologic disorders
Unknown	No reported information on AIDS-defining OIs and no information available on CD4 lymphocyte count or percentage.	No data		

Asian, Middle Eastern, and North African countries.[9] Individuals at greatest risk for contracting HIV include: men who have sex with other men; individuals using intravenous drugs; individuals incarcerated or living in other closed settings; sex workers and their clients; and people who are transgender.[8]

Treatment

Prevention of HIV is a key strategy for those at high risk. Along with general prevention practices such as safe sex (e.g. abstinence, limiting sexual partners, and condom use), *pre-exposure prophylaxis* (PreP) may be prescribed. PreP involves the daily use of antiretroviral (ARV) medications by HIV-negative people to block the acquisition of HIV for those considered at substantial risk of infection (e.g. sexually active gay and bisexual adult men, individuals who inject drugs, partners of infected people). Additionally, *post-exposure prophylaxis* (PEP) is accomplished via a 28-day cycle of ARVs within 72 hours of potential exposure to HIV to prevent infection.[53]

Antiretroviral Therapy (ART), a combination of medications for those with known infection has the goal of reducing the viral load, potentially, to undetectable levels. HIV medication categories include: nucleoside/nucleotide analogs; multi-class drug combinations; non-nucleosides; early inhibitors; and protease inhibitors.[53] Due to immunosuppression, antimicrobial agents may be prescribed prophylactically to supplement the immune system. Monitoring for drug interactions, and potential mutations resulting in drug resistance, is a critical role for the medical team. For those reaching undetectable levels, the chance of infecting others with the disease is virtually negligible. Although medication regimens have improved in efficiency with lowered toxicity, they do still present with potential side effects for individuals living with HIV infection.[53]

In addition to opportunistic infections, impairments associated with its viral infection and HIV treatments occur. Distal Symmetrical Peripheral Neuropathy (DSPN) can affect sensation and deep-tendon reflexes, and cause neuropathic pain and painful night cramps. Risk factors for DSPN include older age, nART (neurotoxic anti-retroviral therapy) use, protease inhibitor use, past medical history of diabetes, and taller height.[54] Screening tools for DSPN can be seen in Table 16.4. Maharaj and Yakasai[55] examined the effects of moderate-intensity aerobic and progressive resistive exercise (PRE) on neuropathic pain for individuals with HIV. The authors identified significant improvement ($p<0.05$) from baseline to six and twelve weeks compared to controls.[55]

Outcome Measures: Function

In a study of physical performance for individuals with HIV by Greene et al.[56] evidence of reduced physical performance on the short physical performance battery (SPPB) predicted mortality in a dose-response manner. Additional functional measures are listed in Table 16.4.

As an intervention, the effectiveness of physical activity for individuals with HIV is increasingly well documented. In a systematic review and meta-analysis of PRE for adult individuals with HIV, it was concluded that PRE, or PRE in combination with aerobic exercise demonstrated improvements in cardiorespiratory fitness, strength, weight, and body composition.[57,58] Individuals with HIV performed the PRE for six weeks with a minimum frequency of three times weekly.[57,58] A meta-analysis by Pérez Chaparro et al.[59] of aerobic and resistance exercise alone, or in combination, found improvements in upper and lower body muscular strength. In spite of the evidence

Table 16.4 Screening Tools for Neuropathy and Function

Tool	Purpose	Description
Single Question Neuropathy Screen (SQNS)	*Neuropathy*	"Do you experience tingling, burning, or numbness in your feet or hands?"
DN4 Questionnaire (Douleur Neuropathique 4)	*Neuropathy*	Also useful in assessing neuropathic pain
Neuropathy Severity Score	*Neuropathy*	Assesses: (1) Presence and severity of symptoms (2) functional limitations (3) ankle reflexes
Self-Administered Leeds Assessment of Neuropathic Symptoms and Signs (S-LANSS)	*Neuropathy*	Seven-item self-report scale developed to identify the pain of predominantly neuropathic origin
Lower Extremity Functional Scale (LEFS)	*Function*	Self-reported questionnaire of lower extremity performance during activities of daily living
Six-minute Walk Test	*Function*	Sub-maximal exercise test for aerobic capacity and endurance
Short Physical Performance Battery (SPPB)	*Function*	Assesses static balance, functional mobility and gait speed

documenting lower levels of meeting recommended exercise guidelines for individuals with HIV, higher levels of physical activity have also been found to be associated with improvements in quality of life.[60] Additionally, physical activity has shown the potential to improve neurocognitive function for individuals with HIV-related neurocognitive impairment.[61] As a modifiable lifestyle behavior, consideration of physical activity should be a recommended standard of care for individuals with HIV.

Early versus Late-stage Disease

Individuals with early stage HIV often live with minimal symptoms and can lead virtually normal lives, aside from their need for ongoing medication and potential side effects. As HIV infection is chronic, the need for adherence to an effective medication regimen is critical and lifelong. Early identification, efforts to lower the viral load, and attention to education to prevent progression of disease (upstaging) and/or disease transmission, are key components for successful medical management. Integrative care for mental, physical, and emotional wellness is also a consideration, with yoga, massage, and acupuncture showing promise as safe strategies, although more research is needed to prove their efficacy.[62–64]

Fortunately, increased public awareness, improved testing capacity, and access to ART have reduced the death rates from AIDS globally. Although improved, the mortality rate in high burden areas such as the continent of Africa remains a key public health issue. In a study of 4,158 decedents with a history of HIV in San Francisco, United States, 87% had an AIDS diagnosis prior to death. Causes of death varied depending on the influence of personal factors such as drug use, and environmental factors such as housing. For individuals not experiencing homelessness, the authors noted a decline in deaths related to AIDS-defining conditions and an increase in causes such as accidents, heart disease, non-AIDS cancers, and drug overdoses. For those experiencing homelessness, deaths associated with mental illness were more likely.[65] In general, there is evidence that homelessness or a lack of stable, secure, adequate housing is associated with poorer outcomes for individuals with HIV.[66]

Individuals with advanced stage disease of AIDS may present with several reasons for referral for palliative care, and with a six-month prognosis, for hospice care. Some will experience AIDS-related cancers such as central nervous system (CNS) lymphoma, Kaposi's sarcoma, and/or systemic lymphoma. Other conditions associated with advanced AIDS include: refractory cachexia; opportunistic infections (e.g. mycobacterium avium complex [MAC], cryptosporidium, cytomegalovirus, toxoplasmosis); renal failure; congestive heart failure; advanced AIDS dementia complex; and progressive multifocal leukoencephalopathy. Eligibility for hospice care for individuals with HIV/AIDS in the United States includes consideration of CD4/viral load levels, concurrently with one of the previously listed conditions associated with advanced disease.[67] Additionally, a Karnofsky Performance Status of <50 also meets hospice eligibility criteria. An interdisciplinary team is needed to manage the multifaceted presentation of advanced AIDS disease. Addressing end-of-life symptoms with a holistic approach can provide for the most peaceful outcomes possible.

Summary

The effects of SUD, intentional self-harm, gun violence, and HIV/AIDS on individuals and societies are complex and often devastating. The co-occurring conditions routinely associated with these conditions require a trained eye and keen observation to draw the deserved attention. Ongoing education and interprofessional collaboration, and the awareness and acknowledgment of the potential long-term effects often observed with these conditions, will allow the treating clinician to provide the most effective plan of care. The involvement of the interdisciplinary team is critical to manage the concurrent needs of these individuals in order to provide the most comprehensive care possible, especially at the end of life.

References

1 Substance Abuse and Mental Health Services Administration. Key substance use and mental health indicators in the United States: Results from the 2017 National Survey on Drug Use and Health (HHS Publication No. SMA

18–5068, NSDUH Series H-53). Rockville, MD: Center for Behavioral Health Statistics and Quality, Substance Abuse and Mental Health Services Administration. https://www. samhsa.gov/data/. Published 2018. Accessed May 5, 2020.

2 Wilson N, Kariisa M, Seth P, Smith H IV, Davis NL. Drug and opioid-involved overdose deaths — United States, 2017–2018. *MMWR Morb Mortal Wkly Rep.* 2020;69:290–297. doi:10.15585/mmwr.mm6911a4.

3 Centers for Disease Control and Prevention. Tobacco. https://www.cdc.gov/tobacco/data_statistics/fact_sheets/health_effects/tobacco_related_mortality/index.htm. Published 2020. Accessed April 9, 2020.

4 World Health Organization. Tobacco. https://www.who.int/news-room/fact-sheets/detail/tobacco. Published May 27, 2020. Accessed May 30, 2020.

5 National Vital Statistics Reports. Deaths: Final data for 2017. https://www.cdc.gov/nchs/data/nvsr/nvsr68/nvsr68_09-508.pdf. 2017;68:9.

6 World Health Organization. Suicide data. https://www.who.int/mental_health/prevention/suicide/estimates/en/. Published 2019. Accessed April 9, 2020.

7 Amnesty International. Gun violence key facts. https://www.amnesty.org/en/what-we-do/arms-control/gun-violence/. Published 2020. Accessed April 9, 2020.

8 HIV.gov. Fast facts. https://www.hiv.gov/hiv-basics/overview/data-and-trends/statistics. Published 2020. Accessed April 9, 2020.

9 World Health Organization. HIV/AIDS. https://www.who.int/news-room/fact-sheets/detail/hiv-aids. Published 2020. Accessed April 9, 2020.

10 World Health Organization. Alcohol. https://www.who.int/substance_abuse/facts/alcohol/en/. Published 2020. Accessed April 9, 2020.

11 World Health Organization. Information sheet on opioid overdose. https://www.who.int/substance_abuse/information-sheet/en/. Published 2018. Accessed April 9, 2020.

12 NIDA. Comorbidity: Substance use disorder and other mental illnesses. National Institute on Drug Abuse website. https://www.drugabuse.gov/node/pdf/1155/common-comorbidities-with-substance-use-disorders. Published August 1, 2018. Accessed May 5, 2020.

13 Najt P, Fusar-Poli P, Brambilla P. Co-occurring mental and substance abuse disorders: A review on the potential predictors and clinical outcomes. *Psychiatry Res.* 2011;186(2–3):159–164. doi:10.1016/j.psychres.2010.07.042.

14 NIDA. Substance use and SUDs in LGBTQ populations. National Institute on Drug Abuse website. https://www.drugabuse.gov/related-topics/substance-use-suds-in-lgbtq-populations. Published September 5, 2017. Accessed May 5, 2020.

15 Scottish Government. Adverse childhood experiences. https://www.gov.scot/publications/adverse-childhood-experiences/. Published July 31, 2018. Accessed April 9, 2020.

16 Fonseca AC. Drug abuse and stroke. *Curr Neurol Rep.* 2013;13(2):325. doi:10.1007/s11910-012-0325-0.

17 National Cancer Institute. Risk factors for cancer. https://www.cancer.gov/about-cancer/causes-prevention/risk. Updated December 23, 2015. Accessed April 9, 2020.

18 Wikipedia. Alcoholic drink. https://en.wikipedia.org/wiki/Alcoholic_drink. Updated April 29, 2020. Accessed April 9, 2020.

19 Our World in Data. Alcohol consumption. https://ourworldindata.org/alcohol-consumption. Published April, 2018. Updated November, 2019. Accessed April 9, 2020.

20 White A, Castle J, Hingson R, Powell P. Using death certificates to explore changes in alcohol-related mortality in the United States, 1999–2017. *Alcohol Clin Exp Res.* 2020;44(1):178–187.

21 Ali SF, Onaivi ES, Dodd PR, et al. Understanding the global problem of drug addiction is a challenge for IDARS scientists. *Curr Neuropharmacol.* 2011;9(1):2–7. doi:10.2174/157015911795017245.

22 Ewing JA. Detecting alcoholism: The CAGE questionnaire. *JAMA.* 1984;252:1905–1907.

23 Selzer ML. The Michigan Alcoholism Screening Test (MAST): The quest for a new diagnostic instrument. *Am J Psych.* 1971;3:176–181.

24 The AUDIT. https://pubs.niaaa.nih.gov/publications/Practitioner/YouthGuide/AUDIT.pdf. Published date unknown. Accessed May 5, 2020.

25 World Health Organization. The WHO ASSIST package for hazardous and harmful substance use. https://www.who.int/publications/i/item/the-who-assist-package-for-hazardous-and-harmful-substance-use. Published date unknown. Accessed December 11, 2020.

26 National Institute on Drug Abuse. CTN. Common Data Elements. https://cde.drugabuse.gov/instrument/e9053390-ee9c-9140-e040-bb89ad433d69. Published date unknown. Accessed May 5, 2020.

27 The American Psychiatric Association Practice Guideline for the Pharmacological Treatment of Patients with Alcohol Use Disorder. https://psychiatryonline.org/doi/book/10.1176/appi.books.9781615371969. Published January 2018. Accessed May 4, 2020.

28 Our world in Data. Smoking. https://ourworldindata.org/smoking. Published 2013. Updated 2019. Accessed May 5, 2020.

29 Centers for Disease Control and Prevention. Understanding the epidemic. Centers for Disease Control and Prevention website. https://www.cdc.gov/drugoverdose/index.html. Updated May, 2020. Accessed April 27, 2020.

30 Centers for Disease Control and Prevention. CDC guideline for prescribing opioids for chronic pain. Centers for Disease Control and Prevention website. https://www.cdc.gov/mmwr/volumes/65/rr/rr6501e1.htm. Published March 16, 2016. Accessed April 27, 2020.

31 Move Forward PT. Avoid addictive opioids. Choose physical therapy for safe pain management. #ChoosePT. American Physical Therapy Association website. http://www.moveforwardpt.com/choose-physical-therapy-over-opioids-for-pain-management-choosept. Updated 2020. Accessed September 27, 2017.

32 Drugs.com. Naloxone injection. https://www.drugs.com/naloxone.html. Published 2020. Accessed May 4, 2020.

33 Wilson C. Naloxone accessibility and use by rehabilitation therapists for opioid overdoses. *Home Healthc Now.* 2020;38(1):50–51.

34 Substance Abuse and Mental Health Services Administration. Recovery and recovery support. https://www.samhsa.gov/find-help/recovery. Updated April 23, 2020. Accessed May 5, 2020.

35 Wang D, Wang Y, Wang Y, Li R, Zhou C. Impact of physical exercise on substance abuse disorders: A meta-analysis. *PLoS One.* 2014;9(10):1–15. doi:10.1371/journal.pone.0110728.

36 Zschucke E, Heinz A, Strohle A. Exercise and physical activity in the therapy of substance abuse disorders. *Scient World J.* 2012;1–19. doi:10.1100/2012/901741.

37 Vancampfort D, De Hert M, Stubbs B, et al. A systematic review of physical activity correlates in alcohol use disorders. *Arch Psychiatr Nurs.* 2015;29(4):196–201. doi:10.1016/j.apnu.2014.08.006.

38 Ebenau A, Dijkstra B, Stal-Klapwijk M, et al. Palliative care for patients with a substance use disorder and multiple problems: A study protocol. *BMC Palliat Care.* 2018;17(1):97. Published August 3, 2018. doi:10.1186/s12904-018-0351-z.

39 National Center for Health Statistics. Increase in suicide in the United States, 1999–2014. https://www.cdc.gov/nchs/products/databriefs/db241.htm. Published April, 2016. Accessed May 5, 2020.

40 World Health Organization. Practice manual for establishing and maintaining surveillance systems for suicide attempts and self-harm. https://www.who.int/mental_health/suicide-prevention/attempts_surveillance_systems/en/. Published date 2016. Accessed May 6, 2020.

41 National Institute of Mental Health. Suicide in America: Frequently asked questions. https://www.nimh.nih.gov/health/publications/suicide-faq/index.shtml. Published date unknown. Accessed May 6, 2020.

42 McEvoy C, Hideg G. Global violent deaths 2017. Time to decide. http://www.smallarmssurvey.org/fileadmin/docs/U-Reports/SAS-Report-GVD2017.pdf. Published 2017. Accessed April 9, 2020.

43 Amnesty International. Gun violence key facts. https://www.amnesty.org/en/what-we-do/arms-control/gun-violence/. Published 2020. Accessed April 9, 2020.

44 Sorenson SB, Schut RA. Nonfatal gun use in intimate partner violence: A systematic review of the literature. *Trauma Violence Abuse*. 2018;19(4):431–442. doi:10.1177/1524838016668589.

45 Iroku-Malize T, Grissom M. Violence and public and personal health: Gun violence. *FP Essent*. 2019;480:16–21.

46 Dougherty PJ, Najibi S, Silverton C, Vaidya R. Gunshot wounds: Epidemiology, wound ballistics, and soft-tissue treatment. *Instr Course Lect*. 2009;58:131–139.

47 Mosenthal AC, Weissman DE, Curtis JR, et al. Integrating palliative care in the surgical and trauma intensive care unit: A report from the Improving Palliative Care in the Intensive Care Unit (IPAL-ICU) Project Advisory Board and the Center to Advance Palliative Care. *Crit Care Med*. 2012;40(4):1199–1206. doi:10.1097/CCM.0b013e31823bc8e7.

48 AIDS.gov. A timeline of HIV/AIDS. Published 2016. Accessed May 7, 2020.

49 CDC. Laboratory testing for the diagnosis of HIV infection: Updated recommendations. https://stacks.cdc.gov/view/cdc/23447. Published 2014. Updated 2018. Accessed May 7, 2020.

50 National HIV Curriculum. Initial evaluation. https://www.hiv.uw.edu/go/basic-primary-care/staging-initial-evaluation-monitoring/core-concept/all. Updated July 3, 2019. Accessed May 8, 2020.

51 Centers for Disease Control and Prevention. Diagnoses of HIV infection in the United States and dependent areas, 2018. https://www.cdc.gov/hiv/library/reports/hiv-surveillance/vol-31/index.html. Published 2018. Accessed May 7, 2020.

52 Centers for Disease Control and Prevention. Revised surveillance case definition for HIV infection—United States, 2014. *MMWR Recomm Rep*. 2014;63(RR-03):1–10.

53 Panel on Antiretroviral Guidelines for Adults and Adolescents. Guidelines for the use of antiretroviral agents in adults and adolescents with HIV. Department of Health and Human Services. https://clinicalinfo.hiv.gov/sites/default/files/guidelines/documents/AdultandAdolescentGL.pdf . Updated December 18, 2019. Accessed December 11, 2020.

54 Evans SR, Ellis RJ, Chen H, et al. Peripheral neuropathy in HIV: Prevalence and risk factors. *AIDS*. 2011;25(7):919–928. doi:10.1097/QAD.0b013e328345889d.

55 Maharaj SS, Yakasai AM. Does a rehabilitation program of aerobic and progressive resisted exercises influence HIV-induced distal neuropathic pain? *Am J Phys Med Rehabil*. 2018;97(5):364–369. doi:10.1097/PHM.0000000000000866.

56 Greene M, Covinsky K, Astemborski J, et al. The relationship of physical performance with HIV disease and mortality. *AIDS*. 2014;28(18):2711–2719. doi:10.1097/QAD.0000000000000507.

57 O'Brien KK, Tynan AM, Nixon SA, Glazier RH. Effectiveness of Progressive Resistive Exercise (PRE) in the context of HIV: Systematic review and meta-analysis using the Cochrane Collaboration protocol. *BMC Infect Dis*. 2017;17(1):268. Published April 12, 2017. doi:10.1186/s12879-017-2342-8.

58 O'Brien KK, Tynan AM, Nixon SA, Glazier RH. Effectiveness of aerobic exercise for adults living with HIV: Systematic review and meta-analysis using the Cochrane Collaboration protocol. *BMC Infect Dis*. 2016;16:182. Published April 26, 2016. doi:10.1186/s12879-016-1478-2.

59 Pérez Chaparro CGA, Zech P, Schuch F, Wolfarth B, Rapp M, Heißel A. Effects of aerobic and resistance exercise alone or combined on strength and hormone outcomes for people living with HIV. A meta-analysis. *PLoS One*. 2018;13(9):e0203384. Published September 4, 2018. doi:10.1371/journal. pone.0203384.

60 Martin K, Naclerio F, Karsten B, Vera JH. Physical activity and quality of life in people living with HIV. *AIDS Care*. 2019;31(5):589–598. doi:10.1080/09540 121.2019.1576848.

61 Dufour CA, Marquine MJ, Fazeli PL, et al. A longitudinal analysis of the impact of physical activity on neurocognitive functioning among HIV-infected adults. *AIDS Behav*. 2018;22(5):1562–1572. doi:10.1007/s10461-016-1643-z.

62 Dunne EM, Balletto BL, Donahue ML, et al. The benefits of yoga for people living with HIV/AIDS: A systematic review and meta-analysis. *Complement Ther Clin Pract*. 2019;34:157–164. doi:10.1016/j.ctcp.2018.11.009.

63 Hillier SL, Louw Q, Morris L, Uwimana J, Statham S. Massage therapy for people with HIV/AIDS. *Cochrane Database Syst Rev*. 2010;2010(1):CD007502. Published January 20, 2010. doi:10.1002/14651858.CD007502.pub2.

64 Dimitrova A, Murchison C, Oken B. Acupuncture for the treatment of peripheral neuropathy: A systematic review and meta-analysis. *J Altern Complement Med*. 2017;23(3):164–179. doi:10.1089/acm.2016.0155.

65 Hessol NA, Eng M, Vu A, Pipkin S, Hsu LC, Scheer S. A longitudinal study assessing differences in causes of death among housed and homeless people diagnosed with HIV in San Francisco. *BMC Public Health*. 2019;19(1):1440. Published November 1, 2019. doi:10.1186/s12889-019-7817-7.

66 Aidala AA, Wilson MG, Shubert V, et al. Housing status, medical care, and health outcomes among people living with HIV/AIDS: A systematic review. *Am J Public Health*. 2016;106(1):e1–e23. doi:10.2105/AJPH.2015.302905.

67 Hospice Guidelines of End-Stage HIV & AIDS. Vitas Healthcare. https://www.vitas.com/for-healthcare-professionals/hospice-and-palliative-care-eligibility-guidelines/hospice-eligibility-guidelines/hiv-and-aids/. Published date unknown. Accessed May 8, 2020.

Part III

Outcome Measures and Interventions

17 Management of Conditions and Symptoms

Amy J. Litterini and Christopher M. Wilson

Introduction

Symptom management for patients at the end of life includes evaluating and identifying underlying causes, addressing reversible conditions, and palliating irreversible conditions. This chapter will explore the therapist's role and management of commonly seen syndromes, conditions, and clinical presentations that individuals experience near or at the end of life.

Frailty

Often accompanying a serious illness, *frailty* is a syndrome characterized by limited physical functional reserve capacity and a function level at or near a vulnerable state of illness or mortality. A clinical syndrome, *frailty* is characterized by a symptom cluster not attributed to normal aging but rather associated with a decline in function and a reduction in biological reserve. Common issues related to frailty include osteoporosis and osteopenia, sarcopenia, failure to thrive, and functional limitations. As defined by Fried et al.,[1] the diagnosis is made with three out of five of the following criteria: (1) unintentional weight loss (4.5 kg [10 lbs]) in the previous year); (2) weak grip strength; (3) low energy/self-reported exhaustion; (4) slow walking speed; and (5) low physical activity. The categorization of *pre-frail* occurs with one or two of the five criteria present and is considered a high-risk for progression to frailty. Frailty has been correlated with the presence of poorer health and concurrent chronic illnesses.[1] *Sarcopenia*, or loss of muscle mass, is considered a contributing factor to the development of frailty and has been identified as the first observed criteria.[2] Additionally, weakness, and exhaustion or weight loss, are initiative of the condition of frailty in elderly women.[3]

A co-occurring condition seen frequently by rehabilitation professionals, frailty often presents with functional deficit sequelae that manifest in poorer health outcomes including falls, disability, hospitalization, and death.[3] A study of 432,828 surgical patients by Shinall et al.,[4] demonstrated elevated mortality risk at 30, 60, 90, and 180 days postoperatively for individuals with frailty. Although frailty can technically occur at any age, and with any serious illness, it increases in prevalence with advancing age and multiple life-threatening illnesses.[4] Patients with frailty lose physiological reserve to accommodate for insults to health, and adaptations to further insults act as contributing factors to progressive decline.

Additional conceptual development has occurred to operationally classify frailty characteristics in patients based on objective scoring methodology by counting accumulating deficits in indices such as the Frailty Risk Index and the Risk Analysis Index (RAI).[4-6] When considering vulnerable patients for aggressive interventions such as surgery, frailty is considered as a preoperative predictor of the likelihood of successful outcomes, and the RAI has been proven effective in measuring frailty in surgical populations.[5,6]

Risk stratification and early identification of frailty should be considered for appropriate referrals to rehabilitation. Concepts such as preoperative optimization of nutritional status, and comprehensive geriatric assessments, are becoming standard of care to identify and address issues for individuals presenting with frailty. Nutritional counseling and exercise prescription are also gaining prominence in the management of individuals with frailty.[7] In a review of systematic reviews of the effectiveness of exercise for community-dwelling pre-frail and frail older adults, the conclusion recommended multi-component exercise of resistance and aerobic training, as well as balance and flexibility exercises, as most beneficial for improving gait speed, strength, balance, and physical performance.[8] Home health referrals often occur for the functional decline observed with frailty. If therapy intervention does not improve the condition, a palliative or hospice referral discussion may be appropriate. For individuals at the end of life when the underlying condition cannot be adequately addressed or reversed, maintaining safe functional mobility and activity tolerance with the highest level of quality of life is the priority.

Immobility and Bed Rest

Reduced activity often accompanies decline with progressive disease. The negative sequelae associated with immobility are well documented; however, an intentional effort can help to mitigate these effects. Prescribed movement and patient-family education are indicated, with attention to safety, in order to promote mobility and maintain autonomy. With the goal to maintain functional mobility as long as possible, as safely as possible, the therapist can collaboratively develop a plan with the patient and family to allow for this important opportunity if desired at the end of life.

Bed rest is a medical order/recommendation to remain in bed secondary to a diagnosis or risk factor, with the exception for some, for trips to the bathroom. Due to the negative consequences of prolonged inactivity, bed rest is rarely used unless absolutely necessary (e.g. high-risk pregnancy, unstable fractures, blood clots). Once thought to be a remedy for diseases, modern-day evidence has disproved any possible benefits of bed rest as a prescribed intervention.[9]

Performance status is routinely defined, in part, by the distribution of time spent out of bed compared to time spent recumbent in bed. The Palliative

Performance Scale (PPS) and the Eastern Cooperative Oncology Group (ECOG) Performance Scale both measure the percentage of time spent in bed daily as criteria for determining performance status, and an indication of prognosis.[10,11] Most life-threatening progressive illnesses lead to increased time spent inactive, resulting in debilitating immobility. In spite of our best efforts, when individuals stay primarily horizontal there are several resulting negative sequelae including, but not limited to, skin breakdown, contractures, reduced organ function (e.g. lung, bladder, and bowel), orthostatic hypotension, infection, and difficult communication. Addressing the underlying medical conditions and sources of fatigue/malaise causing this decreased activity is often the first step. Medication adjustments are often necessary to prevent excessive drowsiness and improve arousal. When an underlying cause cannot be corrected or mitigated, prescribing a schedule for time out of bed can develop a routine to maintain sitting tolerance and improve access to socialization, communication, and activity participation. Durable medical equipment (DME) designed to facilitate independence with bed mobility and transfers, such as half-sized bed rails, trapeze bars, transfer boards, and bed canes, as well as chairs that allow for a degree of reclined comfort in sitting, can help to provide more opportunity for individuals to remain safely out of bed for greater durations of time (see Chapter 20 for Safe Patient Handling and Mobility).

When remaining in bed is the only viable option for an extended period of time, prescribing exercises to be done in supine can provide the individual the opportunity to maintain active range of motion and promote circulation even on bed rest. Active-assisted exercises to be completed by the patient and/or a caregiver can offer a way for the patient and a loved one to maintain motion. Passive exercises can help to maintain joint mobility and reduce the risk for contractures, even when the patient is unable to participate. It is important to offer these activities and then carefully listen to the patient and family responses as to interest and ability to engage in such activities within the context of their disease process and life course. End of life time in bed can be a place of comfort and care when well supported.

Individuals receiving palliative care in a home care setting as well as inpatient settings are at risk for decubitus ulcers. In home care, body mass index, Braden Scale, and Karnofsky Performance Scale are accurate in predicting the risk of the development of pressure ulcers.[12] Additionally, in inpatient palliative care settings, hyponatremia and hypotension have been found to be contributing factors to pressure ulcers.[13] Screening for individual risk factors, and the implementation of mitigation strategies, is appropriate. Evidence points to the greatest benefits from the type of mattress used over other interventions; however, expert opinion should be sought for an appropriate positioning plan.[14] Positioning schedules can promote the redistribution of pressure to skin/superficial tissues throughout the day, and skin inspection should occur during each repositioning. For patients unable to maintain the side-lying (*lateral*) position, wedge pillows can be helpful for propping the back to create a degree of side-lying. The *Sims* position is used for positioning be-tween side-lying and prone, with the use of pillows to the chest and under the flexed top lower extremity. For patients using an adjustable bed, altering the angle into semi-reclined (45°: *Fowler's position*; 30°: *Semi-Fowler's position*) can promote an upright posture for improved lung function; however, caution should be taken as the position can also simultaneously increase pressure on the sacrum. Attention to the angle of flexion between the femur and pelvis is essential to not place the spine in undue flexion; also, elevation of the knees with the bed controls will lessen the tendency to slide down toward the foot of the bed and minimize the need to reposition. Prone positioning has several contraindications (e.g. pelvic fracture, spinal instability, increased intracra-nial pressure, recent cardiac surgery) but has the benefits of shifting fluid from the posterior lung allowing for improved pulmonary capillary perfusion and oxygenation for such individuals as those with acute respiratory distress syn-drome (ARDS), and acute infection with the COVID-19 novel coronavirus (see Chapter 11: Respiratory Diseases).

Caregivers should consider such safe patient-handling tools such as no lift movers and slippery sheets to reduce workload during dependent patient repositioning (see Chapters 5 and 20). DME such as advanced static mat-tresses or advanced static overlays, blanket lifters to reduce pressure on the toes/feet (cardboard boxes can be used at home to similar effect), and foam heel protectors and heel float pressure-relieving boots should be considered to reduce the impact of prolonged bed rest and promote time spent out of bed (similarly, rolled towels can be used as adaptive pressure relief at home). Repeated demonstration, instruction, and review are often needed for family caregivers to become proficient in all of these bed care skills. Communication with the other IDT members can reinforce this information.

Distress

Both chronic and life-threatening illnesses are frequently associated with var-ious levels of distress. *Distress* is defined as feelings associated with extreme levels of anxiety, sorrow, and/or pain; distress can be manifested in physi-cal, emotional, and/or spiritual domains, as well as a combination of distress symptoms occurring simultaneously. According to Morita et al.,[15] *existential distress* pertains to feelings of dependency and being a burden on others, lack of meaning in life, a sense of hopelessness, loss of social role functioning, and feeling emotionally irrelevant. According to a review of the prevalence of existential distress in cancer survivorship, Vehling and Phillip[16] found 33–50% of individuals had existential fears associated with loss of control and identity, and uncertainties about their future.

Distress has the potential for negative impacts on quality of life, particu-larly at the end of life. As the Institute of Medicine's concept of a *good death* has developed and evolved, the inclusion of the goal of *freedom from avoidable distress and suffering* has been emphasized.[17,18] Therefore, appropriate attention should be paid to screening, early detection, and comprehensive distress management. The type of distress identified indicates the types of referrals appropriate to help mitigate the distress levels in the most comprehensive and effective ways possible for each individual.

In cancer survivorship, distress screening is recommended by the National Comprehensive Cancer Network (NCCN) for all patients.[19] Survivors with advanced cancer often experience varying levels of distress, both psychological and physical, from the time of diagnosis and throughout treatment. Distress screening and management have been identified as a standard of care in oncology. Ideally, it should be standardized with universal assessments that translate across care facilities, and should be instituted to recognize, monitor, document, and promptly treat distress at all stages of disease and in all settings.[19] The recommended NCCN *distress thermometer*, also adopted by the Commission on Cancer as a standard for comprehensive cancer centers in the United States, combines the use of a rating from zero (*no distress*) to ten (*extreme distress*) on a graphic of a thermometer with a problem list of practical, family, emotional, spiritual/religious, and physical issues patients can select to indicate issues over the previous week.[20] Many of the physical problems listed fall well within the scope of physical medicine and rehabilitation (e.g. *fatigue, getting around, pain, feeling swollen, tingling in hands and feet, bathing, dressing, eating*).[20] Since many facilities use this tool on a regular basis, there is a viable opportunity to capture deficits and use the responses as a trigger for rehabilitation referrals.

Spiritual well-being is also an important component to health-related quality of life for many, and spiritual beliefs are frequently associated with medical decisions. *Spiritual distress*, or unmet spiritual needs or spiritual pain, can lead to poorer outcomes including unnecessary use of health care resources.[21] The Functional Assessment of Chronic Illness Therapy - Spiritual Well-Being Scale (FACIT-sp), a 12-item questionnaire available in several different languages, was designed to capture levels of spiritual well-being in individuals with cancer or other chronic illnesses with the goal of referral for appropriate care and spiritual counseling.[22]

Individuals with life-limiting diagnoses resulting in distress could conceivably be assessed similarly to cancer survivors for their distress levels secondary to their illness. When assessing distress, the ideal response to the identification of certain types of distress is to follow with appropriate referrals to members of the interdisciplinary care team. Reassessment of distress should also occur at periodic intervals in order to track progress with interventions or necessitate referrals at a later date. Some settings assess distress at the beginning of a visit or interaction, and again at the conclusion of the visit, with the intent to determine the success of the particular intervention and plan established during the visit. Recommendations for integrative medicine strategies can be useful to reduce stress and manage anxiety (see Chapter 6). Prompt, effective, and compassionate responses to changes in existing distress levels, and/or the development of new or worsening distress, is the critical role of the care team for individuals with advanced illness.

Cachexia

Especially in advanced disease, *cachexia* or wasting syndrome, often presents as weight loss, muscle loss, decreased appetite, weakness, and fatigue, and must be closely managed by multiple members of the healthcare team. Physical activity and increasing caloric expenditure, although intuitive and logical, may not initially be the best course of action without addressing the physical and nutritional deficits of these individuals.

Considered a multifactorial paraneoplastic syndrome, *cachexia* was defined by an expert consensus process by Evans et al.[23] as: "a complex metabolic syndrome associated with underlying illness and characterized by loss of muscle with or without loss of fat mass."[pg793] An international consensus in 2011 defined three phases of cachexia, with the first being *pre-cachexia* (loss of up to 5% of body weight).[24] *Cachexia* is defined as weight loss greater than 5%, or weight loss greater than 2% with a body mass index <20 kg/m or sarcopenia. *Refractory cachexia*, considered irreversible, is associated with advanced cancer that is unresponsive to treatment in individuals with low-performance status. Beyond the presence of weight loss and body composition changes, cachexia has been associated with loss of appetite, reduced food intake, and the presence of biochemical abnormalities (e.g. anemia and systemic inflammation). Cachexia has also been associated with reduced physical functioning and quality of life, and increased mortality and susceptibility to treatment-related toxicity.[25] Mortality secondary to cachexia is estimated at 30% or greater for individuals with advanced cancer, while approximately 50% of cancer survivors die with a diagnosis of cachexia.[26] For individuals with other chronic diseases, an estimated 30% of individuals will die annually with a stage of cachexia (i.e. 10–15% with chronic obstructive pulmonary disorder [COPD], 20–30% with congestive heart failure [CHF] and chronic kidney disease [CKD]).[26] Ideally identified early, and recognized by changes in body composition and physical functioning, cachexia should be supported with the implementation of appropriate palliative measures initiated by an interdisciplinary care team.

Currently, there are limited effective management strategies to improve the quality of life and/or survival in individuals suffering from cachexia when the underlying cause cannot be cured or adequately addressed.[26] Pharmacological interventions commonly utilized for cachexia in the United States include megestrol acetate (Megace), dronabinol (Marinol), and somatotropin and serostim (human growth hormone). Much like with the condition of frailty, optimization of nutrition and physical activity should occur in the presence of cachexia. Close attention should be paid to the level of intensity of exercise prescribed so as to not exceed appropriate caloric expenditure in the presence of weight loss. Monitoring tolerance during physical activity, and assessing for side effects following physical activity, is critical for the clinicians caring for individuals with cachexia. Professionals who care for those at the end of life recognize that decreased appetite and eating is often a natural prelude to death. Eating items for pleasure or comfort often becomes a quality of life issue to be supported (e.g. chocolate ice cream or any other favorite dessert). This can be a challenge for family and caregivers who reflexively want to help someone eat, as they understand, even if unable to verbalize, the feared reality that not eating will lead to death.

Breathlessness

A significant number of individuals with terminal illness will experience *breathlessness*, or shortness of breath with activity, and/or at rest. *Dyspnea* is also used to describe shortness of breath, and in particular, on exertion (DOE). Conditions that commonly present with dyspnea include respiratory diseases such as primary and metastatic lung cancer, COPD, and pulmonary fibrosis, and conditions such as pneumonia, pleural effusion, and pneumothorax (see Chapter 11). However, a number of individuals with non-cardiopulmonary life-limiting conditions will also experience breathlessness. Cardiovascular conditions such as recent myocardial infarction, pericardial effusion, and CHF are also associated with dyspnea. Other physiological sources of dyspnea may include anemia, electrolyte imbalances, pulmonary embolism,

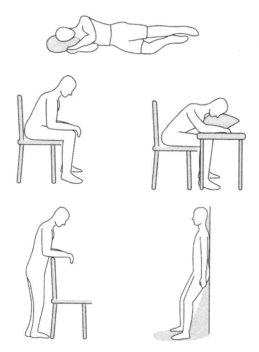

Figure 17.1 Positioning to Relieve Breathlessness.
Source: British Lung Foundation, Cotton Exchange, Bixteth Street, Liverpool, L3 9LQ.

dehydration, anxiety, and/or exacerbations of dyspnea secondary to epi-sodes of severe coughing. New or worsening dyspnea should be evaluated by a medical professional to rule out differential diagnoses such as pulmonary embolism, pneumonia, or pleural effusion.

There are a number of interventions available to clinicians to assist in the control and mitigation of breathlessness. Pharmaceutical strategies may include the use of anticholinergic agents, bronchodilators, anti-anxiety medications, corticosteroids, inhaled steroids, beta-agonists, cough sup-pressants, and decongestants. For individuals suspected to be experiencing infection, antibiotics may be prescribed (and are sometimes offered even in hospice as a comfort, rather than a curative measure), while diuretics may be used for individuals experiencing fluid overload. Palliation for severe dyspnea may include the use of opioids and anxiolytics. In hospice care, liq-uid morphine is often used to relieve dyspnea by nursing. It can be helpful for therapy to help differentiate dyspnea at rest and DOE. Sometimes, just rest can resolve the breathlessness rather than rushing to use medication as the solution.

Oxygen therapy can be used for symptomatic individuals, particularly those whose pulse oxygenation drops below 90% at rest, or with activity. An *incentive spirometer,* a hand-held device with a one-way valve mouthpiece and a piston-type gauge that measures inspiration at levels (units usually range from 2,500 to 5,000 mL volume) with set goals for repetitions, duration, and fre-quency per day, can help promote oxygenation and reduce fluid accumulation in the lungs. Also, controlling and thinning secretions by staying hydrated and using a vaporizer and/or humidifier may help to allow for a productive cough and improved respiratory airflow. Physical activity, and in particular participation in a comprehensive pulmonary rehabilitation program, can be vital to controlling symptoms and maintaining functional mobility for indi-viduals with breathlessness associated with chronic illness.

A critical role for clinicians is patient education related to exacerbations of shortness of breath, and what the individual and family can do to help manage symptoms. A handheld, desktop, or small floor fan directed towards the face can reduce dyspnea or *air hunger.* Elevation of the head of the bed can help reduce breathlessness while attempting to sleep. Reduction of salt in the diet can help reduce fluid retention that can exacerbate breathlessness. Reducing the exposure to environmental allergens such as seasonal pollens, and limiting time out of doors in the presence of high air pollutants, can be beneficial. Good hand hygiene precautions should be utilized to reduce the risk of respiratory infection. Smoking cessation is a key component for indi-viduals with tobacco use disorder (see Chapter 16). Relaxation techniques, and pacing for energy conservation, can be helpful (see Chapter 6 regarding Integrative Medicine). Pursed lip breathing and diaphragmatic breathing can also encourage optimal oxygen utilization and depth of respiration. Leaning forward onto something in sitting (e.g. palms/forearms on thighs or a tray table), also known as the *orthopneic* or *tripod position,* and/or leaning forward on something in standing (e.g. countertop or walker), can also reduce symptoms of breathlessness (see Figure 17.1). Tracking symptoms on a Borg scale can be helpful to keep a record of exacerbations, and/or triggers for exacerbations, associated with breathlessness.[27]

Pathological Fracture Risk

Terminally ill individuals, or those with chronic diseases, often experience demineralization of bones or development of metastatic lesions from cancer that jeopardizes the structural integrity of the skeleton. Based on this fact, rehabilitation professionals must use extreme caution and evidence-based decision-making in establishing when and where rehabilitation interventions should be administered if the individual is at risk of pathologic fracture. Due to the risk of fracture increasing from physical activity and the paradoxical influence of bed rest reducing the stimulus for bone mineralization, a multifactorial assessment of the individual's goals, medical status, and care team concerns must ensue before initiating or modifying physical activity based on the potential for pathologic fracture.

In the application of physical activity, exercise, and rehabilitation, metastatic bone lesions are a commonly encountered and expected issue that must be carefully addressed and understood. In addition to primary bone cancers and metastatic disease, osteoporosis and osteopenia also pose a risk of pathologic fracture. Depending on the therapist's practice setting, there may be a dearth of information beyond a passing mention of osteoporosis, osteopenia, or metastatic disease. As physician team members are often focused on saving their patient's life and optimizing medical and emotional quality of life, the same level of information to establish bony stability may not be available as compared to the interest clinicians who administer physical activity. In these cases where there is a concern for bone stability, advocacy for the patient, and facilitating a diagnostic workup is important to comprehensively manage the individual's physical activity status. If a fall or injury occurred in a high-risk pathologic fracture scenario, it can substantially worsen the remaining quality of life. Conversely, if the pathologic fracture risk is small and the therapist resorts to excessively conservative treatments, their patient may not be able to enjoy an optimal quality of life as their physical status was unnecessarily restricted.

Bone Metastases and Bone Tumors

In cases of metastatic cancer, the incidence of bone metastases varies substantially by tumor type and stage at diagnosis. If a person is diagnosed with stage IV cancer, the risk of development of bony metastases was estimated to be 23.1%.[28] Of all solid tumors, stage IV prostate cancer had the highest likelihood of bone metastases with 71.1% at ten years, followed by stage IV breast cancer with 60.8% at ten years.[28] In addition, there are primary cancers

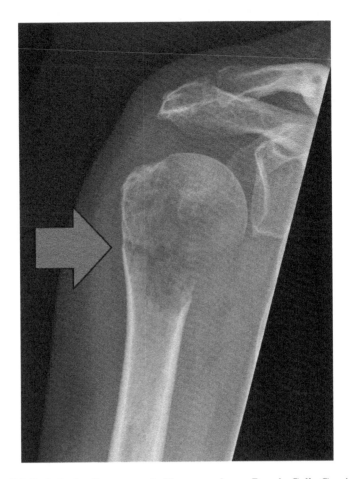

Figure 17.2 Pathologic Fracture of Humerus from Renal Cell Carcinoma. Reprinted under creative common license by Hellerhoff [CC BY-SA 3.0 https://creativecommons.org/licenses/by-sa/3.0)] Original image can be found at https://upload.wikimedia.org/wikipedia/commons/c/ cd/Pathologische_Fraktur_bei_Metastase_Nierencell-Ca_im_ Humerus.jpg.

that can also increase risk of pathologic fracture that also require evaluation and quantification (see Figure 17.2). The most common primary bone tumor in adults is chondrosarcoma (40%), then osteosarcoma (28%), chordoma (10%), Ewing sarcoma (8%), and undifferentiated pleomorphic sarcoma/ fibrosarcoma (4%).[29] In adolescents and children, osteosarcoma (56%) is most common followed by Ewing sarcoma (34%).[29] Especially when providing care for individuals diagnosed with any cancer that may metastasize to the bone, a thorough workup is recommended prior to introduction of physical activity. A positron emission tomography (PET) scan correlated with a computerized tomography (CT) scan is a useful diagnostic test to evaluate the extent and location of bone metastases. To evaluate for metastatic disease, PET scans utilize a glucose analog called fludeoxyglucose (FDG).[30] As neoplasms and metastases are more metabolically active than surrounding tissues, they will reveal areas of increased glucose uptake which will then demonstrate potential areas of metastatic disease, including bone metastases.[30]

In order to establish the stability of metastatic lesions, and to understand the decision-making of the physician care team members, familiarity with oncologic orthopedic stability scales is beneficial. The two most common scales are the Mirels' score (Table 17.1) and the Spinal Instability Neoplastic Score (SINS) scale (Table 17.2). The Mirels' scale is utilized for extremity and long-bone stability, and the SINS scale is designed to establish the stability of the vertebral column. Both scales require identification of whether a lesion is lytic, blastic, or mixed. *Lytic* lesions are characterized by destruction and thinning of bone with ill-defined margins while *blastic* lesions demonstrate bone growth as nodular, rounded lesions, and thick coarse bone.[31] *Mixed* lesions share some

Table 17.1 Mirels' Scale

Scoring	1	2	3
Location	Upper extremity	Lower extremity	Intertrochanteric
Radiographic appearance	Blastic	Mixed	Lytic
Size	<1/3	1/3–2/3	>2/3
Pain	Mild	Moderate	Pain with functional tasks

Table 17.2 Spinal Instability Neoplastic Scale

	Highest Point Score	*Moderate Point Scores*		*Lowest Point Score*
Location	Junctional (occiput-C2, C7-T2, T11-L1, L5-S1) = 3 points	Mobile Spine (C3-C6, L2-L4) = 2 points	Semi rigid (T3-T10) = 1 point	Rigid (S2-S5) = 0 points
Pain	Yes = 3 points	Occasional pain but not mechanical = 1 point		Pain-free lesion = 0 points
Bone lesion	Lytic = 2 points	Mixed (lytic/blastic) = 1 points		Blastic = 0 points
Radiographic spinal alignment	Subluxation/translation present = 4 points	De novo (new) deformity (kyphosis/scoliosis) = 2 points		Normal alignment = 0 points
Vertebral body collapse	>50% collapse = 3 points	<50% collapse = 2 points	No collapse with > 50% body involved =1 point	None of the above = 0 points
Posterolateral involvement of spinal element	Bilateral = 3 points	Unilateral = 1 point		None of the above = 0 points

lytic and blastic qualities. Radiologist reports are beneficial to establish lytic, blastic, or mixed lesions, as well as establishing lesion size and location.

One of the challenges of the scales is that they are best applied for evaluating a single bone metastasis or bone tumor in isolation, and are not as beneficial in evaluating the overall compound risk of an individual's pathologic fracture for multiple or diffuse bone metastases. In addition, the scales are best applied when advanced training or experience evaluating radiologic imaging is needed. Even some therapists with more advanced training in analysis of diagnostic imaging may still experience challenges with an autonomous evaluation of orthopedic oncologic stability. Knowledge and understanding of the scales will assist a therapist during discussions with orthopedic oncologists or other physician team members. Foundational knowledge of the Mirels' and SINS scales can empower a therapist to facilitate (or understand) the decision-making when there is clearly no need for restricted weight bearing or treatment modifications due to a single, small, isolated metastasis. On the other end of the spectrum, these scales will assist therapists when collaboration or workup is necessary before initiating safe, goal-oriented, physical activity.

Established in 1989, Mirels' score remains widely utilized and accepted.[32,33] In the Mirels' score, lesions are evaluated based on location, radiographic appearance, size of the lesion (proportional to the diameter of the cortex), and patient pain report.[33] In Mirels' investigations, all patients with functional pain (mechanical weakness of the bone resulting in pain during performance of daily activities) proceeded to fracture.[33] The Mirels' score demonstrated a sensitivity of 91% and a specificity of 35% and performed better than clinical judgment across various experience levels.[34] After evaluation, the score for the lesion is summed based on the four categories. If the lesion scored less than 7, radiation and observation are recommended. A score of greater than or equal to 9 should prompt a discussion of prophylactic fixation or reduction of weight-bearing. A score of 8 should result in a shared clinical judgment with the care team.[33]

In examination of spinal stability, the SINS score utilizes some of the same principles as the Mirels' score (lytic versus blastic versus mixed), pain, and location. Other components to be evaluated include spinal alignment on imaging, the extent of vertebral body collapse, and whether there is posterolateral involvement of spinal elements.[35] Each domain is scored from 0 to 3 with a best score of 0 and a worst score of 18. The SINS scale demonstrated a sensitivity of 95.7% and specificity of 79.5% to identify an unstable lesion (Table 17.2).[35]

After evaluation of high-risk spinal metastases, categorization can occur to be stable (scores from 0 to 6), indeterminate (possibly impending) instability (scores from 7 to 12), or instability (scores from 13 to 18).[35] Fisher et al.[35] recommends surgical consultation with a SINS score greater than 7. After establishment of orthopedic stability in the presence of metastatic disease, Galvao et al.[36] described general guidelines for initiating upper body or lower body exercise interventions based on the presence of bone metastases. In the study, utilizing these guidelines it was found that the participants tolerated the exercises well without an increase in skeletal complications.[36] Furthermore, Sheill et al.[37] described decision-making in the presence of metastatic disease for exercise prescription (Table 17.3).

Pathologic Fracture Risk Assessment

With individuals with chronic disease or frailty, the risk of pathologic fracture is increased in the presence of osteoporosis or osteopenia. A useful tool to establish the risk of pathologic fracture from osteoporosis/osteopenia is the FRAX (fracture risk assessment) calculator (www.shef.ac.uk/FRAX/).[38] The FRAX calculator is a free service sponsored by the University of Sheffield "developed from studying population-based cohorts from Europe, North America, Asia and Australia."[38] This tool can assist therapists to establish the ten-year risk of pathologic fracture in adults. It incorporates sex, ethnicity, age, menopausal status, hormone replacement status, body mass index, health status, glucocorticoid use, fracture status, and alcohol use to determine the risk of fracture. There is also a FRAX smartphone app available from the iOS Apple Store.

Table 17.3 Exercise Prescription-based on Metastatic Location[37]

Location of Metastasis			Pelvis	Lumbar Spine	Thoracic/ Ribs	Proximal Femur	All Regions of Body
Type of exercise	Resistance exercise	UE	Yes	Yes	Yes (avoid shld flx, ext, abd, add)	Yes	Yes (avoid shld flx, ext, abd, add)
		Trunk	Yes	Avoid	Avoid	Yes	Avoid
		LE	Yes (avoid hip flx/ext but include knee flx/ext)	Yes	Yes	Yes (avoid hip flx/ext but include knee flx/ext)	Yes (avoid hip flx/ext but include knee flx/ext)
	Aerobic exercise		NWB	NWB	NWB or WB	NWB	NWB
	Static flexibility		Yes	Yes (avoid spinal flex, ext, rot)	Yes (avoid spinal flex, ext, rot)	Yes	Yes (avoid spinal flex, ext, rot)

Legend: UE = upper extremity, LE = lower extremity, flx = flexion, ext = extension, shld = shoulder, abd = abduction, add = adduction, NWB = non-weight bearing (e.g. biking, recumbent stepper), WB = weight bearing, rot = rotation

Pain

As modeled by Cicely Saunders, the concept of *Total Pain* encompasses multiple domains, beyond just nociceptive pain from a chemical or mechanical disturbance.[39,40] *Nociceptive* pain (i.e. radicular, somatic, and/or visceral), whether acute or chronic, is a condition commonly treated by rehabilitation professionals. However, due to our routine lack of integration in hospice or palliative care teams, therapist services are less frequently utilized with this patient population. Because of this factor, patients may become increasingly reliant on the use of opioids or other pharmacological agents which may have their own side effects at end of life. In addition, key strategies are required for the management of the other domains of pain including psychological, social, and spiritual pain. These domains may serve to present as, amplify, or exacerbate physical pain, and if the healthcare professional does not address all domains of the individual's total pain, outcomes will be less effective and contribute to unwarranted suffering or anxiety near or at the end of life.

Pain is defined as "an unpleasant sensory or emotional experience associated with actual or potential tissue damage, or an experience described in terms of such damage."[41] *Acute* pain is considered time-limited, while *chronic* pain lasts for three months or longer and beyond the healing phase. *Persistent* pain, often experienced by individuals at the end of life, continues while the causative factors remain. *Recurrent* pain occurs with repeated episodes in the same area, while *breakthrough* pain presents between regularly scheduled long-acting pain medication (e.g. often associated with advanced cancer). The experience of pain from person to person is subjective, quite individualized, and dependent on several personal and environmental factors. Pain perception is affected by several characteristics including past experiences (e.g. previous trauma), spiritual beliefs, cultural influences, psychosocial state, and physical/body structures (e.g. diagnoses and stage of disease). Descriptions of pain are related in terms associated with type and quality of pain, timing (e.g. onset, duration), body region affected/location of pain, pain severity/intensity, and pain tolerance as it pertains to functional limitations. As pain is an individualized and subjective experience, patient self-report is the most commonly utilized method for pain assessment (see Chapter 18). For patients unable to effectively communicate or describe their symptoms, such as children and individuals with a diagnosis of dementia, specialized assessment tools and keen observation skills are required by clinicians to determine the role of nonverbal cues in the communication of pain.

Coping strategies, access to resources, available support, and attitudes toward pain alter the pain response from patient to patient. The experience of pain can result in *pain catastrophizing* (associated with helplessness, pessimism, exaggerated negative reactions) and *fear avoidance* behaviors (associated with pain-related fear, hypervigilance, avoidance/decreased activity) for some patients.[42,43] As maladaptive coping styles, these responses should be recognized by clinicians, identified early, and addressed appropriately so as to empower the individual and avoid further negative sequelae from inactivity, deconditioning, and disability. Education regarding the accurate interpretation of pain sources, as well as teaching the patient self-management techniques, can provide greater opportunity for a patient-therapist alliance for successful pain control.

Pain is a commonly reported symptom for patients at the end of life, both for individuals with cancerous and non-cancerous diagnoses. For cancer survivors, it was found that 35–56% of individuals with metastatic disease, and 76% of patients on hospice experienced pain.[44] In a study by Grond et al.,[45] individuals with advanced head and neck tumors, and gastrointestinal and genitourinary tumors, reported the highest levels of pain. In a study of 277 patients with advanced non-cancerous illnesses in China, pain was reported by 48.8% of the survey respondents.[46]

Goals for pain management at the end of life are to reduce or eliminate pain intensity/severity, control and manage sources of painful stimuli and/or inflammation, and palliate chronic pain (persistent and breakthrough) while limiting associated side effects. Moderate-to-severe pain at the end of life is generally managed with a combination of pharmacological interventions including opioid-based regimens (i.e. oral, transdermal, parenteral [injection], rectal suppository). Due to the concerns with the overuse of opioids in the presence of the opioid crisis and substance use disorder epidemic (see Chapter 16) and their many side effects including constipation, nausea and vomiting, pruritus, delirium, respiratory depression, motor and cognitive impairment, and sedation, non-opioid strategies should be considered when appropriate.[47] Other pain control methods include non-opioid medications (e.g. Ketamine, intravenous lidocaine), corticosteroids, antidepressants, anticonvulsants, topical agents (e.g. lidocaine patch), non-steroidal anti-inflammatory drugs (NSAIDs), and acetaminophen to address both persistent and breakthrough pain.[47] Depending on the legality in a particular jurisdiction, medicinal cannabis/tetrahydrocannabinol (THC) products/edibles are being used with increasing frequency to help manage terminal symptoms, including pain. Interventional pain strategies (e.g. epidural and intrathecal pumps, regional plexus blocks, neurolysis, radiofrequency ablation), surgical interventions (e.g. kyphoplasty for pathological fractures, debulking procedures), and in the instance of metastatic cancer, radiation therapy techniques, are often employed.[47] Integrative medicine techniques have also been advocated for to address symptoms of pain in advanced illness, such as acupuncture, massage, and Reiki (see Chapter 6).

Comprehensive, multidimensional pain management at the end of life includes pain awareness, assessment, and alleviation.[48] Therefore, success with this approach is best observed with an interprofessional pain management team (see Chapter 6). The biopsychosocial-spiritual model framework is most appropriate for the assessment and management of total pain in individuals receiving hospice and palliative care. Referral to key members of the care team to address the different aspects and contributing factors within an individual's pain experience has the greatest likelihood of attaining goals of accurate recognition and effective care planning for successful outcomes in pain management. For therapists, several pain management modalities in our usual treatment toolbox may be appropriate for individuals experiencing pain at the end of life. Typical modalities (often called biophysical agents) used by clinicians are generally considered for nonpharmacologic pain modulation, for the management of inflammation and the promotion of healing, to aid in regulation of muscle tone, to improve collagen tissue extensibility, and to reduce motion restrictions.[49] As for any individual receiving medical care, patient safety must be at the forefront in the clinician's mind with the use of any modality. Assessing risks while considering benefits is a critical balance that matches the right patient with the right modality, and if appropriate, at the right time. Prior to prescribing modality use, consideration of active disease process(es), circulatory status to tolerate fluctuations/changes due to applied modalities, effects of medications on pain perception, the individual's ability to communicate symptoms, and the realistic goals for the modality, all must be cautiously evaluated. Close communication with the medical team is also indicated during care planning and treatment delivery.

With careful attention to screening for safety of the integumentary system, physical agents may be beneficial for certain musculoskeletal and neuromuscular sources of pain for appropriate individuals with advanced diseases. Cancer survivors as a specific patient population have historically had limited and/or cautious access to modalities due to concerns for the potential spread of disease secondary to the ability of certain modalities to increase circulation. Wilson et al.[49] performed an updated literature review which examined sources published between 2001 and 2016 on safety, efficacy, and use of physical agents for cancer survivors based on the original 2001 review (sources 1972–2001) completed by Pfalzer.[50] With the exception of fairly recently introduced modalities such as low-level laser and scrambler therapy, Wilson et al.[49] found no new evidence for thermal, mechanical, electromagnetic, or electrotherapeutic agents. This review is, however, a very valuable source for precautions and considerations for modality use specific to cancer survivors.

Transcutaneous electrical nerve stimulation (TENS) has also been advocated for in clinical practice guidelines as a non-pharmacological intervention for pain management by national associations such as the US NCCN for the management of cancer-related pain.[47] However, the available literature is both of limited research quality and is not definitive on the effects of TENS.[49] In spite of this paucity of evidence, authors such as Cheville and Basford[51] acknowledge this limitation, but recommend consideration for interventions such as TENS for reasonable candidates with localized pain which is: (1) inadequately controlled; (2) have untenable adverse medication side effects; or (3) those who prefer nonpharmacological interventions. These authors also thoughtfully advocate for traditional rehab approaches including prescription of assistive devices and equipment, the use of orthotics, positioning (e.g. bolsters, armrests, cushions, wedges), therapeutic exercise, and manual therapy.[51]

As with most of all conditions and diagnoses, movement can provide comfort, even in the latest stages of disease and weeks/days of life. When individuals spend greater amounts of time recumbent or in bed as they experience physical decline, weakness and potentially painful stiffness will inevitably occur without intervention. To assist patients in avoiding unnecessary joint and soft tissue discomfort associated with inactivity and immobility, thoughtful prescription of therapeutic activities such as bed mobility, activities of daily living (e.g. bathing/grooming/dressing), and range of motion (active/active assisted/passive) should be considered (see section on Immobility/Bed rest earlier in Chapter 17). Comprehensive pain management should be focused, team-based, patient-centered, and intentional with the patient's participation and quality of life in mind.

Delirium, Confusion, Restlessness, Agitation

A common, yet challenging, symptom in end-stage disease is the development of delirium. Although this condition is commonly observed in elderly individuals, it presents a unique challenge for rehabilitation professionals who depend on developing patient-centered goals to optimize quality of life and assure ethical participation in rehabilitation. Although dementia, delirium, and depression, collectively known as the "3 D's", can have somewhat similar presentations, they are distinctly different diagnoses. *Dementia* is a progressive neurodegenerative diagnosis associated with memory loss and behavioral changes (see Chapter 13), while clinical *depression* is a mood disorder associated with the emotion of sadness and loss of interest/apathy. *Delirium*, an acute confusional state, is most frequently associated with: fluctuating consciousness; inattention and distractibility; slurred speech and language difficulties; anxiety; suspicion/fear; agitation; and lethargy. Differential diagnosis should be made as soon as possible to begin appropriate interventions to reverse symptoms and/or address the underlying cause(s) as cognitive deficits with an onset of delirium can become persistent. Precipitating factors potentially associated with the development of delirium include: immobilization; pain; medical lines and tubes (e.g. intravenous lines or indwelling Foley catheters); surgery; sleep deprivation/disruption; medications (e.g. new prescription, withdrawal, or polypharmacy); infection; metabolic derangements; issues with fluids, electrolytes, or nutrition; and changing environment (e.g. unfamiliar people, places, and situations). Early identification of delirium is critical, as it is often unrecognized and underdiagnosed.[52] Delirium should be identified as a serious detrimental neuropsychiatric disorder which can potentially be successfully reversed, mitigated, and palliated.

The development of delirium is an unfortunate scenario that occurs frequently at the end of life, with studies revealing estimates up to 13–42% of patients in palliative care units and up to 88% of individuals at the end of life.[53] A complex, multifactorial medical condition associated with increased medical costs and hospital length-of-stay, delirium is the most frequent symptom requiring palliative sedation in the hospice setting.[54] As the condition is associated with altered mental status, it can, in turn, diminish the awareness of actual symptoms by the treating clinician and contribute to levels of distress for both the patient and caregivers.[55] Clinicians do a disservice by the basic consideration of our patients as just "pleasantly confused" or simply "sleepy," and not following up on presentations of an altered mental status.

In a study by Mercadante et al.,[56] patient presentation and characteristics of individuals with delirium (n = 263) were examined. Patients were more likely men of older age, had a lower Karnofsky score at admission, and were receiving hospice in home care. On admission to hospice, delirium was observed in 41.8%, and the diagnosis was associated with weakness, nausea, drowsiness, and lack of appetite and well-being. For those with normal cognitive status at the time of hospice admission, 27% subsequently developed delirium within one week. For the patients receiving a diagnosis of delirium with appropriate interventions, improvement in the cognitive status corresponded to a significant improvement in weakness, depression, and appetite.[56] Delirium can also be associated with impending death (see the end of this chapter).

There are several standardized tests to identify delirium, including The Edmonton Symptom Assessment Scale (ESAS), the MDAS (Memorial Delirium Assessment Scale), and the Confusion Assessment Method for the Intensive Care Unit (CAM-ICU).[57-59] The CAM-ICU is considered a gold standard due to its psychometric properties and the short time required to administer (five minutes).[60,61]

There are beneficial interventions for healthcare providers to pursue optimal clinical outcomes in the presence of delirium and other confusional states, including referral to interprofessional colleagues and intervention strategies to assist confused patients with care planning and participation in rehabilitation. Medications including antipsychotics (e.g. haloperidol or risperidone) may be considered appropriate. For patients at risk of leaving their bed in an unsafe or disoriented state, a lowered bed closer to the floor or floor mats on the side of the bed can help to reduce the risk of injury. Bed alarms and door alarms can also be used to alert caregivers if a patient is moving from a place of safety and potentially wandering to an unsafe area (e.g. the top of a flight of stairs, outdoors, into a street/traffic, towards a body of water).

Coordinated interventions for individuals presenting with delirium should include consistency with therapist interventions (e.g. timing of sessions, cues), minimizing stimuli (e.g. background music, earplugs), and engaging familiar family members in care and care planning. See Chapter 7 for adaptive communication strategies for individuals with confusion. Additionally, sleep hygiene strategies should be employed (e.g. avoid sleep medications, avoid medication administration or vitals assessment during sleeping hours, minimize daytime naps, toilet use before bed). Regular orientation to time/day/person/place should occur frequently throughout the day via verbal communication and displayed in a visible location in the individual's room. Regular safe mobility and maintenance of hydration should be encouraged. Pain should be adequately managed, and relaxation exercises should be taught and encouraged, to help reduce anxiety and agitation. Assuring availability and access to necessary sensory and communication aids such as glasses, hearing aids, and dentures, can not only improve the patient's quality of life and activity participation but also promote orientation and communication capabilities.

Lymphedema and Edema Management

Advanced diseases are often associated with the conditions of edema and lymphedema due to organ failure and/or damage to the lymphatic system. Although edema management for individuals with non-life-threatening conditions has become the standard of care globally, management of swelling while co-occurring with advanced illness is not a primary focus, nor is it generally addressed as successfully. Progressive swelling conditions can significantly limit comfort and quality of life for those experiencing it, and therefore, proactive management attempts should be prioritized.

The Difference between Edema and Lymphedema

The lymphatic system is responsible for (1) immune defense (e.g. removal of debris from the interstitium, production of lymphocytes, and protection from the spread of malignancy); (2) nutrition (e.g. intestinal lymph vessels absorb digested fats/lipoproteins); and (3) maintenance of fluid balance (i.e. filtration/reabsorption). An estimated 10% of the capillary ultrafiltrate is considered the *lymph obligatory load* which returns to the circulatory system via reabsorption by the lymphatic system.[62] *Edema* is the general term for swelling due to increased fluid collection in the interstitium; it is a visible and palpable sign of injury or a malfunctioning system, and is associated with different etiologies. In the body's initial response to injury, acute edema results from a transfer of fluid (exudate) from the blood into tissue. Edema, which can be either generalized/diffuse or localized, can also result from immobilization, or it can be an initial symptom of an underlying disease such as CHF or other venous system disorders (see Chapter 8).[62] *Lymphedema*, considered a chronic condition, is the abnormal collection of protein-rich lymph fluid in the interstitium that, if left untreated, can cause chronic inflammation, fibrosis of the affected tissues, and/or wounds.

The lymphatic system is considered an accessory route for the transportation of lymph fluid from the tissues into the bloodstream. In this role, the lymphatic system works in parallel with the cardiovascular system to maintain fluid balance throughout the body in a unidirectional fashion.[62] Disruption of this balance, caused by anatomic malformation or trauma, can result in dynamic or mechanical lymphatic insufficiency, leading to localized or generalized edema. *Dynamic insufficiency* occurs when the normal transport capacity of the lymphatic system is ineffective to accommodate the lymphatic load. *Mechanical insufficiency* occurs when transport capacity is reduced due to functional or acquired causes.[62]

Primary and Secondary Lymphedema

Primary lymphedema is attributed to an anatomical malformation within the lymphatic system (e.g. lipedema) and is considered congenital (onset at >2 years of age), lymphedema praecox (onset often near puberty, 2–35 years of age), or lymphedema tarda (older adult onset >35 years of age). *Secondary lymphedema*, associated with mechanical insufficiency, is attributed to causes such as surgery, radiation, trauma, and/or infection. The development of lymphedema in cancer survivorship is often the result of lymphadenectomy during the staging and surgical treatment of cancers, and/or from damage to superficial lymphatics or remaining lymph nodes by radiation therapy techniques (see Chapter 9). Incidence rates of lymphedema in cancer survivorship vary based on diagnosis and treatment modalities used. Shaitelman et al.[63] documented pooled incidence rates for cancer treatment-related secondary lymphedema. They found rates for breast cancer survivors following sentinel lymph node biopsy (SLNB) at 6.3% (0–23%), and following axillary lymph node dissection (ALND) at 22.3% (11–57%); melanoma survivors following SLNB at 4.1%, following ALND 3%, and following inguinofemoral lymph node dissection at 18%; and gynecologic cancer survivors following SLNB at 9% (0–25%). Advanced cancerous tumors can result in *malignant lymphedema* due to active tumor infiltration and compression of lymphatic pathways.

Although commonly observed in cancer survivors, 85% of individuals with advanced non-cancer diagnoses at the end of life have reported the presence of edema among 277 survey respondents from China.[46] Extreme generalized edema, referred to as *anasarca*, is widespread edema throughout the body most often occurring as a result of major organ failure. A separate global health concern arising from a different etiology, *lymphatic filariasis* (LF) is a swelling condition caused by infection with filarial parasites transmitted by mosquitoes, which is estimated to impact 40 million individuals worldwide.[64] The parasitic infection of the lymphatic vessels disrupts normal lymphatic function resulting in increased risk for infection, and lymphedema and/or hydrocele, and in severe cases, disfiguring elephantiasis. The world regions most significantly impacted by LF include the continent of Africa, the Caribbean Islands, South America, the Eastern Mediterranean, Southeast Asia, and the Western Pacific.[64]

The presentation of unilateral edema requires a differential diagnosis to rule out acute medical conditions such as deep vein thrombosis (DVT) and/or cellulitis, and the onset of new or recurrent malignancies. Conditions such as arterial and venous insufficiency must also be evaluated, and co-occurring conditions or scenarios contributing to edema should be considered including allergic reactions, medication-associated edema, and iliac vein obstruction (May-Thurner Syndrome). Diagnostic measures such as Doppler ultrasound, ankle-brachial indices (ABI), and transcutaneous oxygen pressures should be considered, where available and when appropriate, as foundational tests for evaluating any new onset of edema.

Assessment of Lymphedema

There are several objective measures of secondary lymphedema which vary in time to administer, associated costs, necessary equipment, and level of convenience. Current strategies include bioelectrical impedance or bioimpedance analysis (BIA), and volume measurements such as circumferential measurement (CM), water displacement (WD), and perometry. A clinical practice guideline (CPG) on lymphedema assessment from the Academy of Oncologic Physical Therapy of the American Physical Therapy Association by Levenhagen et al.[65] provided recommendations for the assessment of individuals who: (1) are at risk for lymphedema (Norman Questionnaire, the Morbidity Screening Tool, and volume measurements); (2) have subclinical/early stage lymphedema (BIA and volume measurements); (3) are in moderate to late stages (CM and WD); or (4) are in the early/late stages (perometry).[65] Following a diagnosis of lymphedema, severity is labeled based on levels established by the International Society of Lymphology in Table 17.4.[66]

Lymphedema Management

The international standard of care for the traditional management of lymphedema includes complete decongestive therapy (CDT), which consists of the multimodal combination of manual lymphatic drainage, compression (i.e. bandaging, garments, and/or devices), exercise, and patient education on self-management, risk reduction, and skincare. CDT is administered in two phases with phase I focused on reduction of lymphedema, and phase II concentrated on maintenance of reduction. For individuals with advanced illness, the goals of lymphedema management are to improve comfort and function, as well as address quality of life, without excessive intervention. Cheville et al.[67] recommend modifications to traditional CDT for lymphedema management in the palliative care setting, which include considerations such as additional skin protection with buffering materials during compression, lower grade compression/pressure methods, and skin checks with shorter bandaging periods. The authors also recommend an experimental trial of bandaging in the presence of renal or cardiac failure secondary to the occurrence of redistribution of fluid rather than elimination.[67] Consideration of lower-cost devices and bandages, particularly for individuals on hospice, should occur when goals can potentially be met with these rather

Table 17.4 Stages of Lymphedema

Stages of Lymphedema
Stage 0   *Latent, subclinical with no edema visible; only symptoms are present*
Stage I   *Early onset of peripheral edema, soft (pitting); no secondary tissue changes; elevation reduces swelling*
Stage II   *Pitting is present; elevation rarely reduces swelling; progressive tissue fibrosis*
Stage III   *Pitting is absent; skin changes such as thickening, hyperpigmentation, increased skin folds, fat deposits; severe fibrosis*

Source: International Society of Lymphology. The diagnosis and treatment of peripheral lymphedema. 2016 Consensus document of the International Society of Lymphology. *Lymphology.* 2016;49:170–184. https://www.italf.org/wp-content/uploads/2017/09/20106-35060-1-PB.pdf.

than expensive custom compression garments which often take substantial amounts of time and cost for fabrication. Wound management may also be required in the presence of pressure wounds or venous stasis ulcerations associated with chronic lymphedema and venous insufficiency, including management of exudate with absorbent dressings and treatment for the presence of infection.[67] *Lymphorrhea* (leaking of serum fluid through the skin), *lipodermatosclerosis* (inflammation and subcutaneous fibrosis of the legs and ankles), and stasis dermatitis should be documented, monitored, and clinically addressed. For individuals with paralysis, Cheville et al.[67] advocate for the use of pneumatic compression devices, a combination of short stretch and long stretch bandages, and the use of gravitational positioning.

Certified Lymphedema Therapists

A certified lymphedema therapist (CLT) is a healthcare professional who has successfully completed a certification and training process in the diagnosis, treatment, and management of lymphedema. Certified lymphedema therapists are generally licensed physical therapists, physical therapist assistants, occupational therapists, certified occupational therapy assistants, licensed massage therapists, and/or nurses who have received advanced training for a defined number of hours and passed a certification examination. According to the Lymphology Association of North America (LANA), 135 hours of classroom instruction are currently required to sit for their certification exam.[68] Internationally, training programs exist from institutions such as The Vodder Academy International, Casley-Smith International, the Norton School, Foeldi College, and the International Lymphedema & Wound Training Institute. When available and possible, referral to a CLT can assure the highest skill level and knowledge for the management of edema and lymphedema. In the absence of a CLT, appropriate strategies for limb positioning, light compression techniques with skin checks, and retrograde massage can be palliative for symptoms of edema and a logical approach performed safely by the general practitioner for improvement of the individual's quality of life and comfort level, especially at the end of life.

Edema and Lymphedema at the End of Life

For individuals with advanced illness, fluid balance often becomes a challenge. Many conditions, specifically those associated with failure within the cardiopulmonary, renal, and/or hepatic systems, as well as decreased albumin levels (e.g. anorexia, cachexia, ascites), are often complicated by fluid imbalances and overload. Additionally, as patients near the end of life, their food and fluid intake naturally starts to decrease with reduced activity levels and diminished appetite. Appropriate adjustments, with the mindset of preventing dehydration while not overloading the failing system with excessive fluid, are challenging not only for the individuals with advanced illness but also for the caregivers and family. Addressing symptoms of dry mouth are best approached with things such as ice chips or popsicles, as opposed to pushing excessive fluids to a failing system. For individuals in a state of sedation, swallowing may be impossible, and attempts to drink or provide fluids to the patient may cause choking and/or aspiration. Education of the patient and family members is key in this instance.

Medications are the most appropriate strategy for *pulmonary edema* or excess fluid in the lungs. Peripheral edema in the extremities, such as that associated with late-stage heart failure or ascites, may be more challenging to address, however. Diuretics may be helpful initially, but by the nature of the increase in urination they cause, they often become impractical for an individual unable to perform regular toileting safely or conveniently. Modified compression techniques are recommended with appropriate modifications in the palliative and hospice care settings.[67,69] Elevation of the extremities, and light retrograde massage techniques, can be beneficial. Skin care in the presence of swelling is also necessary to address dryness and help prevent infection. The use of moisturizers for the skin, regular gentle cleaning, and frequent position changes can act to protect the integumentary system. Teaching family members and caregivers how to perform light massage techniques to swollen extremities, assist with effective elevated positioning, and provide skincare techniques such as the application of creams and lotions, can be a way to allow them to provide a caring touch and offer comfort to their loved one at the end of life. Oils and lotions with light scents can provide an aromatherapy effect for patients who may enjoy such sensations; however, generally avoid this for individuals with symptoms of nausea.

Abdominal and Pelvic Floor Symptoms

Individuals with advanced illness may present with a multitude of symptoms associated with their disease, progression of disease, and/or treatment-related side effects. Quality of life is often diminished by symptoms and clinical presentations associated with nausea, ascites, constipation, incontinence, and/or diarrhea. Often these issues can limit one's participation in activities of daily living, occupational pursuits, and leisure activities. Most significantly, urinary and fecal incontinence is a direct predictor of falls and injury in frail individuals. The ability to mitigate these symptoms and accommodate for, and around them, can be assisted by the care team and the rehabilitation professional specializing in this area.

Ascites

Progressive liver failure, associated with diagnoses such as cirrhosis, hepatitis, and primary or metastatic liver cancer (see Chapter 9, malignant neoplasms), often results in ascites. *Ascites* is the accumulation of fluid within the abdominal cavity, which in advanced cases, distends the abdomen causing discomfort, pressure, nausea, and bloating for the patient. Shortness of breath can also occur due to increased pressure on the diaphragm; if fluid migrates across the diaphragm, ascites can also cause pleural effusion. Bilateral lower extremity swelling, as well as umbilical hernia are possible with significant ascites. The severe sense of fullness, and tightness in the abdominal cavity and chest, often restricts comfortable range of motion and functional mobility. The diagnosis is typically made by physical exam, ultrasound, and/or MRI or CT scanning. When associated with disseminated cancer, it is referred to as *malignant ascites*.

A condition also seen during liver failure which may accompany ascites is *jaundice*, or icterus, when the skin and the sclera (whites of the eyes) become yellow due to excessive amounts of bilirubin, or hyperbilirubinemia. *Pruritus*, or itchy skin, may also be present. Jaundice can cause significant distress for both the patient and their loved ones due to the rather alarming and disturbing physical appearance that it can cause. Jaundice is typically diagnosed by observation on physical exam, and the source confirmed by liver function tests.

Conservative management of ascites usually involves a low sodium diet, fluid restriction, and the use of diuretics. Therapeutic *paracentesis*, when up to several liters of fluid are removed with a large-gauge needle, can help to relieve painful pressure. For patients with chronic or malignant ascites, paracentesis can be done on a routine basis for palliation for pressure relief and comfort, though it has a side effect of progressive weakness from protein loss. For refractory cases where minor surgery or interventional radiology procedures are a choice and a viable option, transjugular intrahepatic portosystemic shunts (TIPS), peritoneovenous shunts (e.g. Denver) and ports, and implanted catheter vacuum drainage systems (e.g. PleurX) may be considered when severe symptoms are not controlled by other interventions. In the case of malignant ascites, intraperitoneal chemotherapy (including palliative hyperthermic intraperitoneal chemotherapy [HIPEC]) may also be a consideration.[70]

When treating individuals with ascites, caution should be taken with positioning and activity recommendations. Side-lying can be a more comfortable position for many when the abdomen is distended, whereas supine and prone may be poorly tolerated. Trunk rotation and side-bending range of motion may be limited, while excessive trunk and hip flexion should also be avoided. Performing comfortable, available range of motion (e.g. hook-lying trunk rotation), and breathing techniques, may assist patients in reducing feelings of stiffness and dyspnea, resulting in improved comfort. For patients receiving regular palliative paracentesis, scheduling physical activity sessions after fluid reducing procedures may be better tolerated than random attempts at physical activity.

Nausea

Nausea, the unpleasant, queasy sensation within the back of the throat, chest, and/or upper abdomen, can lead to emesis (vomiting) if poorly controlled. Nausea does not always result in vomiting, but when it occurs, the abdominal muscles, diaphragm, and stomach contract to expel the contents of the stomach through the esophagus and mouth. Nausea and vomiting can be influenced by a variety of triggers, including *extra-abdominal* factors (medications, electrolyte imbalances, brain tumors/metastases), or *intra-abdominal* factors (gastroparesis, ileus, gastric outlet obstruction, bowel obstruction). The regions of the body most commonly involved with the onset of nausea include the abdomen and pelvis, the brain and spinal cord, and the vestibular system. Co-occurring conditions including constipation, diarrhea, and pain can contribute to the onset and intensity of nausea symptoms.

There are different types of nausea based on the onset, including: *anticipatory*, a sensation of queasiness that commences with the thought of something unpleasant that is pending; *motion sickness*, with the onset during movement; and *morning sickness*, associated with pregnancy, but also seen with elevated intracranial pressure and uremia. The timing of nausea can be: *acute*, occurring within 24 hours following the onset of a condition (e.g. food poisoning), medical insult, or intervention (e.g. surgical procedure or chemotherapy administration); *delayed*, with an onset beyond 24 hours after an event; *breakthrough*, where symptoms persist despite prophylactic intervention; or *refractory*, unable to be adequately managed despite interventions. Establishing the precipitating cause of nausea can often be challenging, as it is at times undetermined or the result of multiple, concurrent contributing factors.

Nausea and vomiting, the dreaded potential side effects of terminal illness or its treatments, are concerns for many individuals and their loved ones as they near the end of life. According to a systematic review of symptoms in individuals with advanced disease by Solano, Gomes, and Higginson,[71] nausea was reported by 43% of individuals with AIDS, 6% of cancer survivors, and 17% and 30% of patients with heart and renal disease, respectively. The management of nausea and vomiting should be comprehensive and initiated early. Prevention and/or risk reduction are key, when possible. Patient education regarding avoidance of the following can be helpful: large meals; the use of, or proximity to, heavy fragrances (e.g. perfume, aftershave, fragrant flowers); foods with strong aromas during cooking or while eating; consumption of alcohol; food or drink with high levels of acidity (e.g. citrus, tomatoes, coffee); spicy foods or condiments; and/or fried or greasy foods.[72] Clear liquids and small meals of bland foods such as **b**ananas, **r**ice, **a**pplesauce, and **t**oast (white bread or crackers), also known as the BRAT diet, can be well-tolerated for some individuals with nausea.

In instances of recurrent and/or intractable nausea and vomiting, lab work should be performed and patients may require intravenous hydration, antibiotics for infection, and/or hospitalization to manage severe dehydration and/or electrolyte imbalances. First and second-line antiemetics such as ondansetron (Zofran), scopolamine patches, prochlorperazine (Compazine), Metoclopramide (Reglan), and palonosetron (Aloxi) should be considered, as well as other classes of drugs such as cannabinoids tetrahydrocannabinol (Marinol), corticosteroids (dexamethasone), benzodiazepines (Ativan), and off-label use of low-dose haloperidol (Haldol).[73,74] For individuals unable to maintain adequate caloric intake for prolonged periods of time, a nasogastric tube may be inserted for temporary nutritional support if the patient and/ or family wishes (see Appendix 1 for Advance Directives). For individuals experiencing dysphasia, and/or the inability to keep medication down by mouth in pill form, alternate routes of administration for antiemetics (and other prescribed medication) should be considered (i.e. injection, rectal suppository, oral liquid concentrates, sublingual [under the tongue], and buccal [between the gums and cheek]). Signs and symptoms of infection, including elevated body temperature, should be monitored to assess for conditions such as sepsis. In the presence of nausea and vomiting in conjunction with abdominal pain, bloating, and reduced bowel sounds and function, medical evaluation for conditions such as bowel obstruction should be performed.

Physician review of prescribed medications should also occur due to the correlation of opioids to nausea. A systematic review by Sande, Laird, and Fallon[75] of 15 studies with 1,524 patients on the management of nausea and vomiting secondary to opioid use in cancer survivorship found only weak evidence for the benefits of switching opioid regimen, the use of antiemetics, and/ or changing the route of opioid administration. In this instance, non-opioid pain management regimens should be considered. Acupressure and acupuncture have been used in the management of nausea, as have other relaxation techniques within Integrative Medicine (see Chapter 6).

Constipation

Historically, constipation has been considered a medical diagnosis when a patient has infrequent bowel movements of fewer than three per week. However, additional symptoms have been associated with the formal definition in recent years to more completely define the condition of *constipation* including hard stool consistency and physical symptoms such as bloating, discomfort, and distention.[76] In order to enhance patient reporting of bowel function, stool consistency has been outlined with imagery and descriptions in the Bristol Stool Chart (Figure 17.3).[77] Early recognition is key for the management of constipation to allow for active interventions. Standardized questionnaires such as the Bowel Function Index (BFI) and the Bristol Stool Form Scale (BSFS) can be administered to assess bowel function via simple, brief, validated questionnaires.[78,79]

According to Solerno et al.,[71] constipation is reported most frequently by cancer survivors (65%), and patients with renal disease (70%). Mercadante et al.[80] also found two-thirds of advanced cancer survivors presenting to a palliative care service with a diagnosis of constipation, and those with normal bowel function were at risk of developing constipation within one week of admission to service due to lack of recognition or subsequent under-treatment. For individuals who are prescribed opioid pain medications, opioid-induced constipation (OIC) should be anticipated and proactively addressed.

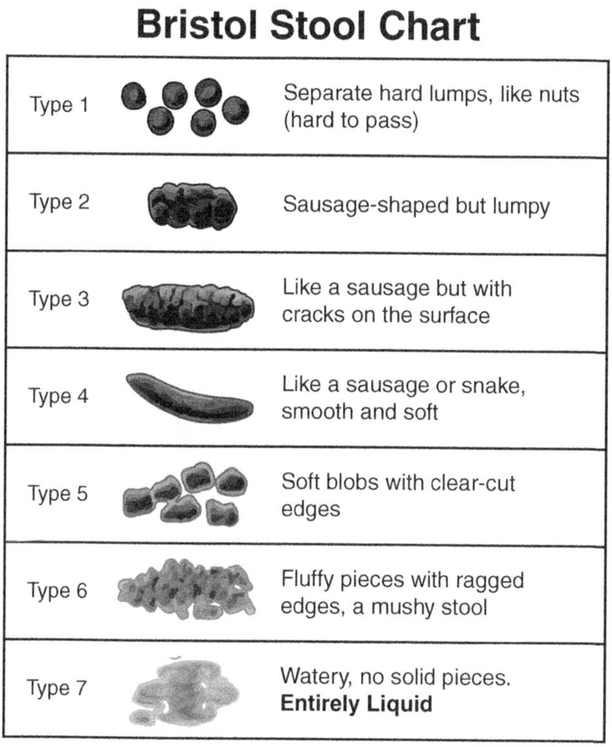

Bristol Stool Chart

Type 1		Separate hard lumps, like nuts (hard to pass)
Type 2		Sausage-shaped but lumpy
Type 3		Like a sausage but with cracks on the surface
Type 4		Like a sausage or snake, smooth and soft
Type 5		Soft blobs with clear-cut edges
Type 6		Fluffy pieces with ragged edges, a mushy stool
Type 7		Watery, no solid pieces. **Entirely Liquid**

Figure 17.3 Bristol Stool Chart.
Source: Bristol Stool Chart reproduced with kind permission of Dr KW Heaton, formerly Reader in Medicine at the University of Bristol. ©2000-2020, Norgine group of companies.

A European expert panel identified opioids as a frequent cause of bowel dysfunction, with constipation being the most frequently reported side effect of opioid use.[81] Opioids have several receptor sites widely distributed throughout the gastrointestinal (GI) tract which, in turn, reduce motility resulting in constipation. In addition to reduced motility, opioids also decrease secretion and increase absorption of fluids within the GI tract, compounding symptoms of constipation. Standard laxatives, including osmotic agents and stimulants such as senna, and stool softeners such as docusate sodium, are commonly recommended over-the-counter (OTC) strategies which are often effective. Additional prescription medications may be required, in combination with OTC medications, in cases of OIC. Consideration of adjustments to the current opioid pain medication regimen, and/or route of administration, may be required in refractory constipation.

For patients known to be at risk for, or experiencing, constipation secondary to either their condition or their medications, a bowel regimen should be initiated as early as possible (e.g. maintaining fluid intake, high-fiber diet/fiber supplementation, regular physical activity, use of stool softeners). In addition to medication, it is recommended to increase fluid intake, when possible and appropriate (e.g. water, juices, soups, and ice creams). When possible, increasing fiber intake, through foods or fiber supplements, can also promote regular, adequate bowel movements. A consultation with a registered dietitian may be beneficial to discuss dietary options for types, timing, and consistency of intake. Patients should also be advised to avoid excessive straining while constipated secondary to the risks for the development of hemorrhoids.

Prolonged immobility contributes to constipation. Regular bodily movement through safe physical activity, both passively and/or actively, should also be incorporated into a bowel regimen. Morisawa, Takahashi, and Nishi[82] demonstrated that several different forms of physiotherapy were successful in improving bowel motility in healthy subjects. Subsequently, Morisawa et al.[83] studied the effect of passive exercise of the lower limbs and trunk (PELT) on bowel sounds for patients in the ICU. They determined ten minutes of alternating passive lower extremity flexion, along with trunk rotation within a comfortable available range of motion, were effective in increasing bowel sounds when compared to a control group of patients at rest.[83]

Positioning can also assist in promoting adequate bowel movements. Gravity can assist in movement of stool towards the rectum in both the seated position, and left side-lying. A footstool in front of the toilet placed under the feet, which elevates the knees above the hips for a more squatted position, encourages more complete evacuation from the bowel in the seated position. Additionally, referral to a pelvic floor therapist may also be of benefit in the management of chronic constipation. Please see the bowel algorithm in Figure 17.4 for the recommended steps.

Unresolved or untreated chronic constipation can lead to fecal impaction and bowel obstruction. For the appropriate patient, and with communication with the medical provider, light abdominal massage may be a beneficial modality to consider for individuals with chronic constipation. Instruction in abdominal massage, particularly for individuals with Parkinson's disease, has shown to be beneficial.[84] Rectal suppositories and oil retention enemas may be successful in mild cases, and in severe cases, manual digital disimpaction (under the order of a physician and within the scope of nursing practice) can potentially address fecal impaction while the source is being evaluated to prevent recurrence. In patients with a suspected bowel obstruction, urgent medical intervention should be recommended and/or provided. For patients still wishing for intensive medical intervention in the presence of a life-threatening illness, strategies such as corticosteroids to relieve the obstruction can often be effective prior to the consideration for surgical intervention.[85]

Diarrhea

Diarrhea, or loose watery stools, can occur for a variety of reasons, including medications, disease processes, and infection (viral or bacterial). Diarrhea is classified in severity by grades from 1 (an increase of up to four stools per day

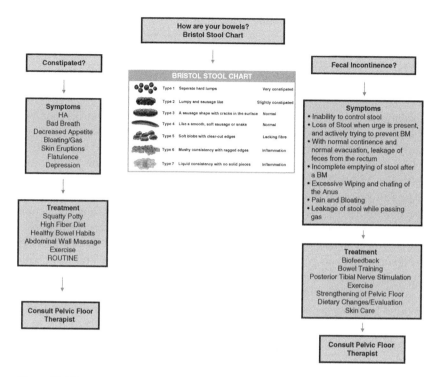

Figure 17.4 Bowel Algorithm.

Source: Reproduced with permission by Nicole Sadeghi, MPT. Bristol Stool Chart reproduced with kind permission of Dr KW Heaton, formerly Reader in Medicine at the University of Bristol. ©2000-2020, Norgine group of companies.

beyond a person's baseline), to 4 (life-threatening, requiring urgent medical care). Stool consistency and the descriptions of diarrhea have been outlined in the Bristol Stool Scale (see Figure 17.4).[77] Diarrhea has been found to be highly prevalent among individuals with AIDS (90%), when compared to cancer survivors (29%) and patients with renal disease (21%).[70]

Medical attention should be provided for recommendations regarding pharmacological intervention such as antidiarrheal medication and intravenous hydration in the presence of dehydration for patients with intractable diarrhea. When possible, stool cultures should be performed to determine the presence of diarrhea-causing bacteria including Clostridium difficile (C-diff), and the presence of vancomycin-resistant enterococci (VRE), with appropriate personal protective equipment precautions and hand hygiene practices used by clinicians and family members. When treating patients experiencing diarrhea, particular attention should be paid to the risk for both dehydration and electrolyte imbalances. Fluid intake with electrolytes should also be increased to help prevent dehydration with ongoing symptoms. Being cognizant of the most recent lab values and chemistry profiles is important for the safety of the patient's plan of care. Furthermore, recommending activities that are the least jarring, and also do not place undue pressure on the lower abdomen, are advisable. Additionally, referral to a pelvic floor therapist may also be beneficial in the management of chronic diarrhea. Please see the bowel algorithm in Figure 17.4 for recommended steps.

Urinary and Fecal Incontinence

Incontinence, the involuntary loss of bladder and/or bowel function, is a common symptom associated with the end of life. Unfortunately, falls are also strongly correlated with incontinence, particularly in elderly hospitalized individuals.[86] Maintenance of safe functional mobility for the greatest duration possible can also allow individuals the autonomy of independent toileting as long as they are able. Fall risk reduction practices in the presence of incontinence include: the use of night lights; avoiding fluids in the evening after dinner time and before bed; avoiding acidic drinks (cranberry juice, coffee); the use of a regular voiding schedule; and access to a bedside commode and/or urinal. Caution should be taken in patients with visual deficits, altered mental status, and those with prescribed diuretic medications. Gait deviations should be addressed with gait training and the appropriate assistive device to improve safe ambulation during trips for toileting. For patients with early or persistent incontinence, referral to a pelvic floor therapist may be beneficial (see Figure 17.5).

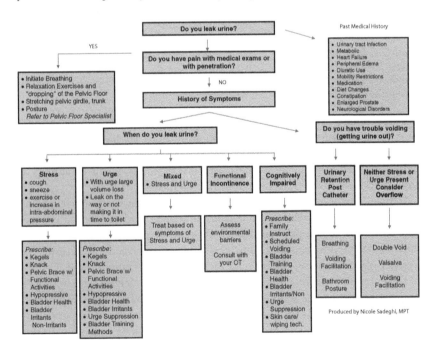

Figure 17.5 Urinary Incontinence Algorithm.
Source: Reproduced with permission by Nicole Sadeghi, MPT.

Appropriate infection precautions and personal protective equipment are necessary for caregivers of an individual experiencing either urinary or fecal incontinence. Appropriate personal hygiene products and garments should be considered, including absorbent briefs and coverage for bed linens, with frequent garment changes recommended. The use of appropriate protective barrier creams and ointments may be needed for the skin of the perineum. Skin checks to the perineal area are also indicated due to the risk for breakdown with chronic exposure of the skin to moisture from urine and/or fecal material.

For individuals with an ostomy (i.e. urostomy or colostomy), awareness of the presence of a stoma and collection pouch device is critical for the treating clinician. Patient education efforts should be geared towards the reduction of intra-abdominal pressure (IAP) through body mechanics training for the reduction of risk of hernia and improved stoma management. Caution should be taken with exercise prescription so as to avoid excessive pressure on the device or stoma, as well as with activities that are excessively jarring which may be poorly tolerated. Patients should avoid Valsalva maneuvers, which can force tissue out and back through the stoma, causing painful irritation and inflammation.

Impending Death

An inevitable but often unpredictable occurrence with every individual facing a life-threatening illness is death, and unless sudden death occurs, it is important for team members to be able to identify when death is approaching. In general, there are key signs and symptoms that may indicate that death may be imminent; sometimes this is called *actively dying*. Once identified, the interdisciplinary team will be able to mobilize resources and take strategic steps to facilitate the dying process with as much comfort and dignity as possible. Often this means providing enough medication to facilitate comfort for some of the key conditions and symptoms. Ideally, this would be organized by a protocol or series of standardized steps; the National Hospice and Palliative Care Organization (NHPCO) terms this as an *imminent death protocol*.[87]

Many of the steps in an imminent death protocol are preparatory, to anticipate comfort and dignity issues near death. Examples cited by NHPCO include procuring supplies and educating caregivers on providing mouth/oral care, utilizing dark sheets (and having dark towels available) if bleeding is expected, anticipating bowel and bladder incontinence, and establishing a plan to discontinue medications that are not essential for comfort or dignity.[87] Medications that may remain applicable include morphine for pain and dyspnea, and medications to manage respiratory secretions.[88] A critical and clinically useful step in an inpatient setting (hospital, nursing facility, inpatient hospice) is to have a nondescript signal for healthcare team members to signify when a patient is near death or has passed away. Institutions use varying signals such as a picture of a leaf or flower posted on the outside of the person's door. This signal will allow all team members to quickly grasp the evolving situation and coordinate with colleagues to establish if services (like physical therapy or occupational therapy) are still warranted or appropriate. In addition, unresolved spiritual or emotional issues may become a higher priority and should be addressed in a timely manner.

When death is nearing, there are often signs or symptoms that present and signify this transition.[88,89] If the person is lucid, the person might verbalize outright that they feel like they are dying. Some individuals also report seeing family or friends who have already passed away. Other behavioral symptoms of impending death may be decreased oral intake of food or drink or withdrawal, restlessness, or agitation beyond the person's normal behavioral responses. Terminal restlessness or agitation can occur and is evidenced by continuous walking or pacing in some cases, and more often trying to get up from bed, needing to move, or verbalizing 'I need to go.' Medications such as Roxanol (liquid morphine sulfate) and Ativan (Lorazepam) are commonly used for sedation by the nursing team. Therapists may help reduce, though not eliminate, inevitable fall risks if the person is up and about. If the person is in bed or trying to get up, teaching the family caregivers to hold and rock them while sitting can provide a sense of 'going,' similar to techniques used to soothe distress and anxiety through such stimulation and without such sedating medication effects.

Clinically, there are some identifiable symptoms of impending death that may be appreciated upon examination.[88] These may include decreased urine output (oliguria) and decreased body temperature or limb temperature. Another key finding or symptom might include a change in limb or skin coloration often termed *mottling*. This is often caused by the physical shunting of blood to vital organs away from the extremities and is usually a sign that death is hours to minutes away. Finally, peripheral cyanosis and diminished pulses may be appreciated upon exam.[90]

Near-death awareness, sometimes labeled as delirium, has been identified as a common occurrence in the dying process and is addressed by Callahan and Kelley in their book *Final Gifts*.[91] The person may be communicating or seeing a deceased loved one or a divine presence, or may speak in metaphoric language. Such behavioral changes are a frequent and natural presentation that could easily be misunderstood if only observed as a medical phenomenon (e.g. delirium or dementia), and thus treated as such.

Another condition noted during imminent death includes respiratory tract changes including *terminal rales* or *death rattle*. This is often a result of fluid buildup in the respiratory tract which may occur when swallowing or coughing are no longer possible.[88] Use of medication such as Levsin can dry these secretions and reduce these sounds, often comforting the caregivers, if not the patient. As impending death progresses, there may be episodes of apnea, Cheyne-Stokes breathing, or gasping.[90] Finally, when impending death is appropriately medically managed, the final hours and minutes of a person's life may be calm or quiet as the person slips into unconsciousness and eventually stops breathing. One consideration during this time is that there is no clear evidence when the physical senses such as hearing and touch are lost. This provides an opportunity for continued engagement by loved ones through speaking to the individual, sharing treasured memories, playing music, singing, holding hands, or any other therapeutic touching. These activities serve to provide purpose, calm, and meaning and comfort for all parties during the remaining time of a person's life.

Questions often arise from family members regarding how long their loved one has to live. The interdisciplinary team may have discussed this in conference or in consultation with one another. This timing is notoriously difficult to predict, so often a range is offered to help guide the preparation of those observing this process. Timeframes such as days-to-weeks, or hours-to-days can provide some surety in the uncertainty of the dying process, and open a conversation about what is occurring. End-of-life caregivers are aware that the life process can go on longer than expected, or end suddenly. It is good to be aware and help the family to understand that the dying will happen in its own time. In some instances, the person will hold on until a certain loved one arrives; in others, the person seems to wait until an often fatigued loved one leaves momentarily, and then slip away. Whatever happens, it is as it was to be, after the best efforts of all involved.

Summary

Individuals face many challenges to their comfort, well-being, and quality of life at the end of life. A thoughtful, compassionate, and deliberate team approach, with keen observation of symptoms and early, evidence-based intervention strategies, is the ideal mechanism to palliate symptoms. A therapist is often well suited to employ their understanding of disability and loss with many of the tools in their clinical toolbox to contribute to easing many of these issues and problem-solving to optimize quality of life. In order to offer these services, therapists must actively advocate for proactive inclusion within the hospice or palliative plan of care.

References

1 Fried L, Tangen C, Walston J, et al. Frailty in older adults: Evidence for a phenotype. *J Gerontol A Biol Sci Med Sci.* 2001;56(3):M146–M156. doi:10.1093/gerona/56.3.m146.
2 Xue Q. The frailty syndrome: Definition and natural history. *Clin Geriatr Med* 27. 2011;1–15. doi:10.1016/j.cger.2010.08.009.
3 Xue Q, Bandeen-Roche K, Varadhan R, et al. Initial manifestations of frailty criteria and the development of frailty phenotype in the Women's Health and Aging Study II. *J Gerontol A Biol Sci Med Sci.* 2008;63(9):984–990.
4 Shinall MC, Arya S, Youk A, et al. Association of preoperative patient frailty and operative stress with postoperative mortality. *JAMA Surg.* 2020;155(1):e194620. doi:10.1001/jamasurg.2019.4620.
5 Ng TP, Feng L, Nyunt MS, Larbi A, Yap KB. Frailty in older persons: Multisystem risk factors and the Frailty Risk Index (FRI). *J Am Med Dir Assoc.* 2014;15(9):635–642.

6   Hall DE, Arya S, Schmid KK, et al. Development and initial validation of the Risk Analysis Index for measuring frailty in surgical populations. *JAMA Surg.* Published online November 23, 2016. doi:10.1001/jamasurg.2016.4202.

7   Cruz-Jentoft AJ. Perspective: Protein and exercise for frailty and sarcopenia: Still learning. *J Am Med Dir Assoc.* 2013;14:69–71.

8   Jadczak AD, Makwana N, Luscombe-Marsh N, Visvanathan R, Schultz TJ. Effectiveness of exercise interventions on physical function in community-dwelling frail older people: An umbrella review of systematic reviews. *JBI Database System Rev Implement Rep.* 2018;16(3):752–775. doi:10.11124/JBISRIR-2017-003551.

9   Allen C, Glasziou P, Del Mar C. Bed rest: A potentially harmful treatment needing more careful evaluation. *Lancet.* 1999;354(9186):1229–1233. doi:10.1016/s0140-6736(98)10063-6.

10   National Palliative Care Research Center. Palliative Performance Scale (PPSv2) http://www.npcrc.org/files/news/palliative_performance_scale_PPSv2.pdf. Published 1996. Accessed February 7, 2020.

11   Eastern Cooperative Oncology Group-ACRIN. ECOG performance status. https://ecog-acrin.org/resources/ecog-performance-status. Published 2020. Accessed February 7, 2020.

12   Artico M, Dante A, D'Angelo D, et al. Prevalence, incidence and associated factors of pressure ulcers in home palliative care patients: A retrospective chart review. *Palliat Med.* January 2018;32(1):299–307. doi:10.1177/0269216317737671.

13   Sternal D, Wilczyński K, Szewieczek J. Pressure ulcers in palliative ward patients: Hyponatremia and low blood pressure as indicators of risk. *Clin Interv Aging.* 2016;12:37–44. Published December 29, 2016. doi:10.2147/CIA.S122464.

14   Chou R, Dana T, Bougatsos C, Blazina I, Starmer A, Reitel K, Buckley D. Pressure Ulcer Risk Assessment and Prevention: Comparative effectiveness. Comparative Effectiveness Review No. 87. (Prepared by Oregon Evidence-based Practice Center under Contract No. 290-2007-10057-I.) AHRQ Publication No. 12(13)-EHC148-EF. Rockville, MD: Agency for Healthcare Research and Quality; May, 2013.

15   Morita T, Tsunoda J, Inoue S, Chihara S. An exploratory factor analysis of existential suffering in Japanese terminally ill cancer patients. *Psycho-Oncology.* 2000;9(2):164–168. doi:10.1002/(sici)1099-1611(200003/04)9:2<164:aid-pon447>3.0.co;2-s.

16   Vehling S, Philipp R. Existential distress and meaning-focused interventions in cancer survivorship. *Curr Opin Support Palliat Care.* 2018;12(1):46–51. doi:10.1097/SPC.0000000000000324.

17   Field M, Cassel CK. *Approaching Death: Improving Care at the End of Life.* Washington, DC: National Academy Press; 1997.

18   Institute of Medicine. *Dying in America: Improving Quality and Honoring Individual Preferences near the End of Life.* 2015. Washington, DC: The National Academies Press. doi:10.17226/18748.

19   National Comprehensive Cancer Network. (v1.2020). *Clinical practice guidelines in oncology: Distress management.* https://www.nccn.org/professionals/physician_gls/pdf/distress.pdf. Published 2020. Accessed May 13, 2020.

20   National Comprehensive Cancer Network. NCCN distress thermometer and problem list for patients. https://www.nccn.org/patients/resources/life_with_cancer/pdf/nccn_distress_thermometer.pdf. Published 2020. Accessed May 13, 2020.

21   Plotnikoff G, Wolpert D, Dandurand D. Chapter 114- integrating spiritual assessment and care. In: Rakel D, ed. *Integrative Medicine.* 4th ed. Elsevier; 2018:1058–1063. doi:10.1016/B978-0-323-35868-2.00114-6.

22 Bredle JM, Salsman JM, Debb SM, Arnold BJ, Cella D. Spiritual well-being as a component of health-related quality of life: The Functional Assessment of Chronic Illness Therapy—Spiritual Well-Being scale (FACIT-Sp). *Religions.* 2011;2:77–94.

23 Evans W, Morley J, Argilés J, Bales C, Baracos V, Guttridge D, et al. Cachexia: A new definition. *Clin Nutr.* December 2008;27(6):793–799. doi:10.1016/j.clnu.2008.06.013.

24 Fearon K, Strasser F, Anker SD, et al. Definition and classification of cancer cachexia: An international consensus. *Lancet Oncol.* 2011;12(5):489–495. doi:10.1016/S1470-2045(10)70218-7.

25 Bruggeman AR, Kamal AH, LeBlanc TW, Ma JD, Baracos VE, Roeland EJ. Cancer cachexia: Beyond weight loss. *J Oncol Pract.* 2016;12(11):1163–1171. doi:10.1200/JOP.2016.016832.

26 von Haehling S, Anker SD. Cachexia as a major underestimated and unmet medical need: Facts and numbers. *J Cachexia Sarcopenia Muscle.* 2010;1(1):1–5. doi:10.1007/s13539-010-0002-6.

27 Borg G. Psychophysical bases of perceived exertion. *Med Sci Sport Exerc.* 1982;14:377–381.

28 American Society of Clinical Oncology. Bone cancer – Statistics. https://www.cancer.net/cancer-types/bone-cancer/statistics. Updated 2017. Accessed Nov 10, 2019.

29 Michael H, Tsai Y, Hoffe SE. Overview of diagnosis and management of metastatic disease to bone. *Cancer Control.* 2012;19(2):84–91. doi:10.1177/107327481201900202.

30 O'Sullivan GJ, Sullivan FLC, Cronin CG. Imaging of bone metastasis: An update. *World J Radiol.* 2015;7(8):202–211. doi:10.4329/wjr.v7.i8.202.

31 Jawad MU, Scully SP. In brief: Classifications in brief: Mirels' classification: Metastatic disease in long bones and impending pathologic fracture. *Clin Orthop Relat Res.* 2010;486(10):2825–2827.

32 Mirels H. Metastatic disease in long bones. A proposed scoring system for diagnosing impending pathologic fractures. *Clin Orthop Relat Res.* 1989;(249):256–264.

33 Damron TA, Morgan H, Prakash D, Grant W, Aronowitz J, Heiner J. Critical evaluation of Mirels' rating system for impending pathologic fractures. *Clin Orthop Relat Res.* 2003;415:S201–S207.

34 Fourney DR, Frangou EM, Ryken TC, et al. Spinal instability neoplastic score: An analysis of reliability and validity from the spine oncology study group. *J Clin Oncol.* 2011;29(22):3072–3077. doi:10.1200/JCO.2010.34.3897.

35 Fisher CG, DiPaola CP, Ryken TC, et al. A novel classification system for spinal instability in neoplastic disease: An evidence-based approach and expert consensus from the spine oncology study group. *Spine.* 2010;35(22):E1221–E1229.

36 Galvao DA, Taaffe DR, Spry N, et al. Exercise preserves physical function in prostate cancer patients with bone metastases. *Med Sci Sports Exerc.* 2018;50(3):393–399. doi:10.1249/MSS.0000000000001454.

37 Sheill G, Guinan EM, Peat N, Hussey J. Considerations for exercise prescription in patients with bone metastases: A comprehensive narrative review. *PM&R.* 2018;10(8):843–864.

38 University of Sheffield. FRAX fracture risk assessment calculator. https://www.sheffield.ac.uk/FRAX/. Updated 2008. Accessed November 10, 2019.

39 Saunders C. A personal therapeutic journey. *BMJ.* 1996;313:1599–1601.

40 Clark D. "Total pain," disciplinary power and the body in the work of Cicely Saunders, 1958–1967. *Soc Sci Med.* 1999;49:727–736.

41 International Association for the Study of Pain: Classification of Chronic Pain, Second Edition (revised). https://www.iasp-pain.org/Publications News/Content.aspx?ItemNumber=1673. Published 2018. Accessed June 3, 2020.

42 Quartana PJ, Campbell CM, Edwards RR. Pain catastrophizing: A critical review. *Expert Rev Neurother.* 2009; 9(5); 745–758. doi:10.1586/ern.09.34.

43 Russek L. Chronic Pain. In: O'Sullivan S, Schmitz T, Fulk G, eds. *Physical Rehabilitation.* 7th ed. Philadelphia, PA: F.A. Davis Company; 2019:1097.

44 Kutner JS, Kassner CT, Nowels DE: Symptom burden at the end of life: Hospice providers' perceptions. *J Pain Symptom Manage.* 2001;21(6):473–480.

45 Grond S, Zech D, Diefenbach C, et al. Assessment of cancer pain: A prospective evaluation in 2266 cancer patients referred to a pain service. *Pain.* 1996;64(1):107–114.

46 Woo J, Lo R, Cheng JO, Wong F, Mak B. Quality of end-of-life care for non-cancer patients in a non-acute hospital. *J Clin Nurs.* 2011;20 (13–14):1834-1841. doi:10.1111/j.1365–2702.2010.03673.x.

47 Swarm RA, Paice JA, Anghelescu DL, et al. Adult cancer pain, version 3.2019, NCCN clinical practice guidelines in oncology. *J Natl Compr Canc Netw.* 2019;17(8):977–1007. doi:10.6004/jnccn.2019.0038.

48 Wachholtz AB, Fitch CE, Makowski S, Tjia J. A Comprehensive Approach to the Patient at End of Life: Assessment of Multidimensional Suffering. *South Med J.* 2016;109(4):200–206. doi:10.14423/SMJ.0000000000000439.

49 Wilson A, Ensign. G, Flyte K, Moore M, Ratliff, K. Physical agents for cancer survivors: An updated literature review. *Rehabil Oncol.* 2018;36(2):132–140. doi:10.1097/01.REO.0000000000000081.

50 Pfalzer L. Physical agents/modalities for survivors of cancer. *Rehabil Oncol.* 2001;19(2):12–24.

51 Cheville AL, Basford JR. Role of rehabilitation medicine and physical agents in the treatment of cancer-associated pain. *J Clin Oncol.* 2014;32(16):1691-1702. doi:10.1200/JCO.2013.53.6680.

52 de la Cruz M, Fan J, Yennu S, Tanco K, Shin S, Wu J, Liu D, Bruera E. The frequency of missed delirium in patients referred to palliative care in a comprehensive cancer center. *Support Care Cancer.* 2015;23:2427–2433.

53 Waterfield K, Weiand D, Dewhurst F, et al. A qualitative study of nursing staff experiences of delirium in the hospice setting. *Int J Palliat Nurs.* 2018;24(11):524–534. doi:10.12968/ijpn.2018.24.11.524.

54 Mercadante S, Porzio G, Valle A, Aielli F, Casuccio A. Home Care-Italy Group. Palliative sedation in patients with advanced cancer followed at home: a prospective study. *J Pain Symptom Manag.* 2014;47:860–866.

55 Kang JH, Shin SH, Bruera E. Comprehensive approaches to managing delirium in patients with advanced cancer. *Cancer Treat Rev.* 2013;39:105–112.

56 Mercadante S, Masedu F, Maltoni M, et al. Symptom expression in advanced cancer patients admitted to hospice or home care with and without delirium. *Intern Emerg Med.* 2019;14:515–520. doi:10.1007/s11739-018-1969-9.

57 Bruera E, Kuehn N, Miller MJ, Selmser P, Macmillan K. The Edmonton Symptom Assessment System (ESAS): a simple method for the assessment of palliative care patients. *J Palliat Care.* 1991;7(2): 6–9.

58 Breitbart W, Rosenfeld B, Roth A, Smith MJ, Cohen K, Passik S. The memorial delirium assessment scale. *J Pain Symptom Manag.* 1997;13:128–137.

59 Gusmao-Flores D, Salluh JI, Chalhub RÁ, Quarantini LC. The Confusion Assessment Method for the Intensive Care Wnit (CAM-ICU) and Intensive Care Delirium Screening Checklist (ICDSC) for the diagnosis of delirium: A systematic review and meta-analysis of clinical studies. *Crit Care.* 2012;16(4):R115. doi:10.1186/cc11407.

60 Wong CL, Holroyd-Leduc J, Simel DL, Straus SE. Does this patient have delirium?: Value of bedside instruments. *JAMA.* 2010;304(7):779–786. doi:10.1001/jama.2010.1182.

61 Gélinas C, Bérubé M, Chevrier A, et al. Delirium assessment tools for use in critically ill adults: A psychometric analysis and systematic review. *Crit Care Nurse.* 2018;38(1):38–49. doi:10.4037/ccn2018633.

62 Zuther, JE, Norton S. *Lymphedema Management: The Comprehensive Guide for Practitioners.* 3rd ed. New York, NY: Thieme Medical Publishers; 2013.

63 Shaitelman SF, Cromwell KD, Rasmussen JC, et al. Recent progress in the treatment and prevention of cancer-related lymphedema. *CA Cancer J Clin.* 2015;65(1):55-81. doi:10.3322/caac.21253.

64 World Health Organization. Morbidity management and disability prevention. https://www.who.int/activities/building-capacity-of-national-programmes-to-implement-who-recommended-strategies/morbidity-management-and-disability-prevention. Published 2020. Accessed June 1, 2020.

65 Levenhagen K, Davies C, Perdomo M, Ryans K, Gilchrist L. Diagnosis of upper-quadrant lymphedema secondary to cancer: Clinical practice guideline from the oncology section of APTA. *Rehabil Oncol.* 2017;35;E1–E18.

66 International Society of Lymphology. The diagnosis and treatment of peripheral lymphedema. 2016 Consensus document of the International Society of Lymphology. *Lymphology.* 2016;49:170–184.

67 Cheville AL, Andrews K, Kollasch J, Schmidt K, Basford J. Adapting lymphedema treatment to the palliative setting. *Am J Hosp Palliat Care.* 2014;31(1):38–44. doi:10.1177/1049909112475297.

68 Lymphology Association of North America (LANA). *LANA Certified Lymphedema Therapist® Candidate Information Brochure.* https://www.clt-lana.org/uploads/2016/3.%20LANA%20Candidate%20Information%20Booklet%20(CIB).pdf. Published date unknown. Accessed June 1, 2020.

69 International Lymphoedema Framework. *Position document: Best practice for the management of lymphoedema – 2nd edition: Compression therapy: A position document on compression bandaging.* http://www.lympho.org/portfolio/compression-therapy-a-position-document-on-compression-bandaging/. Published 2012:57–61.

70 Hodge C, Badgwell BD. Palliation of malignant ascites. *J Surg Oncol.* 2019;120(1):67–73. doi:10.1002/jso.25453.

71 Solano JP, Gomes B, Higginson IJ. A comparison of symptom prevalence in far advanced cancer, AIDS, heart disease, chronic obstructive pulmonary disease and renal disease. *J Pain Symptom Manage.* 2006;31(1):58–69. doi:10.1016/j.jpainsymman.2005.06.007.

72 Glare P, Miller J, Nikolova T, Tickoo R. Treating nausea and vomiting in palliative care: A review. *Clin Interv Aging.* 2011;6:243–259. doi:10.2147/CIA.S13109.

73 Albert RH. End-of-life care: Managing common symptoms. *Am Fam Physician.* 2017;95(6):356–361.

74 Buttner M, Walder B, von Elm E, et al. Is low-dose haloperidol a useful antiemetic: A meta-analysis of published and unpublished randomized trials. In: *Database of Abstracts of Reviews of Effects (DARE): Quality-assessed Reviews* [Internet]. York (UK): Centre for Reviews and Dissemination (UK); Published 2004. https://www.ncbi.nlm.nih.gov/books/NBK71116/

75 Sande TA, Laird BJA, Fallon MT. The management of opioid-induced nausea and vomiting in patients with cancer: A systematic review. *J Palliat Med.* 2019;22(1):90–97. doi:10.1089/jpm.2018.0260.

76 Bharucha AE, Dorn SD, Lembo A, Pressman A. American Gastroenterological Association medical position statement on constipation. *Gastroenterology.* January 1, 2013;144(1):211–217.

77 Bristol Stool Chart. Reproduced with kind permission of Dr KW Heaton, formerly Reader in Medicine at the University of Bristol. ©2000–2020, Norgine group of companies.
78 Ueberall MA, Muller-Lissner S, Buschmann-Kramm C, et al. The Bowel Function Index for evaluating constipation in pain patients: Definition of a reference range for a non-constipated population of pain patients. *J Int Med Res.* 2011;39:41–50.
79 Lewis SJ, Heaton KW. Stool form scale as a useful guide to intestinal transit time. *Scand J Gastroenterol.* 1997;32:920–924.
80 Mercadante S, Masedu F, Maltoni M, et al. The prevalence of constipation at admission and after 1 week of palliative care: a multi-center study. *Curr Med Res Opin.* 2018;34(7):1187–1192. doi:10.1080/03007995.2017.1358702.
81 Farmer AD, Drewes AM, Chiarioni G, et al. Pathophysiology and management of opioid-induced constipation: European expert consensus statement [published correction appears in United European Gastroenterol J. March 2019;7(2):178]. *United European Gastroenterol J.* 2019;7(1):7–20. doi:10.1177/2050640618818305.
82 Morisawa T, Takahashi T, Nishi S. The effect of a physiotherapy intervention on intestinal motility. *J Phys Ther Sci.* 2015;27(1):165-168. doi:10.1589/jpts.27.165.
83 Morisawa T, Takahashi T, Sasanuma N, et al. Passive exercise of the lower limbs and trunk alleviates decreased intestinal motility in patients in the intensive care unit after cardiovascular surgery. *J Phys Ther Sci.* 2017;29(2):312–316. doi:10.1589/jpts.29.312.
84 McClurg D, Walker K, Aitchison P, et al. Abdominal massage for the relief of constipation in people with Parkinson's: A qualitative study. *Parkinsons Dis.* 2016; 4842090. doi:10.1155/2016/4842090.
85 Feuer DJ, Broadley KE. Corticosteroids for the resolution of malignant bowel obstruction in advanced gynaecological and gastrointestinal cancer. *Cochrane Database Syst Rev.* 2000;3:CD001219.
86 Falcão RMM, Costa KNFM, Fernandes MDGM, Pontes MLF, Vasconcelos JMB, Oliveira JDS. Risk of falls in hospitalized elderly people. Risco de quedas em pessoas idosas hospitalizadas. *Rev Gaucha Enferm.* 2019;40(spe):e20180266. doi:10.1590/1983-1447.2019.20180266.
87 National Hospice and Palliative Care Organization. Management of Imminent Death in Hospice Care. National Hospice and Palliative Care Organization website. https://www.nhpco.org/wp-content/uploads/2019/05/Imminent_Death_Management_Resource.pdf. Published May 2019. Accessed June 13, 2020.
88 LeGrand SB, Walsh D. Comfort measures: Practical care of the dying cancer patient. *Am J Hospice Palliat Med.* 2010;27(7):488–493.
89 Cable-Williams B, Wilson D. Awareness of impending death for residents of long-term care facilities. *Int J Older People Nurs.* 2014;9:169–179. doi:10.1111/opn.12045.
90 Hui D, dos Santos R, Chisholm G, et al. Clinical signs of impending death in cancer patients. *The Oncologist.* June 2014;19(6):681–687.
91 Callahan M, Kelley P. *Final Gifts.* New York, NY: Poseidon Press; 1992.

18 Measuring and Quantifying Outcomes

Amy J. Litterini and Christopher M. Wilson

Introduction

Outcome measures have become an increasingly necessary component of skilled rehabilitation over the last few decades. They serve several purposes, including: (1) an evidence-based method of objective assessment of progress; (2) a way to demonstrate value to the patient; (3) a unified language among therapists locally, regionally, nationally, and internationally to promote outcome data collection in multicenter studies; and (4) justification for payment by third-party payers. Outcome measures are typically categorized as either patient-reported outcome measures (PROMs), such as questionnaires, or performance-based outcome measures (PBOMs), such as the Timed Up and Go Test, administered by a clinician. In the palliative care setting, outcomes such as performance status (e.g. physical functioning), pain, fatigue, balance and fall risk, self-efficacy, activities of daily living (ADL) performance, and quality of life (QoL), are critical measures which have a significant impact on individuals with life-threatening illnesses, as well as the end-of-life experience of their families.

Choosing an Appropriate Outcome Measure

The intentional selection of measurements with good psychometric properties is the *gold standard* to ensure the appropriate reliability, validity, specificity, and sensitivity of the selected measures. Furthermore, a scale of measurement with a comparison of results to the reported minimum important change (MIC) and minimally clinically important difference (MCID), allows the clinician to make evidence-based informed decisions about initial treatment planning and subsequent modifications. For individuals at the end of life, test burden should also be a serious consideration for therapists as they select PROMs and PBOMs, and the frequency with which they administer them. Time to complete (e.g. total number of survey questions, required duration to perform requested skills), complexity, and energy expenditure should be at the forefront of the selection process. Short-form versions of surveys, containing the fewest number of questions while maintaining psychometric properties, are the ideal choice when possible in order to not fatigue the patient or excessively distract from the effectiveness of a therapeutic session.

Performance Status

When caring for individuals with life-limiting illnesses, the measurement of performance status is a critical indicator of current and future disease trajectory, disease-treatment decisions, as well as change in status. Various performance status scales measure parameters such as ADLs/self-care, time spent out of bed, ambulatory status, activity participation, nutritional/fluid intake, and level of consciousness, while labeling the results with a value (i.e. numbers or percentages). Poorer performance status scores are indicative of poorer prognoses, including mortality rates;[1] widely used performance status scales include the Karnofsky Performance Status Scale (100 [normal]–0 [dead]), the Eastern Cooperative Oncology Group (ECOG) Scale of Performance Status (0 [fully active]–5 [dead]), and the Palliative Performance Scale, or PPS (100% [normal]–10% [bed confined/total care]).[2–4] Some hospice organizations utilize performance status, such as that classified by the PPS, as an indicator of eligibility for enrollment.

In the absence of a temporary and reversible medical insult, a documented reduction in performance status is generally indicative of progressive decline. For the interdisciplinary team (IDT), changes in performance status scores may be appropriately utilized as indicators for a referral to rehabilitation services for interventions such as adaptive equipment training, gait training with or without the fitting of new assistive devices, and bed mobility and transfer training (see Chapter 4).

Pain

As mentioned previously, pain is one of the most frequently experienced symptoms of individuals receiving palliative care, and/or for those at the end of life (see Chapter 17). Accurate assessment of pain allows for more appropriate individualized care planning, as well as necessary adjustments to existing treatment regimens. Several different methods can be used to quantify pain, including numeric scales, verbal descriptors, visual scales (paper or electronic), clinician-family observation, and multidimensional pain assessments. When possible, the ideal pain assessment is one that is comprehensive and addresses various aspects of the pain experience including intensity, location, and quality, as well as appropriateness for the patient's level of cognition. The Numeric Pain Rating Scale (NPRS) and visual analog scale (VAS) for pain are commonly utilized pain assessments; however, as unidimensional and highly subjective tools, they are limited in their role as a sole representation of pain intensity.[5] Multidimensional pain assessments that incorporate components such as body diagrams, and pain descriptors indicative of quality of pain (e.g. the Brief Pain Inventory [Short Form] and the Short Form McGill Pain Questionnaire), capture various domains of pain and pain interference dimensions, rather than a simple snapshot of intensity.[6,7]

Specialized pain assessment tools, appropriate for specific patient populations, allow the clinician to better assess an individual's pain presentation. Originally developed for pediatric patients in a burn unit, the Wong-Baker FACES® Pain Rating Scale is an appropriate pain measure for pediatric patients on palliative care (https://wongbakerfaces.org/).[8]

Additionally, the Oucher is a pediatric pain assessment tool designed for relatability to different cultures, and is available with facial images of children of different races (http://www.oucher.org/order.html).[9] A systematic review on cancer pain measurements in pediatrics by Miale et al.[10] concluded that Wong-Baker FACES® and Oucher scales were *highly recommended*, while the Adolescent Pediatric Pain Tool and the Pieces of Hurt Assessment Tool Poler Chip Tool were *recommended*.

For individuals with a diagnosis of mild-to-moderate cognitive impairment and/or dementia, a pain distress intensity scale using a thermometer, which visually represents pain intensity from a low-level (cool color blue) to a high level (bright red), may be appropriate for individuals able to self-report pain through imagery.[11] For individuals with advanced dementia, observational pain assessment tools, such as the Pain Assessment in Advanced Dementia scale (PAINAD), are necessary for clinicians to interpret a patient's nonverbal behaviors (e.g. breathing, negative vocalizations, facial expressions, body language, and consolability).[12]

Considering pain is such a significant experience for individuals with advanced diseases, the need to assess and reassess pain on a regular basis is critical to comprehensive care at the end of life. The selection of appropriate pain assessment tools is also vital to obtaining accurate information in order to devise the most beneficial pain management plan of care (see Chapter 17).

Fatigue

Fatigue, which often becomes progressively more profound and debilitating with advanced illness, is a common source of activity limitation and participation restriction for individuals with life-limiting diseases. When compared to other diagnoses, perhaps the most well-documented phenomenon of fatigue presenting concurrently with illness is cancer-related fatigue (CRF). In a study by Tsai et al.[13] of terminally ill cancer survivors within an inpatient hospice in Taiwan, the symptom of fatigue was "...associated with the overall symptom distress, depression, anxiety, and performance status. Furthermore, fatigue was significantly correlated with 8 (eight) individual distressful symptoms: nausea, vomiting, lack of appetite, sleep disturbance, dyspnea, dry mouth, restlessness, and problems of concentration." Similarly, a systematic review and meta-analysis of CRF by Oh and Seo[14] found similar associations as those documented by Tsai et al.[13] They found a higher correlation of CRF with nausea and vomiting when compared to symptoms of pain and dyspnea, and advocated for the medical management of the combined symptom burden rather than symptom management in isolation (see Chapter 17).[13]

Regarding fatigue assessment, there are various tools available. Much like pain assessment, fatigue intensity can be assessed with appropriate unidimensional measures such as a visual analog scale and a 10-point numeric scale (analogous to the NPRS). When attempting to assess interference of fatigue with function and QoL, assessments such as the Fatigue Severity Scale, the Brief Fatigue Inventory, and the Functional Assessment of Chronic Illness Therapy - Fatigue (FACIT-F) can be utilized.[15] A systematic review by Fisher, Davies, Lacy, and Doherty[16] for fatigue assessment in cancer survivorship concluded the unidimensional questionnaires of the Modified Brief Fatigue Inventory (mBFI), the Cancer-Related Fatigue Distress Scale, and the 10-point Rating Scale for Fatigue were *highly recommended*, while the MD Anderson Symptom Inventory and Wu Cancer Fatigue Scale were *recommended*. Regarding multidimensional questionnaires, Fisher et al.[16] found the Multidimensional Fatigue Symptom Inventory to be *highly recommended*.

Balance Deficits and Fall Risk

One of the most detrimental and traumatic experiences for an individual with terminal illness is the fear of falls, or the occurrence of an actual fall. For individuals who may sustain a fall injury that impacts their QoL and increases pain for their remaining days, to anticipate and reduce the risk of such issues is ideal when feasible. This opportunity provides a unique role for rehabilitation professionals due to primary and comorbid disease processes, as well as the physical effects of inactivity, which place this patient population at a high risk of falls. In addition, the patient's medical status or cognitive status may decline quickly or fluctuate dramatically, further limiting the patient's judgment and safety awareness. The situation offers an opportunity to open the critical conversation of when the rehabilitation professional feels it is no longer safe to perform an activity because of the risk outweighing the benefit to the patient or client.

Patient safety for individuals at the end of life is a critical concern for the IDT. A qualitative study was conducted by Schmucker et al.[17] of home hospice providers regarding perspectives on patient safety incidents causing unnecessary harm across 17 hospices in 13 of the United States. Injuries from falls and inadequate symptom control were the most frequently reported concerns. The most frequently cited contributing factors to injurious falls for individuals on hospice included: (1) frail/debilitated patients living alone, or being left alone by caregivers; (2) the caregivers' physical and cognitive limitations; (3) the patients' physical and cognitive limitations; (4) the patients' or families' inability to understand, disagreement with, or non-adherence to the hospice teams' care plan; (5) the family not accepting the short prognosis, and forcing activity on a dying patient; (6) family overwhelmed with the caregiver role; (7) poor or physically hazardous living conditions; and (8) rapid increases in patient weakness and debility (see Chapter 5 for caregiver information).[17]

There are several options for determining static and dynamic balance, and indicators of fall risk. In the simplest of ways, perhaps the most brief and convenient observation by any member of the IDT is a patient's inability to perform single leg stance (static balance) and/or move outside of their base of support in standing (dynamic balance). The inability to do so is an indicator of poor gait ability (ambulation is repeated single leg stance) and/or to maintain balance during ADLs. Regarding prediction of future risk of falls in community-dwelling individuals, Lusardi et al.[18] determined the "Berg Balance Scale score (≤50 points), Timed Up and Go times (≥12 seconds), and 5 times sit-to-stand times (≥12 seconds) are currently the most evidence-supported functional measures and results to determine individual risk of future falls." From the oncology literature, a systematic review by Huang et al.[19] determined the Fullerton Advanced Balance Scale, and usual and fast gait speed, were *highly recommended*, while the Balance Evaluation Systems Test, Timed Up and Go, and Five Times Sit to Stand were *recommended*.

Following assessment revealing balance deficits and/or increased fall risk, the evidence for interventions to address risk reduction is limited. As the actual mechanisms leading to falls are complex and multifaceted individual scenarios for each patient, accurately targeting and mitigating the risk can prove to be elusive. In a systematic review of 95 randomized control trials examining falls in older patients in residential settings, nursing care facilities, and hospitals, the quality of evidence was generally classified as either low or very low.[20] The authors were uncertain of the effect of interventions such as exercise, physiotherapy, the use of bed alarm sensors, medication review, and/or multifactorial interventions. They determined supplemental vitamin D most likely reduces the rate of falls, but not the risk of falling.[20]

Gait Speed

A critical indicator of physical performance, *gait speed*, or *walking speed* (i.e. self-selected/usual [indicative of current function] or fast/maximal [indicative of community ambulation capabilities]), is a relatively quick and easy assessment that yields extremely valuable information. In a pooled analysis of nine cohort studies with individual data from 34,485 community-dwelling adults aged 65 years or older, Studenski et al.[21] determined gait speed was associated with survival in all studies (pooled hazard ratio per 0.1 m/sec, 0.88; 95% confidence interval, 0.87–0.90; $P < 0.001$). Increased survival was noted across the full range of gait speeds for older adults (mean age 73.5, SD 5.9), with significant increments per 0.1 m/sec; therefore, reduced gait speed is predictive of mortality. Middleton, Fritz, and Lusardi[22] highlighted the common clinical perspective of gait speed as a "functional vital sign," and summarized the literature including the predictive capabilities, responsiveness, and recommended assessment techniques (i.e. 5–10-meter distances). Specifically, the 10-meter walk test (10MWT) is a frequently utilized performance measure of physical function with indications for patients with

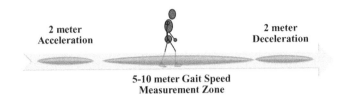

2 meter
Acceleration

2 meter
Deceleration

5-10 meter Gait Speed
Measurement Zone

Figure 18.1 Measurement of Gait Speed.

progressive neurologic disorders, brain injury, spinal cord injury, limb loss, and stroke recovery.[23] Additionally, the 10MWT has been found to have indications for patients with prostate and breast cancer.[24,25]

An assessment of gait speed in meters per second (m/sec), over a defined distance, with two-three meters each for acceleration and deceleration phases, can be a brief, easy way to monitor for functional decline over time for individuals in inpatient, outpatient, and/or home care settings (see Figure 18.1). Within facilities, having a designated area with the distance clearly marked increases the convenience. With such a sensitive measure, subtle declines could potentially be identified over time for individuals with advanced illness. This could be established as an indicator for referrals for rehabilitation interventions (e.g. a documented reduction of gait speed of 0.1 m/sec in an outpatient/ambulatory care setting).

Self-Efficacy

Looney et al.[26] described challenges in the inpatient setting to utilizing traditional functional outcome measures, especially near or at the end of life, when a person's physical functioning is progressively impaired and physical status is highly variable. Due to this, another useful area to demonstrate the effectiveness of therapist care is through the application of valid and reliable self-efficacy scales. The concept of self-efficacy reflects the empowerment of the patient to have confidence in managing a specific aspect of their overall health care.[27] In the domain of pain self-efficacy, there are two commonly utilized scales, the Pain Self-Efficacy Questionnaire (PSEQ)[28,29] and the Chronic Pain Self-Efficacy Scale.[30] Looking specifically at the PSEQ, its test-retest reliability was reported to be 0.73.[28] It has been demonstrated to be responsive to change, and a 9-point change has been determined to be the MCID.[31]

The importance of quantifying pain self-efficacy is exemplified when considering the long-term management of an individual with intractable bone cancer, for example. It may not be an achievable goal for this patient to have a 0/10 pain on the NPRS as the bone neoplasms are no longer amenable to curative treatments. In this scenario, the therapist may focus on teaching several different interventions, equipping the patient to assist in managing their inevitable ongoing pain as well as pain crises. If this patient were to have a pain crisis, examples of therapist education or interventions may be teaching the patient offloading or unweighting techniques to reduce the stress forces on a metastatic bone lesion, education on protective weight-bearing, and avoiding end ranges of motion.[32] In addition, if coordinated with the physician and patient, the compassionate use of therapeutic modalities may be warranted.[33] Wilson and Stanczak,[34] as well as Cameron,[35] described that in cases of advanced disease where cure is not an option and the treatment focus is QoL, a trial of biophysical agents may be appropriate and may assist an individual in performing their daily activities with comfort, requiring fewer pain medications (see Chapter 17). In order to quantify this newfound self-efficacy, a quantitative scale would be beneficial to clarify that although the therapist did not immediately impact the patient's pain severity, the patient now has "tools in their toolbox" to manage their pain more independently and confidently. This may empower them to not need to call emergency services or require hospitalization for intractable pain.

Another example of the use of self-efficacy scales is with falls efficacy, measuring confidence in walking and/or fear of falling. As safety in PC is a priority among health professions, falls efficacy may be a beneficial quantification via the Modified Falls Efficacy Scale or the Falls Efficacy Scale-International (FES-I).[36] In addition, the Activities-specific Balance Confidence (ABC) scale may be employed to reflect improved confidence in balance.[37] This may be a useful quantification in the event that objective performance scales do not adequately reflect the improvement in global balance and fall risk reduction.

One of the most commonly cited group of scales is called the Functional Assessment of Chronic Illness Therapy (FACIT, www.facit.org). The FACIT scales group includes "...90 questionnaires and translated and linguistically validated...into over 70 languages for use in over 100 countries."[38] As with EORTC QoL scales,[39] there are a number of diagnosis-specific QoL scales which also quantify "fatigue, treatment satisfaction, spiritual well-being, HIV, multiple sclerosis, arthritis, and other chronic conditions." Many of the FACIT scales share the same foundational questions from the FACT-G (Functional Assessment of Cancer Therapy-General). The FACT-G is a PROM utilizing a zero through four scale to quantify domains including physical, social, functional, and emotional.[40] In order to assess other diagnoses or health domains, a series of additional question items are administered that may be an adjunct to the base FACT-G questions or used on their own.

Activities of Daily Living

ADLs include the basic, routine tasks individuals perform every day, ideally without assistance. Typical categories of ADLs include: bathing; grooming; dressing (i.e. upper and lower body); eating; transferring; toileting; continence; and mobility (i.e. ambulation on even and uneven surfaces). Categories of instrumental activities of daily living (IADL) include: use of technology to communicate; medication management; meal preparation; housekeeping;

managing personal finances; shopping; accessing transportation; and pet care. Measurement of ADL performance provides critical information regarding how much skilled care an individual requires, and/or the need for discharge to a step-down unit (e.g. skilled nursing facility/nursing home) versus home with the appropriate level of assistance. Referral for occupational therapy, consideration of home health aide assistance, and the acquisition of adaptive equipment to improve the level of independence, are appropriate strategies for ADL training and planning to meet care needs.

Although the ability of a patient to perform ADLs is often a subcategory of performance status, there are specific measures designed to capture the level of performance in each of the specific ADL categories. The Functional Independence Measure (FIM, 18-items rated on a 7-point ordinal scale [1: total assist to 7: complete independence]), Katz Index of Independence in ADL (6: high, 0: low), and the Barthel Index (0–100) are frequently used ADL assessments.[41–43]

Quality of Life

As a patient with a terminal illness may have weeks, months, or years to live, a significant focus of care should be toward optimizing remaining quality of life. A central philosophy of palliative and hospice care is the focus on health-related QoL (HRQoL); therefore, regular assessment and dedicated treatment are cornerstones of advanced care planning. This shift in focus toward QoL away from aggressive rehabilitative procedures is a change in care philosophy for many rehabilitation professionals. Changes may include being more willing to accept a patient refusal, emphasizing comfort instead of "no pain, no gain," or providing rehabilitative procedures to optimize safety even if physical function allows for higher activity levels but the risk outweighs the benefit to long-term QoL (i.e. a fall and fracture). An informed, collaborative, and patient-centered treatment plan should be a priority in this instance.

Specific to QoL in palliative care, there is an original FACIT-Pal scale and the shortened tool, the FACIT-Pal-14.[44] The original FACIT-Pal includes 46 questions in categories including physical well-being, social/family well-being, emotional well-being, functional well-being, and additional concerns, with the patient-reported responses ranked from 0: *not at all*, to 4: *very much*, within the past seven days. The FACIT-Pal-14 eliminates the grouped categories but retains the scoring structure and questions targeting physical (e.g. energy, nausea, pain, dyspnea, constipation), psychosocial (e.g. QoL satisfaction, attitudes towards prognosis), emotional (e.g. feelings of sadness, hopefulness), and support-related domains (e.g. ability to discuss concerns, level of emotional support). Both demonstrate adequate psychometric properties, with the FACIT-Pal "able to discriminate between participants who died within three months of completing the baseline and participants who lived for at least one year after completing the baseline assessment (t = −4.05, P < 0.001)."[45] Shinall et al.[46] found the FACIT-Pal-14 had good internal consistency and evidence of construct validity. King et al.[47] determined the EORTC QLQ-C15-PAL was also an appropriate PROM for QoL assessment in the palliative care setting, which is a shortened version from the original EORTC QLQ-C30.[48]

It may seem intuitive that individuals with a terminal illness facing the end of life would have poor QoL, but with appropriate care and support that need not always be the case. By reducing total symptom burden, empowering the individual with strategies, and honoring their end-of-life choices, the IDT can work in partnership with the patient-family to maximize QoL. A key focus of the IDT should be optimizing the remaining quality of life by coordinating and strategically employing the unique talents of the IDT members. Therapists should embrace their key role to provide care that takes QoL into consideration and make necessary adjustments to prioritize QoL for the remainder of an individual's life.

Summary

Accurate outcomes assessment takes careful consideration in the selection and utilization of the appropriate measure for the right patient at the right time. Mindfulness of psychometric properties, clinical utility, test burden, and the intended purpose with the application of the measure, is vital in the palliative and hospice care setting. As these tools often are a determinant of provisions of care, such as the type of interventions prescribed, necessary referrals ordered, level/intensity of care required, and discharge destination, the correct measure selection, and proper utilization is key to obtaining the optimal outcome for the individual at the end of life.

References

1 Tas F, Sen F, Odabas H, Kılıc L, Keskın S, Yıldız I. Performance status of patients is the major prognostic factor at all stages of pancreatic cancer. *Int J Clin Oncol.* 2013;18(5):839–846. doi:10.1007/s10147-012-0474-9.

2 Karnofsky D, Burchenal J. The clinical evaluation of chemotherapeutic agents in cancer. In: MacLeod C, ed. *Evaluation of Chemotherapeutic Agents.* New York, NY: Columbia University Press; 1949:191–205.

3 Oken M, Creech R, Tormey D, et al. Toxicity and response criteria of the Eastern Cooperative Oncology Group. *Am J Clin Oncol.* 1982;5:649–655.

4 Anderson F, Downing GM, Hill J, et al. PPS: A new tool. *J Palliative Care.* 1996;12(1):5.

5 Kang Y, Demiris G. Self-report pain assessment tools for cognitively intact older adults: Integrative review. *Int J Older People Nurs.* 2018;13(2):e12170. doi:10.1111/opn.12170.

6 Miettinen T, Kautiainen H, Mäntyselkä P, Linton SJ, Kalso E. Pain interference type and level guide the assessment process in chronic pain: Categorizing pain patients entering tertiary pain treatment with the Brief Pain Inventory. *PLoS One.* 2019;14(8):e0221437. Published August 20, 2019. doi:10.1371/journal.pone.0221437.

7 U Jumbo S, C MacDermid J, E Kalu M, L Packham T, S Athwal G, J Faber K. Measurement properties of the Brief Pain Inventory-Short Form (BPI-SF)

and the Revised Short McGill Pain Questionnaire-Version-2 (SF-MPQ-2) in pain-related musculoskeletal conditions: A systematic review protocol. *Arch Bone Jt Surg.* 2020;8(2):131–141. doi:10.22038/abjs.2020.36779.1973.

8   Garra G, Singer AJ, Domingo A, Thode HC Jr. The Wong-Baker pain FACES scale measures pain, not fear. *Pediatr Emerg Care.* 2013;29(1):17–20. doi:10.1097/PEC.0b013e31827b2299.

9   Tomlinson D, von Baeyer CL, Stinson JN, Sung L. A systematic review of faces scales for the self-report of pain intensity in children. *Pediatrics.* 2010;126(5):e1168–e1198. doi:10.1542/peds.2010-1609.

10 Miale S, Harrington S, Brown K, Braswell A, Cannoy J, Krisch N, Rock K. Academy of Oncologic Physical Therapy EDGE Task Force on Cancer: A systematic review of outcome measures for pain in children. *Rehabil Oncol.* 2019;37:47–54. doi:10.1097/01.REO.0000000000000165.

11 Ware LJ, Herr KA, Booker SS, et al. Psychometric evaluation of the revised Iowa Pain Thermometer (IPT-R) in a sample of diverse cognitively intact and impaired older adults: A pilot study. *Pain Manag Nurs.* 2015;16(4):475–482. doi:10.1016/j.pmn.2014.09.004.

12 Warden V, Hurley AC, Volicer L. Development and psychometric evaluation of the Pain Assessment in Advanced Dementia (PAINAD) scale. *J Am Med Dir Assoc.* 2003;4(1):9–15. doi:10.1097/01.JAM.0000043422.31640.F7.

13 Tsai LY, Li IF, Lai YH, Liu CP, Chang TY, Tu CT. Fatigue and its associated factors in hospice cancer patients in Taiwan. *Cancer Nurs.* 2007;30(1):24–30. doi:10.1097/00002820-200701000-00005.

14 Oh HS, Seo WS. Systematic review and meta-analysis of the correlates of cancer-related fatigue. *Worldviews Evid Based Nurs.* 2011;8(4):191–201. doi:10.1111/j.1741-6787.2011.00214.x.

15 Fisher M, Davies C, Lacy H, Doherty D. Oncology Section EDGE Task Force on Cancer: Measures of cancer-related fatigue—A systematic review. *Rehabil Oncol.* 2018;36(2):93–105.

16 Hewlett S, Dures E, Almeida C. Measures of fatigue: Bristol Rheumatoid Arthritis Fatigue Multi-Dimensional Questionnaire (BRAF MDQ), Bristol Rheumatoid Arthritis Fatigue Numerical Rating Scales (BRAF NRS) for severity, effect, and coping, Chalder Fatigue Questionnaire (CFQ), Checklist Individual Strength (CIS20R and CIS8R), Fatigue Severity Scale (FSS), Functional Assessment Chronic Illness Therapy (Fatigue) (FACIT-F), Multi-Dimensional Assessment of Fatigue (MAF), Multi-Dimensional Fatigue Inventory (MFI), Pediatric Quality Of Life (PedsQL) Multi-Dimensional Fatigue Scale, Profile of Fatigue (ProF), Short Form 36 Vitality Subscale (SF-36 VT), and Visual Analog Scales (VAS). *Arthritis Care Res (Hoboken).* 2011;63(Supplement 11):S263–S286. doi:10.1002/acr.20579.

17 Smucker DR, Regan S, Elder NC, Gerrety E. Patient safety incidents in home hospice care: the experiences of hospice interdisciplinary team members. *J Palliat Med.* 2014;17(5):540–544. doi:10.1089/jpm.2013.0111.

18 Lusardi MM, Fritz S, Middleton A, et al. Determining risk of falls in community dwelling older adults: A systematic review and meta-analysis using posttest probability. *J Geriatr Phys Ther.* 2017;40(1):1–36. doi:10.1519/JPT.0000000000000099.

19 Huang M, Hile E, Croarkin E, Wampler-Kuhn M, Blackwood J, Colon G, Pfalzer L. Academy of Oncologic Physical Therapy EDGE Task Force: A systematic review of measures of balance in adult cancer survivors. *Rehabil Oncol.* 2019;37(3):92–103. doi:10.1097/01.REO.0000000000000177.

20 Cameron ID, Dyer SM, Panagoda CE, et al. Interventions for preventing falls in older people in care facilities and hospitals. *Cochrane Database Syst Rev.*

2018;9(9):CD005465. Published September 7, 2018. doi:10.1002/14651858. CD005465.pub4.

21 Studenski S, Perera S, Patel K, et al. Gait speed and survival in older adults. *JAMA.* 2011;305(1):50–58. doi:10.1001/jama.2010.1923.

22 Middleton A, Fritz SL, Lusardi M. Walking speed: The functional vital sign. *J Aging Phys Act.* 2015;23(2):314–322. doi:10.1123/japa.2013-0236.

23 Shirley Ryan Ability Lab. 10 Meter Walk Test. https://www.sralab.org/rehabilitation-measures/10-meter-walk-test. Updated January 22, 2014. Accessed June 10, 2020.

24 Huang M, Blackwood J, Croarkin E, Wampler-Kuhn M, Colon G, Pfalzer L. Outcomes: Clinical measures of balance a systematic review. *Rehabil Oncol.* 2015;33(1):18–27.

25 Davies C, Colon G, Geyer H, Pfalzer L, Fisher M. Oncology EDGE Task Force on Prostate Cancer Outcomes: A systematic review of outcome measures for functional mobility. *Rehabil Oncol.* 2016;34(3):82–96.

26 Looney F, Cobbe S, Ryan A, Barriscale I, McMahon A. The search for a functional outcome measure for physical therapy in specialist palliative care: An ongoing journey. *Rehabil Oncol.* 2020;38(1):22–29.

27 Mystakidou K, Tsilika E, Parpa E, Gogou P, Theodorakis P, Vlahos L. Self-efficacy beliefs and levels of anxiety in advanced cancer patients. *Eur J Cancer Care.* 2010;19(2):205–211.

28 Nicholas MK. The pain self-efficacy questionnaire: Taking pain into account. *Eu J Pain.* 2007;11(2):153–163.

29 Di Pietro F, Catley MJ, McAuley JH, et al. Rasch analysis supports the use of the pain self-efficacy questionnaire. *Phys Ther.* 2014;94(1):91–100. doi:10.2522/ptj.20130217.

30 Anderson KO, Dowds BN, Pelletz RE, Edwards WT, Peeters-Asdourian C. Development and initial validation of a scale to measure self-efficacy beliefs in patients with chronic pain. *Pain.* 1995;63(1):77–83.

31 Maughan EF, Lewis JS. Outcome measures in chronic low back pain. *Eur Spine J.* 2010;19(9):1484–1494.

32 Albrecht TA, Taylor AG. Physical activity in patients with advanced-stage cancer: A systematic review of the literature. *Clin J Oncol Nurs.* 2012;16(3):293–300. doi:10.1188/12.CJON.293-300.

33 Cheville AL, Basford JR. Role of rehabilitation medicine and physical agents in the treatment of cancer-associated pain. *J Clin Oncol.* 2014;32(16): 1691–1702. doi:10.1200/JCO.2013.53.6680.

34 Wilson CM, Stanczak JF. Palliative pain management using transcutaneous electrical nerve stimulation (TENS). *Rehabil Oncol.* 2020;38(1): E1–E6. doi:10.1097/01.REO.0000000000000188.

35 Cameron MH. *Physical Agents in Rehabilitation.* St. Louis, MO: Elsevier:231.

36 Pua YH, Ong PH, Clark RA, Matcher DB, Lim EC. Falls efficacy, postural balance, and risk for falls in older adults with falls-related emergency department visits: Prospective cohort study. *BMC Geriatr.* 2017;17(1):291. Published December 21, 2017. doi:10.1186/s12877-017-0682-2.

37 Powell LE, Myers AM. The activities-specific balance confidence (ABC) scale. *J Gerontol A Biol Sci Med Sci.* 1995;50(1):M28–M34.

38 FACIT.org. About us - FACIT.org. https://www.facit.org/FACITOrg/AboutUs. Accessed June 11, 2020.

39 Groenvold M, Klee MC, Sprangers MA, Aaronson NK. Validation of the EO-RTC QLQ-C30 quality of life questionnaire through combined qualitative and quantitative assessment of patient-observer agreement. *J Clin Epidemiol.* 1997;50(4):441–450.

40 Brucker PS, Yost K, Cashy J, Webster K, Cella D. General population and cancer patient norms for the functional assessment of cancer therapy-general (FACT-G). *Eval Health Prof.* 2005;28(2):192–211.

41 Shirley Ryan Ability Lab. Functional independence measure. https://www.sralab.org/rehabilitation-measures/fimr-instrument-fim-fimr-trademark-uniform-data-system-fro-medical. Updated October 6, 2015. Accessed June 10, 2020.

42 Shirley Ryan Ability Lab. Katz index of independence in activities of daily living. https://www.sralab.org/rehabilitation-measures/katz-index-independence-activities-daily-living Updated January 22, 2014. Accessed June 10, 2020.

43 Shirley Ryan Ability Lab. Barthel index. https://www.sralab.org/rehabilitation-measures/barthel-index. Updated May 21, 2020. Accessed June 10, 2020.

44 Zeng L, Bedard G, Cella D, et al. Preliminary results of the generation of a shortened quality-of-life assessment for patients with advanced cancer: The FACIT-Pal-14. *J Palliat Med.* 2013;16(5):509–515. doi:10.1089/jpm.2012.0595.

45 Lyons KD, Bakitas M, Hegel MT, Hanscom B, Hull J, Ahles TA. Reliability and validity of the Functional Assessment of Chronic Illness Therapy-Palliative care (FACIT-Pal) scale. *J Pain Symptom Manage.* 2009;37(1):23–32. doi:10.1016/j.jpainsymman.2007.12.015.

46 Shinall MC, Ely EW, Karlekar M, Robbins SG, Chandrasekhar R, Martin SF. Psychometric properties of the FACIT-Pal 14 administered in an out-patient palliative care clinic. *Am J Hosp Palliat Care.* 2018;35(10):1292–1294. doi:10.1177/1049909118763793.

47 King MT, Agar M, Currow DC, Hardy J, Fazekas B, McCaffrey N. Assessing quality of life in palliative care settings: Head-to-head comparison of four patient-reported outcome measures (EORTC QLQ-C15-PAL, FACT-Pal, FACT-Pal-14, FACT-G7). *Support Care Cancer.* 2020;28(1):141–153. doi:10.1007/s00520-019-04754-9.

48 Groenvold M, Petersen MA, Aaronson NK, et al. The development of the EORTC QLQ-C15-PAL: A shortened questionnaire for cancer patients in palliative care. *Eur J Cancer.* 2006;42(1):55–64. doi:10.1016/j.ejca.2005.06.022.

19 Therapists' Interventions among Practice Settings

Christopher M. Wilson and Amy J. Litterini

Introduction

Individuals with chronic, life-threatening, or terminal illnesses will be encountered in every practice setting from community exercise programs to hospitals, inpatient rehabilitation (IPR), and nursing facilities, in their own homes, and finally hospice organizations. As many physical activity providers and therapists generally only practice in one setting, it is an added (but necessary) challenge to have a comprehensive understanding of the patient's journey and the therapist's role and treatment techniques across the entire disease journey. In order to provide patient-centered, proactive, preventative care, an understanding of the varying therapist intervention strategies and unique clinical adaptations employed in each practice setting is warranted. As each of these clinical settings are unique with a wide variety of required skills and knowledge, this chapter is not intended to capture all aspects of mastery within a specific clinical setting but to provide unique nuances and insights into how each of these settings may help to optimize quality of life (QoL) for the individual with a terminal illness.

Unique Interventions in Diverse Practice Settings

Upon initial diagnosis, an individual's symptom burden may not be significant, and the disease trajectory will transition from more ambulatory, community-based services, to more hospitalizations and, in some cases, a hospice facility or home health hospice services. As each person's disease journey is highly unique, some individuals may not receive care in every setting and depending on the pathology and circumstances, timeframes and clinical needs in a specific setting are highly variable. This chapter discusses the variety of common and unique clinical interventions performed by therapists with individuals with life-threatening illnesses in these settings.

Community Exercise and Wellness

In the early stages of the disease, individuals newly diagnosed with a life-threatening illness may pursue community-based physical activity and health services. These may be through a municipal community center, private healthcare fitness center, or personal trainers. Although these community healthcare services may not be tailored specifically to the unique needs of the individual's medical situation, they still play an important role in maintaining health, engaging socially with others, and providing purpose to life during this difficult time.

At all stages of the disease process, individuals should be encouraged to reach out to condition-specific public-focused organizations (e.g. Alzheimer's Association, Living Beyond Breast Cancer, National Multiple Sclerosis Society). Most organizations maintain a comprehensive website aimed towards community members/individuals with the disease, as well as families and healthcare providers. Beneficial resources on these websites include frequently asked questions by trustworthy sources, support groups, and myriad special events, webinars, and meetings. These organizations' websites may be useful resources for condition-specific exercise programs or health-related activities that may be a better fit than programming aimed at the general public.

As has been established throughout this text, physical activity is important to an individual's physical, mental, and emotional well-being. As a key component of community-based exercise and support programs is reducing barriers to access, individuals with chronic or life-threatening diseases may inquire or attempt to attend programs intended for the general public. As progressive medical complexity and safety issues are a reality for these individuals, due diligence should be taken to assure that the program is safe and appropriate and will not exacerbate symptoms or cause undue health issues. Written medical clearance from the individual's physician is highly recommended (and often required by institutional policy). Once medical clearance has been established, the community physical activity provider may need to anticipate the needs of this individual. This may include encouraging frequent rest breaks, having a place to sit down during group exercise, or proactively modifying exercises based on an individual's needs. Finally, not every exercise program is appropriate for everyone's health level. A community exercise provider must have an awareness of what concerns elevate to the level of contacting the referring provider and be prepared to refer the individual to a lower-level class, if indicated, or to a trained medical professional such as a physical therapist (PT).

Outpatient or Ambulatory Therapist Services

As with the community-based physical activity programs, outpatient or ambulatory therapist services play a critical role in long-term management and care of individuals with a chronic or life-threatening illness. As therapists in the inpatient settings may only provide care for patients during one relatively short stay, delivering ongoing professional guidance to the individual is not a feasible option. The outpatient therapist, however, can build a long-term, sustainable relationship with the individual. They can be a consistent resource and guide throughout the disease process. With some diagnoses or conditions, there may already be a robust process for providing condition-specific physical activity for those with chronic, degenerative, or terminal conditions. Examples include neurologic PT or occupational therapist (OT) services, cardiac rehabilitation for individuals with congestive heart failure, or pulmonary rehabilitation for individuals with chronic obstructive pulmonary disorder (COPD). Although these programs are well established and often available in many locations, their use and availability are inconsistent and dependent on a physician, or patient preference, or inadequate funding.[1]

Although the outpatient therapist may not physically treat their clients consistently for their entire disease journey, best practice would include maintaining consistent contact via telehealth or scheduling periodic consultations. This would allow the therapist to employ their evaluative skills to identify an underlying problem or subtle decline in function and proactively provide advice or interventions before an issue causes substantial harm or dysfunction. In essence, these individuals with a chronic or life-threatening illness need a *therapist for life*. Especially as their symptoms will wax and wane, and have a progressively negative effect on their physical and functional performance, it is anticipated that therapist services are more frequently needed.

One of the challenges reported by outpatient therapists includes feeling disconnected from the rest of the chronic disease or palliative care (PC) interdisciplinary team (IDT), especially as most PC or chronic disease management teams are hospital-based or within a specific home care agency. It is highly recommended that the outpatient therapist works to build a relationship and proactively reaches out to their patient's currently established PC team or collaborate with the patient's primary care physician. Within the United States, one of the common misconceptions is that older adults who require the services of a skilled therapist to maintain or slow the decline of their chronic condition are not able to receive it. As was discussed in Chapter 4, the Jimmo versus Sebelius settlement clarified that if a patient requires skilled services to maintain or slow the decline of their condition, as long as the documentation can justify the skilled need, the services would be eligible for payment.[2] In general, other outpatient or ambulatory care services may also be eligible for these preventative/maintenance services, especially in nations with a nationalized or government-supported healthcare systems such as Canada, the United Kingdom, or Australia. In the outpatient setting in these nations, ambulatory healthcare services may not be as contingent upon consistent physical or functional gains, as payment is not as closely tied to clinical improvement, although individual private insurance companies may still have this requirement.

An additional challenge to the ambulatory setting is the potential for limited access to critical medical information due to the lack of a systematic, integrated electronic medical record. For example, if an outpatient PT practices in a private clinic with their own medical record system (that is not connected to their patient's hospital or physician medical record), the PT may not have access to the history of vital signs, surgical reports, diagnostic imaging reports, emergency room physician notes, or other key pieces of information. In some cases, a therapist may be able to glean some of this information via taking a thorough oral patient history; however, unless the patient is an exceptionally competent and detailed historian, there may be gaps in the information or key data may not be received by the PT. Box 19.1 depicts questions that may help garner critical information about the state of the disease process for the outpatient therapist.

Box 19.1 Key History Taking Questions for the Individual with a Chronic or Life-Threatening Disease

1   Who is the physician who you would consider to be primarily managing your health condition?
2   How often do you see this physician and when is your next appointment?
3   What clinical values or symptoms does your physician tell you to keep a close eye on?
4   In your opinion, what issue or problem might cause you to need to call emergency services or go to the hospital emergently?
5   Are there any important medications or regimens that you and your doctor have established?
6   Are there any early warning signs that your health condition might need closer medical care?

Acute Care Hospitalization

Inherent to an acute hospitalization is a change in medical status, new onset of symptoms, or other events that preclude an individual's ability to remain at home. As has been described in previous chapters, the individual may be in emotional distress where their symptoms are less well-controlled and require more medical management. Notably, the majority of individuals prefer not to spend the end of their life in an acute hospital setting. In a meta-analysis of 26 articles, it was found that up to 79% of individuals preferred home as their location of death.[3] For physical activity professionals and therapists practicing in an acute hospital system, a confounding variable is the frequent and abrupt changes to the care goals and medical status. Due to the sudden and dramatic medical or physical changes that occur during an acute hospitalization, patients may experience distress and are forced to consider goals and life changes that they may have not previously considered. For example, if a person was living independently at home alone with stable COPD and had an acute exacerbation, his dyspnea on exertion may limit his ability to return home safely and he may need to consider admission to an extended care facility (ECF) or discharge to live with family. Either choice represents an abrupt loss of independence and locus of control, both of which can result in further emotional distress.

Another commonly encountered scenario in the acute hospital setting is the challenging family dynamics. During serious illness, especially hospitalizations, many family members may travel long distances to assist in the decision-making and to support the person through this change in their illness. In some cases, this brings up difficult family dynamics that may impact therapist care.[4] These may include family members wishing to pursue continued life-sustaining measures and rehabilitation while other family members may wish to pursue comfort and QoL measures. Further compounding this already complicated situation is the varied abilities of each individual family member to understand and cope with the disease process abruptly.[4] This includes potentially considering the mortality of their loved one, a situation that they may not have previously considered.[4]

As discussed in Chapter 6, navigating and integrating with the care team can be an essential component of therapist care during a hospitalization. Close communication between OT, PT, and speech language pathology is necessary to provide the best care for the patient. In addition, integrating information learned from the other IDT members will assist in the provision of goal-oriented, patient-centered, and QoL-focused care.

Within the acute care setting, another important challenge that requires the skill of a therapist is establishing medical stability prior to therapeutic interventions. This may also require modification of the interventions if stabilization of a medical issue is not feasible.[5] Although not solely encountered in the acute care setting, abnormal vital signs and lab values are areas that require close monitoring and collaboration. One of the key challenges with recommending standard parameters and guidelines is that situations will always arise that require the clinical judgment of the therapist and care team that vary from established guidelines.[5] For example, some institutions have a hemoglobin value of 7.0 mg/dL as the cutoff point to defer moderate-intensity aerobic exercise or out-of-bed activity, yet in some cases, mobilization or physical activity may be unavoidable despite a lower hemoglobin value.[5,6] Illustrative of this is a patient with acute blood loss from a gastrointestinal bleed from colon cancer who was a Jehovah's Witness. Within this religion, acceptance of blood products for transfusions is often considered to be prohibited.[7] During an intensive care unit stay, the PT facilitated early out-of-bed mobility with hemoglobin at 5.0 mg/dL because a transfusion was not a feasible option. Upon discussion of the risks and benefits of bed rest with the entire care team, it was determined that bed rest would likely make the patient's condition worse as opposed to improving it. In this case, the therapist modified interventions to closely monitor for signs and symptoms of near syncope and constantly evaluated the patient's vital signs during the therapy to avoid a syncopal episode or any other adverse medical event.

Vital sign and lab value parameters for therapeutic interventions vary from institution to institution; however, the American Physical Therapy

Association's Acute Care Lab Values Guide does provide some guidance to clinicians as to best practices based on current research evidence (https://www.acutept.org/page/ResourceGuides#labvalinterp).[5] One notable consideration for therapists interpreting lab values is the consideration of trends in results. For example, an individual with anemia from chronic illness may be asymptomatic during exercise, while an individual who has experienced acute blood loss may be pre-syncopal during that same exercise at the same degree of anemia. In addition, lab values and their symptomatic clinical presentations often are compounded by other clinical findings. For example, anemia on its own may not be as significant as anemia in the presence of hypoglycemia, hypotension, or impaired oxygen exchange.

It remains best practice in the acute care setting to do a thorough chart review before initiating an evaluation or treatment. When caring for an individual with a life-threatening illness, establishing a baseline activity level and social history are important. Although this information may be gathered from the medical records, this should be verified via a subjective interview. A thorough depiction is warranted of the patient's living environment, prior level of function, number of stairs to enter the home, and stairs up to the bedroom or bathroom (if applicable). In addition, data should include the layout of the bathroom including information on whether they have a walk-in shower or a tub shower, and whether handrails or other home modifications have been implemented. Especially if the patient's overarching desire is to return home, that goal is dependent on the therapist's understanding of the patient's previous, current, *and future* functional capacity as it relates to the environment to which they hope to return. When considering the patient's previous functional capacity, a clear understanding must be achieved related to the individual's customary functional status and their more recent functional changes immediately prior to the hospitalization.

Details of the patient's social network and support system will be essential information to gather. *Does the patient have a family in the area? If they are in the area, do they have other obligations (e.g. work or childcare) that may compete with their ability to help the family member?* In addition, the therapist must have a clear understanding of the individual's primary disease process, extent of disease, current treatment regimens, and their effectiveness. Furthermore, a thorough review of co-morbid disease processes and surgery is needed to establish whether they may affect the individual's physical activity performance. In cases of PC or other chronic disease processes, the care notes from the IDT are relevant and important. These would include the overall medical opinion from the attending physicians, an admission note (often known as a history and physical [H&P]), and consultants' opinions of any symptoms or side effects of treatment. Useful consultation notes to review include those from oncologists, cardiologists, pulmonologists, physical medicine and rehabilitation, and orthopedics. For example, if the patient was having chest pain or experiencing new lower extremity pain after a fall, the therapist should thoroughly review the cardiologist's or orthopedic surgeon's notes, respectively, to determine whether physical activity may worsen an evolving or undiagnosed medical condition.

As many healthcare providers, including physicians, may only document once daily about the patient, it is imperative that the therapist in acute care has a strong understanding of the interpretation of lab values, diagnostic tests, and imaging studies to determine whether they will affect the intended intervention plan for that day. As therapy professions are growing in academic preparation and professional autonomy, it is increasingly expected that therapists perform a critical review of these components of the medical record (and perform their own assessment of vital signs) to make an autonomous clinical decision as opposed to relying solely on the information from verbal consultations of other healthcare professions. It is important to also identify when collaboration with other professionals is necessary in the event that the medical record does not provide enough information, or if the information is conflicting or evolving.

Eight days (range 2–16) has been found to be the average hospital length of stay across nations who report data to the Organisation for Economic Co-operation and Development (OECD).[8] As this has been documented to be longer for patients in PC, with a median length of stay of 14.1 days (range 4.7–35.8),[9] a critical role for the therapist is related to discharge planning. This transition from the hospital to the next level of care is a challenging and multifaceted process. The PTs and OTs role in, and contribution to, discharge planning is well documented in the literature; evidence points toward increased readmission rate, and less successful discharge home, when a PT or OT are not consulted to provide their input, or their input is not followed.[10–13] In palliative scenarios, there are several options for discharge from the hospital once medical stability has been achieved, and are described below. A key consideration in discharge planning or transition from one setting to another is the patient's realistic prognosis of life expectancy, rehabilitation potential, and likely outcomes. The responsibility of initiating this discussion with the IDT members may reside with the therapist due to the key insights related to current and predicted functional performance status.

Inpatient Rehabilitation

Discharge to IPR often requires a person to be able to tolerate a substantial amount of aggressive physical rehabilitation for several hours per day. In the IPR setting, functional decline is a confounding variable. Often perceived to be the most rigorous, structured setting for rehabilitation, IPR may not always be a good fit for individuals with a life-threatening illness or in PC. In many instances, patients with advanced cancer or advanced incurable illnesses have been found to require re-hospitalization during an IPR stay. For individuals facing an advanced life-threatening disease, their success in IPR may be limited due to low physiologic reserve and poor tolerance for conventional rehabilitation in IPR. In 2008, Guo et al.[14] found that approximately 70% of oncology patients completed traditional IPR with an average length of stay of ten days and discharge to the community, though this varied greatly by the stage and extent of disease. In this study, the 30% that transferred off IPR to return to the medical floor had (1) an increased chance of dying in hospital; (2) a decreased chance of discharge home directly from hospital; (3) progressive weakness due to disease process; (4) unmanaged symptoms (pain, breathlessness, nausea/vomiting); (5) increased risk of readmission after eventual discharge; and (6) the patient and family goals were found to not consistently match the medical trajectory. Of the patients who transferred back to the hospital units from IPR, 88% were due to a worsening medical condition and 52% were eventually discharged home. Conversely, patients who were able to complete their IPR course of rehabilitation, 90% were able to discharge home.[14] For those individuals who can tolerate the approximately three hours of physical rehabilitation interventions, IPR offers an option to improve function at a relatively rapid rate; however, some individuals who may not tolerate IPR could demonstrate worsening of symptoms and require readmission. This readmission may have negative consequences for the patient, family, and the operations of the IPR. As discussed in Chapter 5, an IPR-based short-stay family training program may be a feasible option for those individuals who wish to return home but whose family does not yet have the skills to support them at home. Although IPR is often a hopeful and appealing choice for individuals with an advanced life-threatening disease, therapists must consider all aspects of the patient's disease trajectory and tolerance for intensive rehabilitation before making this recommendation.

Depending on the admission regulations and payment stipulations for nations, jurisdictions, and individual institutions, the opportunity for providing care for those in PC in an IPR setting varies substantially and is quite circumstantial. For example, in the United States, a requirement for admission into the IPR setting is that the individual be able to tolerate three hours of PT and OT and, if needed, speech language pathology (aka speech therapy). Depending on the individual's condition, if speech language pathology is not needed for this patient's condition, generally the three hours are divided up between PT and OT. Additionally, in the IPR setting, other healthcare team members may provide care. These include rehabilitation nurses who assist and reinforce the new skills learned by the patient during therapy. Recreation therapy is also frequently an integral member of the IPR care team, assisting with reintegration and adaptation of recreational activities. A critical role for individuals in PC is the role of the IPR social worker who can help individuals in IPR to cope and adapt to dramatic changes in their physical, cognitive, and emotional states. Finally, there is often a physiatrist (aka physical medicine and rehabilitation physician) whose primary tasks include coordination of rehabilitation care and medical management during IPR admission. When IPR is an appropriate choice, the IDT, resources, and time-intensive rehabilitation can facilitate optimal outcomes and improve the functioning and QoL of the individual with a life-threatening illness.

Extended Care Facility/Skilled Nursing Facility

After hospitalization, some individuals may require continued nursing care that may be too complex to complete at home by the individual or their family caregivers. They may also require additional rehabilitation to improve strength, functional mobility, or use of adaptive medical equipment before discharge home. In broad terms, an ECF or a skilled nursing facility (SNF) may provide rehabilitation services but at a slower pace, and generally includes a longer length of stay, as compared to an IPR. As compared to a hospital or an IPR, there may be decreased medical staffing for pain or symptom control, though this may vary by location. A key consideration of SNFs or ECFs is that some individuals with a terminal illness are not likely to prefer spending the last months of their life in this type of institution, so like IPR, it should be considered a transitional placement for care until returning home.

Sometimes an SNF or ECF is perceived negatively as a "nursing home" by the patient or family, which may result in them arbitrarily declining discharge to this location, even though the setting may be a conducive environment for receiving care. Although SNF/ECF may be a good fit for symptom management and receiving care, the perceived advantage of being at home in a place of comfort often outweighs this benefit. The individual's preferred discharge disposition is a key point for an acute care therapist to consider during discharge planning. In palliative scenarios, a therapist should endeavor to have a conversation with the patient and family member before making a recommendation for discharge to an SNF/ECF; given that if the patient and family are not open to this care setting, time and efforts would be better spent by all involved to procure the needed equipment and training for a safe discharge to home (see Chapters 5 and 20). In addition, there is evidence that home care services (even with an extensive amount of equipment), may be more cost-effective than discharge to an SNF or ECF.[15]

Conversely, there is a subset of individuals in PC who do prefer the skilled services and assistance provided by an SNF/ECF; when having this conversation, it is important to ask probing, open-ended questions about the patient's ultimate goals of care as to not bias the patient toward a particular disposition. Finally, a commonly cited concern among therapists when considering discharge home or to an SNF/ECF is "how will the patient get out of the bed to perform dressing, bathing, and toileting activities at home?" This is often a significant consideration in determining whether a recommendation to discharge to an ECF is warranted as these therapists wonder, "How can this person go home if they can't even get out of their own bed?" In reality, in some end-of-life scenarios, the answer may be that the person may not need to get out of bed and hospice care will be provided in a bed more frequently as the disease process advances.

Home Health Setting and Home Hospice

As stated previously, home is most frequently cited as the preferred location of living in the months preceding death. There are several key considerations for discharge home including accessibility, performance of basic ADLs, comfort, and safety. As it is fairly uncommon in advanced palliative scenarios for an individual to be completely independent in all daily tasks, training caregivers will be necessary, and often essential to success. If the person is relatively in-dependent with basic ADL, the caregiver or family support may simply entail assisting with higher-level activities such as home maintenance or meal prepa-ration, or may only require a periodic phone call to check in. Durable medical equipment should be procured for the patient's current functional status, as well as anticipated future equipment needs such as a wheelchair in the case of a currently ambulatory patient. In addition to provision of this equipment, the patient and family should be trained in its proper use using the principles of *Rehab in Reverse* as described in Chapter 4; insurance coverage in the United States for such anticipated equipment is a challenge unless the person is going to home hospice care, as traditional home care insurers will likely support only current use needs.

A key component of any safe transition home is validating means of entry into the home and accessing the location where the person will be sleeping. A clear understanding or description of this is imperative, and technology may be able to assist. Instead of simply obtaining a verbal description of a patient's home setting, an alternative means may be for the therapist to request the family to photograph or video record the home set up and layout to assist in the tailoring of equipment recommendations and practicing home entry scenarios.[16]

One of the key barriers to home entry is often steps or stairs. If there are several stairs to ascend to enter the home or a flight of stairs up to a bedroom or bathroom, this likely becomes a primary barrier to safe discharge home and must be addressed. In some scenarios, an individual may not be able to ascend stairs even with the skill and training of a therapist. Alternative means of entry may be necessary, including teaching select family members to assist with ascending/descending the stairs with the patient in the chair. Other op-tions include having emergency medical services to transport into the home up the stairs while on a gurney, or building or renting a temporary wheelchair ramp. If the primary barrier to home entry is ascending stairs up to a bed-room, alternatives may include a hospital bed rental or moving the person's bed frame and mattress onto the main floor. Although some individuals may not want to have this level of home modification, a thorough conversation of the options including discharge to an ECF may assist the patient in making a fully informed decision. Keglovits, Somerville, and Stark[16] found that the most commonly cited home safety deficiencies included: (1) lack of hand support (no grab bars in key locations); (2) characteristics of transfer surface (surfaces too low or too high); (3) malfunctioning or lack of adaptive equipment; (4) weight of items (walkers, commodes or wheelchairs too heavy); (5) steps (steps too high or too many); and (6) lack of signals or cues in the environment (beneficial reminders to perform exercises or safety techniques).[17]

Caution may be warranted when considering extensive or expensive home modifications in a rapidly advancing disease trajectory. One therapist described another well-intentioned therapist's recommendations for safe discharge home but then did not consider the patient's disease trajectory or forthcoming physical capacity.

> "The therapist needs to be ready for the patient's condition to change and fluctuate over days and therapists may be ordering things that are inappropriate. A therapist got the family to put in a stair glide for a dying patient and the therapist didn't realize the disease progression. The family used the glide once, but the patient couldn't get off it. The rehab therapist didn't do the wrong thing. He had good intentions, but the family was in a jumble. Education and communication are critical."[18p5]

A specific intervention required for safety and comfort within the home setting is establishing a safe and accessible environment. In order to accomplish this, there are several standardized home safety evaluations to identify and quantify the level of home accessibility and safety. See Table 19.1 for commonly accepted and utilized home environment assessments.

As described in Chapter 4, the astute therapist should also consider the patient's current level of performance, concurrent functional limitations, as well as the anticipated future disease trajectory. In addition to identifying key home modification recommendations, the execution or completion of these modifications is a key and ongoing role for the therapist practicing in the home health setting. Again, a valid, reliable outcome measure to quantify in-home performance is warranted such as the I-HOPE or the SAFER-HOME assessment.[19,20] Home modification recommendations will often require advocacy for the patient including assisting in identification of needed equipment and coordination with the individual's support network to facilitate installation. In some scenarios, this may be inherent in the living location if the person lives in an independent living facility or any other senior apartment where modifications may be regulated or facilitated through the institution's administrators. If an individual resides in their own home, this may be completed by family or friends to accomplish things like installing rails or grab bars. Finally, the proactive therapist can also work closely with their local municipal senior center or local governmental or non-governmental organizations to procure and sometimes even install recommended equipment. This may include local fire departments, city halls, or religious institutions that operate a loan closet for equipment. Some organizations even have volunteers or funding mechanisms to assist with an installation of these devices (see Chapter 5).

A successful transition and experience at home is an integral component to optimizing QoL and comfort in the presence of a chronic disease or terminal

Table 19.1 Home Environment Assessments

	Domains and Format

In-Home Occupational Performance Evaluation (I–HOPE)[18]	• A performance-based measure
	• Takes 30 minutes to complete
	• Evaluates 44 activities in the home. Four subscales
	
	  1 Activity Participation
	  2 Client's Rating of Performance
	  3 Client's Satisfaction with Performance
	  4 Severity of Environmental Barriers
	
	• The subscales' internal consistency ranged from 0.77 to 0.85, and intraclass correlation coefficients (ICC) ranged from 0.99 to 1.0.

Safety Assessment of Function and the Environment for Rehabilitation-Health Outcome Measurement and Evaluation (SAFER-HOME v2)[19]	• SAFER HOME v2 assesses performance of 93 items around the home divided into ten domains. • Level of safety concern is rated on a 4-point scale • Shown to be valid and reliable • Good internal consistency with a Cronbach's alpha value = 0.859
Home Falls and Accidents Screening Tool (Home FAST)[20]	• Twenty-five item home safety environmental assessment • Some predictive validity and responsive to change • Has utility both as falls screen and post-test • Intrarater reliability (IRR) ICC = 0.82, Test-Retest ICC = 0.77
Westmead Home Safety Assessment (WeHSA)[21,22]	• Four-page checklist of potential hazards around home • Seventy-two hazard categories • Each category has individualized descriptors for hazards • Content validity was 0.80 and IRR kappa all items > 0.40
Rebuilding Together's Safe At Home Checklist[23]	• Checklist to identify home safety, fall hazards and accessibility issues Modification recommendations also included to prioritize interventions • Twelve domains of hazard identification and 83 recommended interventions • Validity and reliability not available

illness. For this to be accomplished, the entire care team must reconsider how to best coordinate and reconfigure the services and interventions delivered in the home. In most healthcare environments, there is often a clear division of labor where disciplines generally have their commonly accepted tasks that are done by certain disciplines. In home PC, supporting the client may require members of the care team to work to the fullest extent of their license and perform tasks that are less commonly performed by that discipline. This might include a home care PT assisting with showering, bathing, or nursing care activities while the registered nurses may assist with physical mobility. This blurring of the lines can assist in facilitating safety and comfort for the individual and their families within the home.

As the patient is often less supported by direct interaction with the caregiver team in home care, anxiety can increase in the event of an unexpected situation. In cases like this, the individual and their families should be thoroughly educated on the possible disease-related challenges and symptom exacerbations including the plan to have the patient and family navigate these situations to prevent difficulty at home. Supportive listening and conversations around both observed and anticipated changes often become the focal point of the education process in end-of-life care.

As outlined in Chapter 23, telehealth and smart devices can be a lifeline and support service for the individual living at home, especially those living in rural areas. Through access to the patient's Wi-Fi or other internet connections, a healthcare system or home health agency can monitor medication and home oxygen administration, vital sign responses, and compliance to and performance of home exercise programs. One of the more recent challenges to the home health setting is the COVID-19 pandemic, which resulted in a substantial disruption and reconfiguration of home health services. Things that were not consistently used, such as telehealth and an extensive amount of personal protective equipment, have become standard of practice when caring for individuals in the home health setting. Unfortunately, inconsistent internet coverage in rural communities and remote countries can pose a barrier to virtual access to healthcare services such as telehealth.

Summary

Therapist practice settings are diverse, and each practice setting requires a unique skill set and modes of interacting with the rest of the IDT. Within the acute hospital setting, access to the IDT is often regularly available, but the patients are rarely medically stable. Conversely, in the outpatient, community, and home health settings, the therapist may have different barriers in coordination with the IDT, but the patient is generally more medically stable. In order for the therapist to provide patient-centered care in their specific practice area, knowledge of the person's journey at other points in their care continuum will provide for improved transitions in care and quality outcomes.

References

1 Pack QR, Squires RW, Lopez-Jimenez F, et al. The current and potential capacity for cardiac rehabilitation utilization in the United States. *J Cardiopulm Rehabil.* 2014;34(5):318–326.

2 Gladieux JE, Basile M. Jimmo and the improvement standard: Implementing medicare coverage through regulations, policy manuals and other guidance. *Am J Law Med.* 2014;40(1):7–25. doi:10.1177/009885881404000101.

3 Billingham MJ, Billingham S. Congruence between preferred and actual place of death according to the presence of malignant or non-malignant disease: A systematic review and meta-analysis. *BMJ Support Palliat Care.* 2013;3(2):144. doi:10.1136/bmjspcare-2012-000292.

4 Su CT, McMahan RD, Williams BA, Sharma RK, Sudore RL. Family matters: Effects of birth order, culture, and family dynamics on surrogate decision-making. *J Am Geriatr Soc.* 2014;62(1):175–182. doi:10.1111/jgs.12610.

5 Tompkins J, Norris T, Levenhagen K, et al. Laboratory values interpretation resource. Academy of Acute Care Physical Therapy – APTA Task Force on Lab Values. https://www.acutept.org/page/ResourceGuides. Published 2017. Accessed June 28, 2020.
6 Fischbach FT, Dunning MB. *A Manual of Laboratory and Diagnostic Tests*. 9th ed. Philadelphia, PA: Wolters Kluwer Health; 2015.
7 West JM. Ethical issues in the care of Jehovah's Witnesses. *Curr Opin Anaesthesiol*. 2014;27(2):170–176. doi:10.1097/ACO.0000000000000053.
8 Organisation for Economic Co-operation and Development. Length of hospital stay (indicator). Organisation for Economic Co-operation and Development website. doi:10.1787/8dda6b7a-en. Published 2019. Accessed on June 28, 2020.
9 Cassel JB, Kerr K, Pantilat S, Smith TJ. PC consultation and hospital length of stay. *J Palliat Med*. 2010;13(6):761–767.
10 Smith BA, Fields CJ, Fernandez N. Physical therapists make accurate and appropriate discharge recommendations for patients who are acutely ill. *Phys Ther*. 2010;90(5):693–703.
11 Falvey JR, Burke RE, Malone D, Ridgeway KJ, McManus BM, Stevens-Lapsley JE. Role of physical therapists in reducing hospital readmissions: Optimizing outcomes for older adults during care transitions from hospital to community. *Phys Ther*. 2016;96(8):1125–1134.
12 Shoemaker MJ, Gutowski A, Mallgren M, et al. Physical therapist determination of discharge disposition in the acute care setting. *J Acute Care Phys Ther*. 2019;10(3):93–106.
13 Holm SE, Mu K. Discharge planning for the elderly in acute care: The perceptions of experienced occupational therapists. *Phys Occup Ther Geriatr*. 2012;30(3):214–228.
14 Guo Y, Persyn L, Palmer JL, Bruera E. Incidence of and risk factors for transferring cancer patients from rehabilitation to acute care units. *Am J Phys Med Rehabil*. 2008;87(8):647–653.
15 Tian W. An all-payer view of hospital discharge to postacute care, 2013. *HCUP Statistical Brief*. 2016;205:1–17.
16 Breeden LE. Occupational therapy home safety intervention via telehealth. *Int J Telerehabil*. 2016;8(1):29.
17 Keglovits M, Somerville E, Stark S. In-home occupational performance evaluation for providing assistance (I–HOPE assist): An assessment for informal caregivers. *Am J Occup Ther*. 2015;69(5):6905290010p1-6905290010p9.
18 Wilson CM, Stiller CH, Doherty DJ, Thompson KA. The role of physical therapists within hospice and PC in the United States and Canada. *Am J Hosp Palliat Med*. 2017;34(1):34–41. doi:10.1177/1049909115604668.
19 Stark SL, Somerville EK, Morris JC. In-home occupational performance evaluation (I–HOPE). *Am J Occup Ther*. 2010;64(4):580–589.
20 Chiu T, Oliver R. Factor analysis and construct validity of the SAFER-HOME. *OTJR*. 2006;26(4):132–142.
21 Mackenzie L, Byles J, Higginbotham N. Reliability of the home falls and accidents screening tool (HOME FAST) for identifying older people at increased risk of falls. *Disabil Rehabil*. 2002;24(5):266–274.
22 Clemson L, Fitzgerald MH, Heard R, Cumming RG. Inter-rater reliability of a home fall hazards assessment tool. *OTJR*. 1999;19(2):83–98. doi:10.1177/153944929901900201.
23 Clemson L, Fitzgerald MH, Heard R. Content validity of an assessment tool to identify home fall hazards: The Westmead home safety assessment. *Br J Occup Ther*. 1999;62(4):171–179. doi:10.1177/030802269906200407.

20 Safe Patient Handling and Mobility

Christopher M. Wilson and Amy J. Litterini

Introduction

In cases of advanced illness or disability, individuals may present with fluctuating, declining, or unpredictable physical performance and yet still wish to participate in out-of-bed activity, or require assistance with physical tasks such as scooting up in bed or getting into a chair. In order to accomplish this physical mobility, specific devices and techniques are available to assist caregivers and patients in optimizing quality of life (QoL). *Safe patient handling and mobility* (SPHM) "involves the use of assistive devices to ensure that patients can be mobilized safely and that care providers avoid performing high-risk manual patient handling tasks."[1] Using these devices reduces a care provider's risk of injury and improves the safety and quality of patient care. Each of these devices and techniques has its own set of benefits and risks. This chapter will discuss options for patient mobility at a variety of physical levels, in order for the therapist to facilitate safe mobility.

Promoting Activity within the Context Physical Variability

Among occupations, healthcare professionals such as nurses and therapists experience some of the highest rates of work-related musculoskeletal disorders.[2-4] Most of these injuries are sustained in the back, neck, and shoulders, but areas such as knees and elbows may also be affected.[5] Often this occurs while assisting patient mobility with higher forces than otherwise advisable. Unfortunately, in the culture of some healthcare institutions, protecting healthcare providers from injuries remains a lower priority than expediency or other concerns. In some jurisdictions, institutions, or nations, a significant push for a "minimal lift environment" or "no lift environment" has begun over the past several decades.[6] As an example, the Canadian Centre for Occupational Health and Safety defines this as

> "A no-lift policy would state that all manual handling tasks are to be avoided where ever possible. No-lift policies successfully reduce the risk only if the organization has the infrastructure in place (e.g., technical

solutions, lifts, equipment, and administrative commitment) to support the initiative. Training is also necessary for caregivers to recognize the risk in activities, and how to follow appropriate steps to move or transfer a patient safely, including use of a gait belt or transfer belt."[7]

Although this is not yet universal, there are significant gains in implementing a minimal/no lift environment. Despite this, there are many administrative and financial barriers to institutions adopting more consistent use of SPHM.

In addition to safe patient handling, using mechanical equipment, some manual transfers, and mobility assistance may be required by healthcare providers and caregivers. A key principle in transfers is carefully avoiding

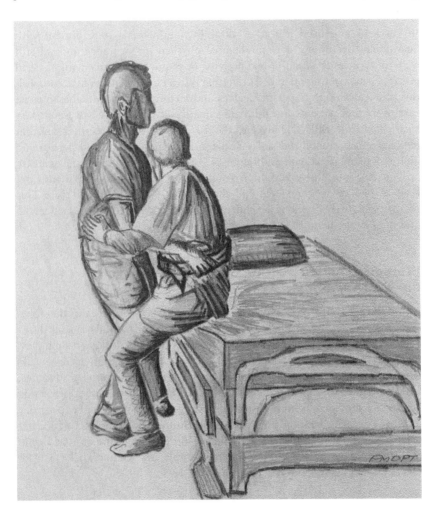

Figure 20.1 Gait Belt and Body Mechanics during Transfers. Illustration by Paul Mangiafico PT, DPT.

lifting more weight than is safe. In a seminal article entitled "When is it Safe to Manually Lift a Patient?" published in 2007, Waters[8] established a benchmark of 35 lbs. (16 kg) as a safe lifting capacity for healthcare workers. Although potentially useful as a guideline, an arbitrary lifting limit has engendered controversy, as this limit may even be excessive in biomechanically disadvantageous environments such as lifting from a low surface or with arms extended. For example, the United States National Institute for Occupational Safety and Health "shares in the consensus among patient handling professionals that the goal of safe patient handling programs should be to eliminate all manual lifting whenever possible."[9p1]

Other key principles of safe patient mobility include: getting as close to the patient as possible (short lever arms); avoid twisting at the spinal column, maintaining a neutral spine (not too flexed, extended, or rotated); bending at the knees during a lift, using a gait or transfer belt; both individuals should have proper footwear (Figure 20.1). If it is anticipated that the healthcare worker may be nearing the limits of what is safe to lift alone, assistance should be requested from a colleague, but generally, mechanical lifting equipment should be considered before requesting more assistance. Finally, the individual being transferred should be well aware of what is happening, what they can expect during the transfer, and how they can assist after thorough instruction beforehand. Finally, a therapist training a caregiver on how to transfer someone should also consider the physical capabilities and limitations of the caregiver before initiating transfer training. For example, it may not be advisable to have an elderly spouse with a history of back pain attempt to transfer their significant other and risk injury to both parties.

One of the key challenges for therapists who are providing restorative or adaptive services to individuals with a life-threatening illness is that there may be two levels of physical mobility: one in which the therapist is working to progress or train the patient, and the other routinely performed by nursing staff and caregivers, considering the patient's current functional and physical capacity. In some cases, this may cause confusion as there may be instances where the nursing team or caregivers observe an individual ambulating to the bathroom one time with the PT or OT, and logically assumes that the patient can consistently make it to the bathroom without difficulty. This may result in the nursing team attempting such ambulation and not being successful (possibly leading to a safety event) as it was not clearly communicated between PT/OT and nursing that this ambulation occurred in highly engineered circumstances under the unique skills, monitoring, and guidance of the PT or OT. This is a scenario where clear communication, verbally and within the medical record, are imperative to clearly state what the individual's current mobility status is in order to avoid falls or other mobility-related issues.

One mechanism to address this issue is having a PT or OT update the activity level orders within the medical record or facilitating the physician to do so, as allowable by institutional policy and jurisdictional laws. Additionally, an easy-to-read, accessible handoff sign that is posted in the individual's room which is updated regularly can help all disciplines to know the person's daily mobility capacity.[10] This handoff sheet could be laminated and posted in patient rooms and updated regularly via a dry-erase marker so that anyone who assists with mobility knows how much activity an individual is able to perform.

Safe Mobility Emergency Techniques

As noted above, physical and medical variability is to be expected when caring for those with a life-threatening illness and several extra safety principles are warranted. These may include following behind the patient with a chair or having a family or caregiver follow with a chair in case an individual becomes unexpectedly fatigued or short of breath during ambulation or mobility (Figure 20.2).

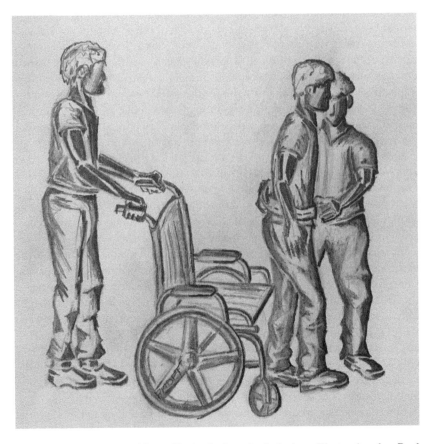

Figure 20.2 Following with a Chair during Ambulation. Illustration by Paul Mangiafico PT, DPT.

Orthostatic Hypotension and Physical Counterpressure Maneuvers

A relatively common event when working with individuals who are medically unstable is orthostatic hypotension. This condition is characterized by an acute drop in blood pressure when changing position, most commonly from lying down to sitting to standing in a rapid manner. There are a number of potential causes of orthostatic hypotension including neurologic disorders (Parkinson's disease, multiple sclerosis), oncologic conditions (spinal cord tumors), autonomic neuropathies, as well as sustained bed rest (from delayed or failed baroreceptor reflexes).[11] In addition, anemia and dehydration can cause orthostatic hypotension.[10] Prevention and early identification of these hypotensive episodes is an important step in preventing a fall or emergency intervention (e.g. lowering a patient to a floor or needing to emergently call out for assistance to get a chair). In some cases, despite the vigilant screening and efforts by a therapist, a patient may experience progressive hypotension without any precursor symptoms. In these situations, interventions such as physical counterpressure maneuvers (PCMs) can be the difference between

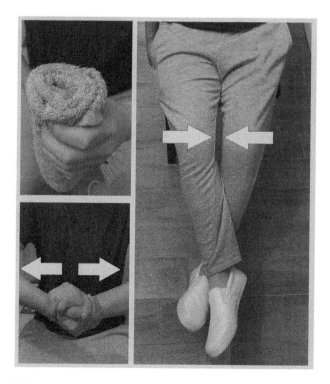

Figure 20.3 Physical Counterpressure Maneuvers.

needing to lower a patient to the ground or coaching the patient through these emergency procedures until a safe, secure place to sit or lie is encountered.

After identifying that a syncopal event is imminent, the therapist quickly selects one out of the three PCM maneuvers that is applicable based on the patient's condition and location (e.g. choosing an upper extremity maneuver when in a standing position or after lower extremity surgery) (Figure 20.3). The therapist rapidly uses concise verbal commands to have the patient maintain this sustained isometric contraction for as long as possible. Meanwhile, immediate actions should be pursued to return the patient to a stable location (e.g. a chair or bed). Finally, further medical evaluation is warranted after PCMs are applied in the event that the precipitating cause is an evolving medical event (e.g. cardiac arrest). Although uncommon, application of PCMs may help to quickly and safely physically stabilize a patient and reduce the risk of injury during physical mobility.

Use Bed Mechanics to Your Advantage

As most therapists are aware, having the patient assist with generating forces to move and transfer can also minimize the risk of injury to the therapist and/ or the patient, and instructing the patient to use their arms or legs to assist is warranted. In addition, there are some bed mechanical systems that experienced therapists have employed to minimize the amount of force transmitted through the therapist's body. One example is when working to sit at the edge of the bed, instead of having the patient pull on the therapist or be manually lifted into a sitting position, mechanically elevating the head of the bed may assist with this procedure. Once the bed is in a full seated and upright position, then the therapist only has to provide steadying support of the upper body while assisting by laterally moving the legs one at a time to the edge of the bed.

One mobility activity that healthcare providers can always anticipate is a patient needing to scoot up toward the head of the bed, as with any elevation of the head of the bed, gravity will over time slide them downwards. During this procedure, friction and shear forces must be mitigated. Especially as an individual becomes progressively bedbound, this repeated boosting and scooting up in bed can result in skin tears and wounds from the frequent shearing forces. There are a number of friction-reducing devices that can assist with this that will be described in the next section on safe patient handling; however, if these are not available, putting the bed flat then into a tilt position with the head lower than the feet (aka the Trendelenburg position) can assist the caregivers in boosting an individual up (Figure 20.4). The use of a folded draw sheet under the patient's trunk across the bed can also help eliminate friction and is useful, especially in home environments.

For patients who may have difficulty with ascending from a seated to a standing position, it may be beneficial to use the bed elevation mechanism to assist with improving the mechanical advantage of a sit to stand transfer. This technique should be used with extreme caution because if the patient

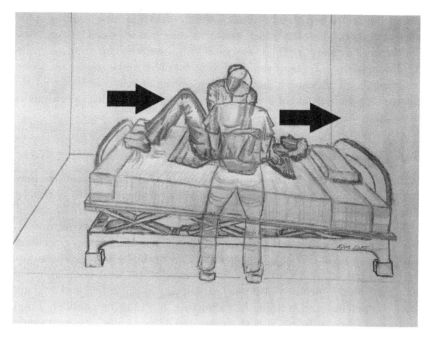

Figure 20.4 Boosting Up in Bed Using Trendelenburg Position. Illustration by Paul Mangiafico PT, DPT.

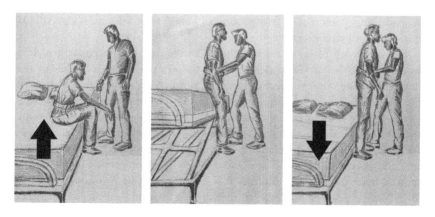

Figure 20.5 Using Bed Elevation Mode to Assist to Stand and Immediate Lowering of the Bed. Illustration by Paul Mangiafico PT, DPT.

does not have enough strength to ascend from sit to stand, his or her standing tolerance may be quite limited. It is highly recommended that after the person achieves a standing position, the bed immediately be lowered down so that the individual does not attempt to sit down on an elevated bed and slide onto the floor (Figure 20.5). In addition, this also places the patient's backside more completely on the bed (a more secure position) when returning to sitting at the edge of the bed. There is a subset of patients, after being assisted into standing via therapist support or via bed elevation assistance, who can stand and walk a substantial distance; however, this is quite variable and it should always be assumed that a patient will not be able to safely ambulate and appropriate safety precautions would be warranted, such as following with a wheelchair as depicted in Figure 20.2).

Safe Patient Handling and Mobility Devices

Within therapy, there are four main domains of SPHM equipment that may be readily applied in situations while working with those with advanced disability or weakness. They are as follows: (1) devices to assist with ambulation; (2) standing frames; (3) mechanical dependent lift systems; and (4) bed mobility, scooting and boosting devices. Each of these devices comes with its own set of unique challenges and opportunities for patient comfort and clinician safety. Issues like infection control, physical accessibility of machines on the specified care unit, patient weight capacities, and ongoing staff competency and training, are domains that must be considered and addressed when utilizing SPHM equipment. For example, one commonly encountered technical issue in the communal use of SPHM equipment is proper storage and charging of portable batteries, or plugging in units that have a full battery charge. If a hurried provider neglects to perform this step, the next provider who attempts to utilize this device may be met with a dead battery, increased frustration, and loss of confidence in the SPHM devices for all parties involved.

For nearly all of these devices there are varying weight capacities. It is essential that the provider identifies and follows the weight capacity of the device to assure that the individual does not exceed the weight capacity of the specified device. Different manufacturers have different weight capacities and there is no universal code or size limit that therapists can refer to by default. Each individual machine from a different manufacturer has unique weight capacities. For dependent mechanical lifts, there are battery-powered lifts and there are non-electrical lifts that elevate using screw mechanisms, cranks, hydraulics, or pneumatics. It is rare that private insurances will pay for a battery-powered or electrical-mechanical lift, and these devices are generally cost-prohibitive for families paying for them out of their own pocket. Some insurance companies will cover the non-electric mechanical lift with appropriate documentation and justification of medical necessity by the care team. This often includes the therapist writing a letter of medical necessity to the patient's insurance company to approve the payment.

One important consideration when prescribing or obtaining SPHM devices includes a clear understanding of the individual's anticipated lifespan. If the person has only days to live with a rapidly advancing disease process, working through the logistics of a mechanical lift purchase that an individual may only use once or twice may not be the best use of time and resources of the patient, family, and care team. Resources may be better applied in establishing other ways to accomplish the same goal of optimizing the remaining QoL.

Devices to Assist with Ambulation

A useful set of devices to assist individuals with mobility include ambulation vests and mechanical supports that partially or completely unweight an individual when they are generally able to propel themselves in a horizontal direction under some amount of their own power (Figure 20.6). Often this device utilizes a vest or cloth sling placed between the legs to assist with physical unweighting. With each of these devices, the therapist must carefully consider the patient's physical status in local anatomic areas as well as any tubes and lines, injuries, wounds, or continence issues.

For example, if a patient has rib fractures or rib metastases, a vest that cinches tightly around the rib cage may not be appropriate. Conversely, a patient who is incontinent of urine or feces may not be a good candidate for utilizing a sling between the legs without additional protection or adaptations. As individuals with advanced life-threatening illness often have unpredictable ambulatory performance, this device will provide a safety net if a patient's legs buckle unexpectedly or the patient has ataxia, spasticity, or choreiform movements. These ambulation devices can provide extra support and safety to reduce the risk of falls and give patients confidence in performing potentially fear-inducing tasks, and are most commonly used in an inpatient setting.

Standing Frames

There are two main types of standing frames: mechanical and non-mechanical. A non-mechanical standing frame generally utilizes a patient's upper body strength to leverage their body from a seated to a standing position (Figure 20.7). Once the individual is standing, the seat pads are rotated downward so that the patient can rest upon them in a semi-seated/semi-standing position. In order to utilize this type of standing frame, the person should have adequate trunk strength and sitting balance to control their upper body while in the upright position. This device has several advantages as it is on wheels and once upright, the person can be mobilized to another seated surface like a toilet or remain in a semi-standing position with little to no lower extremity muscle force.

Case Example: A unique application of SPHM equipment was with a 25-year-old male presenting with lower extremity paralysis after a traumatic lumbar spinal cord injury at the L3 level. After lumbar stabilization surgery, he became very withdrawn and exhibited symptoms of depression. The therapists utilized this device to help him achieve an upright standing position and once achieved, the therapist assisted him by propelling the standing frame

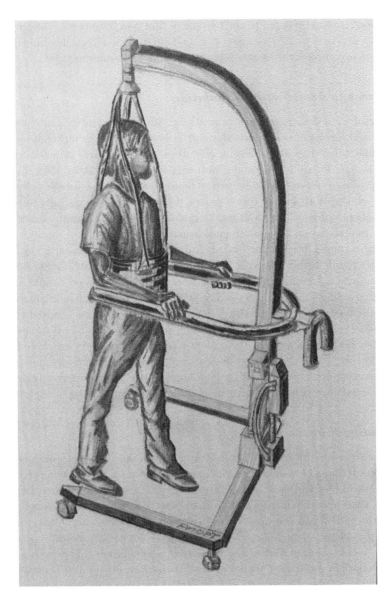

Figure 20.6 Mechanical Lift with a Walking Vest. Illustration by Paul Mangiafico PT, DPT.

around the unit. He was able to stand and talk with the nurses at the nurses' station. Later, he credited this moment to demonstrate to him that there was hope for his functional status and his ongoing ability to live a life of meaning and substance. Although the transfer with the mechanical standing frame was a dependent transfer and essentially did not require much physical or

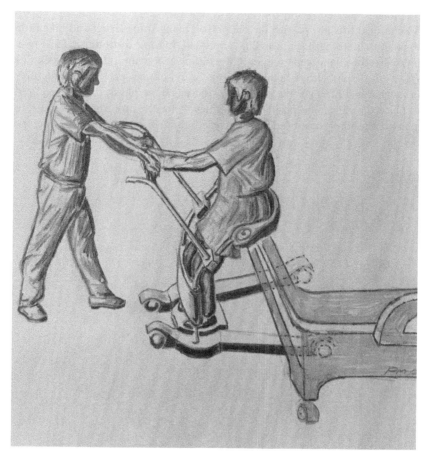

Figure 20.7 Non-mechanical Standing Frame. Illustration by Paul Mangiafico PT, DPT.

rehabilitative support from the therapist, this therapeutic intervention had a substantial impact on his mental and emotional status. This newfound hope encouraged him to return home and live a fulfilling life.

The other type of standing frame is mechanical. In general, this device has a belt that wraps around the person's waist and fastens to a platform to assist with standing. As with the ambulation devices, depending on the location of the forces transmitted through the body, this device may be contraindicated in certain disorders or conditions. For example, both standing frames require both anterior proximal tibias and knees to sustain nearly the person's entire body weight. If the patient has lower extremity fractures, extensive bone metastases, or other conditions that would be exacerbated from this force transmission, this may not be a viable option to assist with upright activities or out-of-bed activities. If life expectancy is long enough, standing frames can be considered for home use.

Mechanical Dependent Lift Systems

Mechanical lifts are passive for the person being transported and take little to no muscle strength (Figures 20.8 and 20.9). In some institutions, these may be referred to by a trade name – for example, these are often referred to as *Hoyer lifts* despite Hoyer being the name brand of one specific manufacturer of mechanical lifts. For the caregivers, there is some physical effort required to place the slings and position the lift device for the procedure; however, in general the forces required are much less than pivot-transferring a person

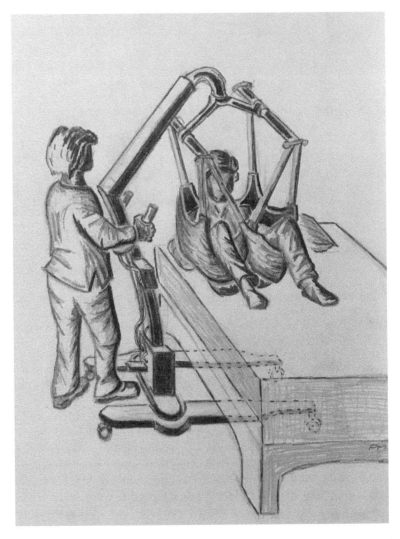

Figure 20.8 Mechanical Lift to or from Bed. Illustration by Paul Mangiafico PT, DPT.

using two or three caregivers. Sling placement and positioning also require some level of mechanical aptitude, physical dexterity, and fine motor coordination. Some sling devices can be placed under a person seated in a chair by leaning them forward and placing straps under the person's legs before fastening it to the device. This type of sling also has the added advantage of keeping the patient's perineal area accessible if toileting, cleansing, or skin inspection activities are required. Practical use of these lifts at home often still requires two-person assist and can be limited by environmental space and surface considerations.

With these devices, there may be certain conditions or diagnoses that also may warrant further investigation before application. Often these devices

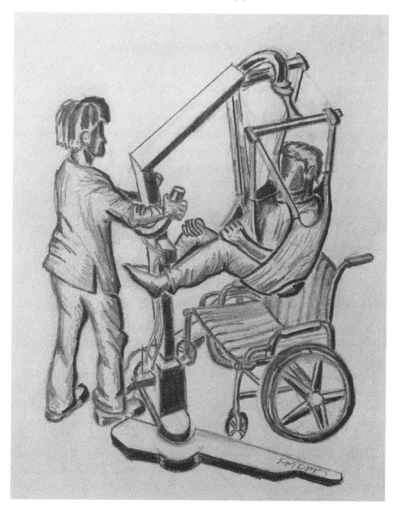

Figure 20.9 Mechanical Lift to or from Wheelchair. Illustration by Paul Mangiafico PT, DPT.

apply some amount of forward flexion (kyphotic) positioning of the lower and middle back. If the individual has bony metastasis, compression fractures, or has had spinal surgery, a discussion with an orthopedic physician or neurosurgeon may be indicated before the use of a mechanical lift. In addition, as the leg portion of the slings may place torsional stress on the hips and femurs, a patient with a pelvic, hip, or femur issue may not be a candidate for a mechanical lift. When used safely and appropriately, these devices can allow an individual and their families to safely achieve upright positioning to access wheelchairs and commodes. This upright, seated positioning can improve QoL by facilitating active social engagement and improved ability to eat meals in a sitting position, which may improve nutrient intake and allow for more efficient swallowing while reducing the risk of aspiration.

Bed Mobility, Scooting, and Boosting Devices

In addition to the devices described earlier, individuals with a terminal illness or chronic condition may encounter temporary or permanent difficulty with changing positions or moving around in bed. When turning or boosting patients up in bed, it generally requires at least two individuals exerting a substantial amount of force and has been documented as one of the main care activities that can result in a musculoskeletal injury.[12] This task is also often challenging because it requires healthcare providers to lean forward and places excessive strain on their back musculature and spinal column while performing a shifting or boosting motion. If possible, elevation of the bed surface is a primary option to reduce potential strain. In order to reduce the physical load on the caregiver's muscles, bones, and joints, several options for improving bed mobility tasks are available and may be used in a variety of situational circumstances.

Passive Friction-Reducing Devices

In order to reduce friction and shear, there are friction-reducing devices that can be placed underneath the patient in preparation for repositioning activities such as boosting up in bed or sliding from one surface to the other (e.g. stretcher/gurney to bed). There are several models available from different manufacturers, but in general, these consist of either one or two separate sheets made of plastic or some other slippery material. The other commonly encountered bed mobility device is an inflatable air cushion that is placed under the patient. Some of the advantages of these devices are that they greatly reduce the amount of force required to move a patient in a laying position. As with some of the other devices, infection control and cost containment are important considerations. In general, these devices are not designed to be kept underneath the patient, as they are typically not moisture permeable. Sweat and other bodily fluids may build up if they remain underneath the person causing infections or skin breakdown. Finally, one of the disadvantages of these devices is that they still require the healthcare providers to have the person roll from side to side (aka logrolling) to be able to get the device underneath them. This may be an added task that was not otherwise required if two providers were simply coming in to boost a patient up in bed using a previously placed cloth draw sheet. Biomechanically, rolling side to side is generally less strenuous on caregivers than the actual boosting, but the logrolling and then boosting tends to take a little more time.

When two slide sheets are laid on top of each other, they result in a decrease in friction. Some of the slide sheets are for dedicated patient use where one patient will use it for their entire stay and then it is disposed of, while others are reusable after decontamination. At a longer term care facility (e.g. extended care facility or skilled nursing facility), there may be more benefit from the dedicated single patient use devices; conversely, it may not be cost economical to utilize these single patient use devices in a hospital setting with a generally short length of stay.

Air Cushion Bed Mobility Devices

Utilizing a similar methodology of placing a device under a supine person in bed is the concept of air cushion lateral transfer devices. These devices are designed to be placed under the patient via the logroll technique and there is an attachable air compressor device. This device, when attached and activated, will inflate the air cushion underneath the patient and allow for a safe, efficient, low-effort in-bed repositioning (Figure 20.10). This is most frequently and efficiently applied during lateral slide transfers (e.g. sliding a person from a bed to a stretcher/gurney/recliner wheelchair). Instead of using a cloth draw sheet and three to four people for this lateral transfer, it can be safely done by two individuals with an overall decreased risk of injury.

Finally, there are specialized air cushion devices that can lift individuals over a meter in the vertical direction. One example of this is the HoverJack (http://www.hovermatt.com/hoverjack.html). This may be useful if a person is unexpectedly found on the floor and is unable to return to bed without assistance. If one of these devices is available, the cushions can be inflated to the bed height and a lateral slide transfer can be accomplished. This is a safer technique than having four to five people manually lift a person off the floor and place them in bed. Innovations like these devices can accomplish the goals of safe in-bed mobility without excessive strain or forces on caregivers.

Summary

In any setting, patient functional status and performance may fluctuate and thus requires the therapist to consider alternative means to accomplish mobility-related tasks and interventions. In order to protect the safety of the patient, therapist, and caregivers, application of SPHM equipment should be considered. In order to determine the most appropriate technique and device,

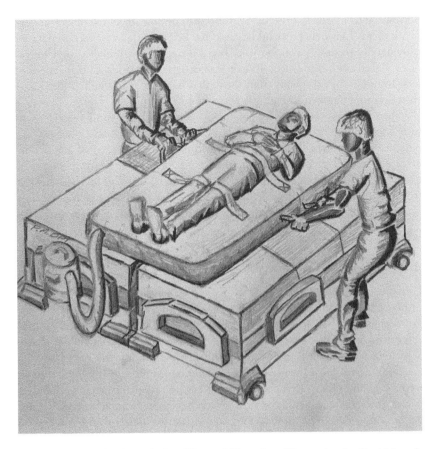

Figure 20.10 Air Cushion Assisted Lateral Transfers. Illustration by Paul Mangi-afico PT, DPT.

the therapist must perform a critical analysis of the task, the patient's current and future physical status, and the capacity of those assisting with the mobility task. Mobility-assist devices, when applied appropriately and judiciously, can help individuals and their families with mobility to engage in daily tasks and enriching life activities.

References

1 US Department of Veterans Affairs. Safe patient handling and mobility (SPHM). https://www.publichealth.va.gov/employeehealth/patient-handling/index.asp. Updated 2016. Accessed June 1, 2020.
2 Rozenfeld V, Ribak J, Danziger J, Tsamir J, Carmeli E. Prevalence, risk factors and preventive strategies in work-related musculoskeletal disorders among Israeli physical therapists. *Physiother Res Int.* 2010;15(3):176–184.

3 Yasobant S, Rajkumar P. Health of the healthcare professionals: A risk assessment study on work-related musculoskeletal disorders in a tertiary hospital, Chennai, India. *Int J Med Public Health*. 2015;5(2):189–195.

4 Hong J, Koo J. Work-related musculoskeletal diseases and occupational injuries in health care workers. *J Korean Med Assoc*. 2010;53(6):446–453.

5 Pompeii LA, Lipscomb HJ, Schoenfisch AL, Dement JM. Musculoskeletal injuries resulting from patient handling tasks among hospital workers. *Am J Ind Med*. 2009;52(7):571–578. doi:10.1002/ajim.20704.

6 de Ruiter H, Liaschenko J. To lift or not to lift: Patient-handling practices. *AAOHN J*. 2011;59(8):337–343. doi:10.1177/216507991105900802.

7 Government of Canada, Canadian Centre for Occupational Health and Safety. Ergonomic safe patient handling program: OSH answers. https://www.ccohs.ca/oshanswers/hsprograms/patient_handling.html. Updated June 1, 2020. Accessed June 1, 2020.

8 Waters TR. When is it safe to manually lift a patient? *Am J Nurs*. 2007;107(8):53–58.

9 Centers for Disease Control and Prevention. Safe Patient Handling and Mobility (SPHM). The National Institute for Occupational Safety and Health (NIOSH) website. https://www.cdc.gov/niosh/topics/safepatient/default.html. Updated August 2, 2013. Accessed August 16, 2020.

10 Wilson CM, Richards NL, Slavin B, et al. Nursing staff perceptions and fall rates with a quality improvement project for mobility screening and written bedside communication: A pretest-posttest design. *Am J SPHM*. 2015;5(2):55–65.

11 Low PA, Tomalia VA. Orthostatic hypotension: Mechanisms, causes, management. *J Clin Neurol*. 2015;11(3):220–226.

12 Weiner C, Alperovitch-Najenson D, Ribak J, Kalichman L. Prevention of nurses' work-related musculoskeletal disorders resulting from repositioning patients in bed: Comprehensive narrative review. *Workplace Health Saf*. 2015;63(5):226–232. doi:10.1177/2165079915580037.

Part IV

Policy, Research, and Education

21 Education on Palliative and End-of-Life Care

Christopher M. Wilson and Amy J. Litterini

Introduction

Every intervention, clinical skill, and assessment technique provided by a therapist was a pearl of knowledge that was taught to them or was gathered by experience. The core skills of providing palliative care (PC) and physical activity to an individual with a life-threatening illness are no different. As this care approach is relatively new, the concepts are not well integrated within entry-level or postgraduate therapist educational offerings, which may even limit basic awareness of this care approach. This chapter will discuss best practices and describe useful resources to assist therapists to learn and teach key PC skills. Finally, in this chapter there are specific examples of educational contributions by a variety of institutions for the reader to consider when beginning to further their own education or that of their colleagues.

How Much Palliative Care to Teach?

Although assisting in the physical activity and rehabilitative goals of those with incurable physical impairments are within the scope of many therapists' practice and are strongly embedded in the entry-level curriculum, there is very little education concentrated toward the late-stage, palliative management of an individual with a life-threatening illness. This begets the question, how much PC should we include in entry-level training of the therapists, as much of this book has established the importance of this clinical approach in the overall improvement of a nation's healthcare system. In 2017, Wilson et al.[1] interviewed therapists from the United States and Canada working in hospice and PC and the overall theme identified was that an introduction to the role of the therapist in PC is important, as well as educating them on some basic concepts and treatment paradigms. However, it was found that an in-depth, competency-based mastery of the topic was not an effective use of the limited amount of time, as most therapy curriculums are extremely full with the various technical aspects of becoming a therapist.[1] It was discussed that resources and time may be better spent introducing the topic in a case-based format to increase the overall awareness of the therapist's role in PC, and where to obtain additional mentoring or continuing education after graduation.[1]

When considering the occupational therapist's (OT's) unique role and contribution toward focusing on adapting activities of daily living (ADLs) and optimizing occupation, Meredith[2] examined entry-level occupational therapy programs in Australia and New Zealand and also surveyed OTs currently practicing in PC. The investigator found that OT schools provided between 2 and 10 hours of PC-specific content. Only 45.8% of OTs recalled receiving undergraduate content in PC, and 75% reported not feeling prepared to practice in PC. OTs who received PC training reported feeling more prepared to practice in PC as compared to those who did not receive PC-specific content. In this study, recommendations were made to establish foundational PC content in OT curriculums.[2] These included OT-specific interventions such as energy conservation, stress management, goal setting, and problem-solving. Participants also recommended education on communication skills, medical aspects of PC, and the unique focus of service delivery in PC such as individualized, client-focused interventions. Finally, OTs practicing in PC also recommended education in the OT's role in bereavement, end-of-life (EoL) care, and psychosocial aspects, and emphasized the importance of "real life learning" via clinical case studies and fieldwork placements. Other relevant topics included self-care, ethical and cultural factors, defining PC, and interprofessional roles.

Proposed within this chapter will be a potential framework for establishing an introductory didactic learning module for therapist students enrolled in entry-level curriculum (Table 21.1). This module is aimed toward generalist therapists who are only periodically providing care for individuals in PC or with life-threatening illnesses. Within an entry-level program, this may entail a one- to three-hour lecture on the specifics of PC and EoL care for the individual profession's role in this practice area, although some institutions with an increased volume of this population may elect to increase the

Table 21.1 Palliative Care and End-of-Life Example Lesson Plan – Two Hours

Minutes	Topic
0–5	Review learning objectives and play Mrs. Dubois Videos 1 + 2
5–20	Detailed history of hospice, palliative care, and impact on healthcare (reducing readmissions, quality of life)
20–35	Discuss care team members and highlight the importance of interdisciplinary team meetings
35–60	Communication skills for therapists including VitalTalk videos. Participants practice in partners with case JP using GUIDE steps
60–75	Describe disease trajectories with case examples
75–90	Outline Briggs' models for therapist services in palliative care with discussion on case examples. Mrs. Dubois videos of various stages of the disease process.
90–110	Five small groups. Activity matching patient cases with Briggs' models including practicing writing a goal for a chosen case
110–120	Question and answer session

curriculum content or duration. Embedded throughout most therapist curricula are discussions of common incurable conditions (i.e. cerebrovascular accident, Parkinson's disease, spinal cord injury), and the subsequent impairments, activity limitations, and participation restrictions. However, an overall understanding of the therapists' role in PC is not always immediately understandable until a solid foundation of rehabilitation or "traditional" therapist skills is established. This module is likely most appropriate in the final portion of a didactic curriculum, ideally before therapist students begin their final clinical affiliations or fieldwork training.

Some sample learning objectives from this session may include

1   The participant will be able to identify when individuals with terminal illness may be appropriate for PC or hospice/EoL care and how to initiate a referral to an appropriate provider.
2   The participant will be able to adapt their clinical documentation procedures and goal writing when providing care for those with a life-threatening illness and varying stages of the disease process.
3   The participant will be able to list three best practices for having a difficult conversation and identify one resource where they could learn more about this topic.
4   The participant will be able to competently and confidently initiate a simulated difficult conversation with a peer to convey bad news followed by self-reflection on improving their approach during patient care.
5   The participant will be able to, after reflection on their own previous practice experience or current practice setting, identify three areas where adaptations to the administrative infrastructure and care team integration would be necessary to provide care for those with life-threatening illnesses.

Based on the aforementioned learning objectives, recommendations for a curriculum include introducing a client in the early stage of a newly diagnosed disease process. This may be done by video vignette, role play, or a paper case report. One example of a useful video vignette was published in the Portal of Geriatrics Online Education (www.pogoe.org) by the Medical College of Wisconsin. This vignette features actors playing a physician and his patient, Mrs. Dubois, who are shown in various stages of a breast cancer diagnosis (Figure 21.1).[3] These videos also demonstrate physical changes and psychosocial/emotional issues from initial diagnosis through death (https://pogoe.org/productid/18397). In the initial diagnosis stage, the case may be discussed within the context of a therapist's preventative or exercise-based interventions. By this point in their careers, most students ending their didactic curriculum or experienced clinicians should be able to identify early therapeutic interventions, as cancer symptoms will not have

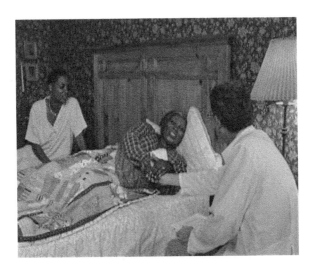

Figure 21.1 Mrs. Dubois End-of-Life Training Video. Medical College of Wisconsin licensed to the Portal of Geriatrics Online Education. https://pogoe.org/productid/18397.

substantially evolved. After this and subsequent discussion of breast cancer treatment and sequelae issues relevant to physical therapy, a useful approach would be to detail the care philosophy of PC and hospice practice/EoL practice. This will include similarities, differences, and interactions with care team members.

Following this introduction, an exercise may be implemented in small groups based on a case scenario and a therapist practicing the skills of how to deliver difficult news. A useful resource for this may be playing videos from a PC organization such as Vital Talk (www.vitaltalk.org). There are several video examples and a variety of important and useful conversation guides which include delivering difficult news, dealing with emotion, facilitating such conversations, and EoL discussions. After this introduction and education in the conversation guides, participants can be presented with a case scenario where they use one of these guides (see Appendix 4).

A helpful case example to employ was one discussed in Chapter 6. *JP is a 59-year-old male who is an executive in an automobile manufacturing company. He has been previously diagnosed with lung cancer with spinal metastases. At the level of the T12 vertebrae, the spinal metastases have begun to encroach on the spinal cord causing progressive lower extremity paralysis and an inability to walk. As the therapist, you continue to identify that JP is exacerbating his pain substantially by performing in therapy and physical activity, however, JP's goals are to continue to work on ambulation. In your professional experience, you feel that ambulation may not be an achievable goal and that he may be making his quality of life worse by increasing his pain and potentially exacerbating his lower extremity paralysis.*

Utilizing the GUIDE steps as outlined on VitalTalk.org,[4] with a partner, practice communicating this information and delivering difficult news as the therapist to this patient, and that a new plan must be set forth. Following this practice conversation, an extensive group discussion on the challenges and best practices that participants experienced will assist with the synthesis and internalization of the concepts.

After introducing the topic of communication skills and having difficult conversations, the content can then shift to the specifics of the therapist's role in disease processes. Again, an additional video (e.g. Mrs. Dubois) or paper vignette of the initial patient's disease process may be beneficial, including symptom advancement and beginning stages of symptoms affecting body structures and functions, activities, and participation. This will lay the framework for the next content area of discussing varying disease trajectories and anticipating functional performance decline. The content on this area as described in Chapter 4, including the disease trajectory figures, would be beneficial to assist learners in understanding varying functional declines and how the therapist can adapt a treatment plan around these circumstances. After an introduction, and case examples of different disease trajectories and functional declines, participants would then be able to identify the specific functional decline of the previously introduced case. Having a group discussion about potential future functional impairments, activity limitations, and participation restrictions, and what a therapist could potentially do to anticipate and mitigate these issues could follow.

The next topic can transition toward different models of therapist care. For example, the description of Briggs' models of *rehabilitation light, case management, rehabilitation in reverse, skilled maintenance,* and *supportive care* would all be appropriate for discussion (Chapter 4).[5] In order to establish these abstract concepts within a clinical context, specific case vignettes could be presented by the instructor or solicited from the learners. Through these vignettes, additional examples of functional decline and disease trajectory with our previously introduced case can be detailed, including EoL issues and how a therapist could apply their skills and knowledge to provide optimum circumstances for a good death with dignity. Finally, patient case scenarios of each of Briggs' models can be assigned to participants with the aim of having the participants match a patient scenario with one of Briggs' treatment models. In addition, participants should practice goal-writing for these individual cases to reinforce writing patient-centered goals that are mindful of a declining disease trajectory.

Experiential Learning Opportunities

There is evidence of benefit for therapy students' participation in experiential PC seminars. In 2011, Kumar, Jim, and Sisodia[6] provided registration to physiotherapy students to participate in a six-hour interactive seminar. Content was delivered via lectures, case examples, and active demonstrations. Topics included the World Health Organization's definition of PC, "spiritual aspects of life, death and healing, principles, levels and models of palliative care, and role of physiotherapists in a palliative care team."[7] Physiotherapist-specific content included principles and models of assessment and care of persons at, or near, the EoL, goal setting, and strategic implementation of physiotherapy treatment. In order to evaluate efficacy of the students' experience with this activity, before and immediately after the session, students completed a 37-item self-report measure entitled the Physical Therapy in Palliative Care-Knowledge, Attitudes, Beliefs and Experiences scale (PTiPC-KABE Scale). The PTiPC-KABE consisted of both qualitative and quantitative data and statistically significant improvements were noted in PC knowledge, attitudes, beliefs, and experiences after the exercise with an overall total score improvement of 35.2%.[7]

Integrated clinical experiences (ICE) have grown in popularity in PT education programs. Shorter than traditional clinical rotations, ICE's allow for brief exposures to different settings where a full, multi-week rotation would be logistically challenging. Some programs have ICE's within their curriculum which allow for observation within unique settings such as inpatient hospice facilities and home care agencies providing hospice services.

Formal hospice volunteer training, with certification standards often mandated nationally (e.g. minimum of 20 hours of training in the United States), is an avenue for healthcare students wishing to learn about, and experience more, in a hospice setting. The additional benefit of experience interacting with individuals receiving hospice and their families, while providing service to the local region, provides a win-win opportunity for both healthcare major education programs and their local community partner hospice providers.

Since in-person experiences with patients at the EoL is often logistically difficult, and not feasible to provide for large cohorts of students across multiple programs, another experiential method some institutions and health care education programs are instituting is virtual reality (VR) patient simulation experiences. A VR simulation allows the student user to experience the perspective of a patient in hospice care through a scenario while wearing VR technology (i.e. audio headset and video goggles). At the University of New England (UNE), students enrolled in the medical professions (i.e. doctor of osteopathy, nursing, physician's assistant, PT, social work, and OT) are provided the simulation experience through the library within their coursework, with the goal of increasing awareness of the dying process and developing empathy through their VR experience as the dying patient

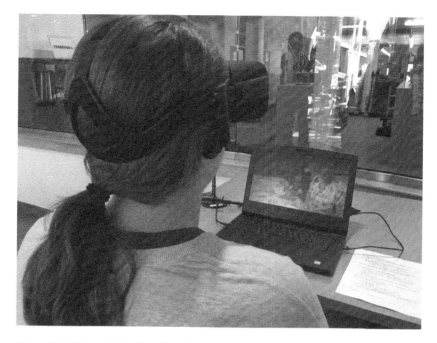

Figure 21.2 Virtual Reality Simulation. University of New England medical student Emily S uses the virtual reality lab to experience the end of life as "Clay." UNE students who use the lab experience the end of life as Clay in three stages. First, they meet with a doctor and receive the news that their diagnosis is terminal. Second, they are in the hospital after a fall, and a nurse begins the discussion about hospice care. In the third and final act, they experience the final moments of life in hospice care, surrounded by family and health workers as their senses fade away. Photo credit: University of New England.

(https://www.une.edu/news/2019/boston-globe-nbc-npr-feature-end-life-virtual-reality-simulation). See Chapter 23 for patient-specific clinical applications of VR (Figure 21.2).

Finally, for smaller cohorts of medical and other healthcare students, UNE's *Learning by Living 48-Hour Hospice Home Immersion*, a program created at UNE's College of Osteopathic Medicine, involves students participating in an immersive learning activity into the Gosnell Memorial Hospice Home in Scarborough, Maine, USA. As opposed to a traditional immersion experience where a student assumes the role of patient/resident in a particular setting (e.g. a skilled nursing facility), the students in the hospice immersion are active participants in patient, family, and post-mortem care during the 48-hours at the inpatient hospice (https://www.une.edu/news/2016/une-osteopathic-medical-students-publish-innovative-immersion-research).

Interprofessional Education

Recently, there has been a substantial growth in interprofessional educational experiences, which provides the added benefit of facilitating collaborative relationships to provide client-centered care. In 2010, the World Health Organization developed a Framework for Action on Interprofessional Education and Collaborative Practice to describe how successful collaborative teamwork is shaped (Figure 21.3). In addition, this framework outlined key changes to policies to facilitate interprofessional healthcare education (Table 21.2).[8]

"Interprofessional healthcare teams understand how to optimize the skills of their members, share case management, and provide better health services to patients and the community. The resulting strengthened health system leads to improved health outcomes."[9] As interdisciplinary, collaborative care is a key component of PC provision, educational endeavors that include an interprofessional component would facilitate improved collaborative-ready practitioners.

Campbell, Trojanowski, and Smith[10] described a 70-minute interprofessional EoL simulation and its impact on knowledge and attitudes among nursing and physical therapy students. Students were presented with a scenario with a patient diagnosed with end-stage lung cancer who was transitioning to hospice. Two of the patient's five children were in the room and a conflict arose related to meeting the patient's wishes related to EoL care that the healthcare student had to navigate. In addition to participating as a healthcare provider, students also role-played as the patient and family members. The healthcare

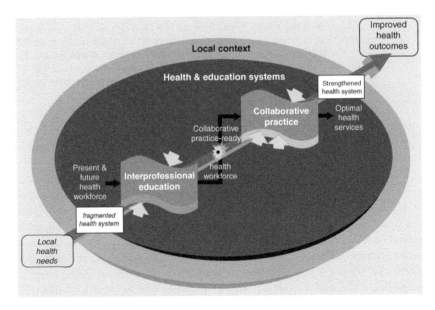

Figure 21.3 World Health Organization's Framework for Action on Interprofessional Education & Collaborative Practice. Reprinted with permission. https://www.who.int/hrh/resources/framework_action/en/.

Table 21.2 WHO Interprofessional Education Framework Suggested
Mechanisms[8]

Educator Mechanisms	Curricular Mechanisms
• Academic staff training in interprofessional education • Educational champions • Institutional support of educational experience • Managerial commitment • Clear learning outcomes	• Detailed plan for logistics and scheduling • Customized and applicable program content • Compulsory attendance • Shared learning objectives • Application of adult learning principles • Contextual learning • Formal learning assessments

Reprinted with Permission. https://www.who.int/hrh/resources/framework_action/en/.

members provided family training and discharge planning in preparation for discharge as well. Both disciplines facilitated discharge planning, the nursing student provided information on comfort measures and medications, and the PT student educated the family on transfer techniques prior to discharge home.

In order to examine the effectiveness of this learning activity, investigators utilized the Frommelt Attitudes Toward Care of the Dying Scale – form B (FATCOD-B), a valid, reliable questionnaire that has a Pearson's Coefficient of 0.90.[11] The FATCOD-B is a self-reported questionnaire consisting of 30 items using a 5-point Likert scale that evaluated the attitudes of healthcare students related to the dying patient and the family. Nursing and PT students (n=83) participated in the EoL simulation and 58 of those students (11 nursing, 47 PT) completed the FATCOD-B before and after the simulation. All students completed a reflection after the simulation.

The following two items on the FATCOD-B showed the greatest improvement of mean scores: (1) "Death is not the worst thing that can happen to a person" improved from 3.62 to 4.09 (p = 0.0018); and (2) "When a patient asks, 'Am I dying?' I think it best to change the subject to something more cheerful" demonstrated an improvement from 2.14 to 1.78 (p = 0.0001).[10] In addition, statistically significant improvements were found in mean scores for the following questions: "The length of time required to give care to a dying person would frustrate me," and "I would be upset when the dying person I was caring for gave up hope of getting better."[10]

Certification in Palliative Care

As PC is a relatively new subspecialty for therapists and physical activity professionals, there is not a widely accepted professional certification to clearly establish standards of practice and provide qualification for optimal PC competency. There are certifications available for other interdisciplinary team members such as physicians, nurses, social workers, chaplains, and counselors that may provide value to therapist providers (https://www.capc.org/jobs/palliative-care-certification/). Additionally, general training in PC concepts may be obtained by programs such as the European Certificate in Essential Palliative Care (ECEPC) (https://www.pah.org.uk/courses/european-certificate-in-essential-palliative-care/). This is an eight-week distance learning, interprofessional program that covers topics, including: (1) What is PC and who is it for?; (2) Symptom issues in PC; (3) Patients with emergency conditions; (4) Patients in the last 48-hours of life; (5) Breaking bad news to patients and families; (6) Bereavement and support; and (7) Common ethical issues. The course was developed at the Princess Alice Hospice in the United Kingdom in 2001. It is now offered at a range of sites internationally. A therapist may also benefit from foundational knowledge in exercise concepts for chronic or life-threatening diseases. The American College of Sports Medicine in collaboration with the American Cancer Society developed the Certified Cancer Exercise Trainer program to improve the application and individualization of exercise concepts for those facing cancer (https://www.acsm.org/get-stay-certified/get-certified/specialization/cet). As this certification is focused on general cancer concepts, it may not provide a thorough enough focus on advanced cancer, or the terminal stages of the disease.

As of this publication, the distance education provider, Medbridge, offers an online certification entitled *Hospice and Palliative Care for Therapists* (https://www.medbridgeeducation.com/certificate-program/13698-hospice-and-palliative-care-for-therapists/). This series of online continuing education courses entails 18 hours that describes clinical adaptations, palliative/hospice care concepts, and self-care concepts for therapists. Although offered by a private educational provider, this certification will likely be the first of a growing list of postgraduate certifications for therapists to improve the patient-centered, specialized care for those facing a life-threatening illness.

Summary

For therapists, entry-level training is often inadequate to ensure confidence and competence in providing PC. An introduction to PC concepts and providing physical activity and care for individuals facing the EoL should be included in the therapist entry-level training programs. As most programs have limited ability to add additional content, a one- to three-hour session may be a sufficient foundation to educate therapists on their role within PC. Experiential learning activities, especially when provided in an interprofessional format, can provide substantial value to prepare therapists to be collaborative providers to best utilize their skills to optimize quality of life.

References

1 Wilson CM, Stiller CH, Doherty DJ, Thompson KA. The role of physical therapists within hospice and palliative care in the United States and Canada. *Am J Hosp Palliat Med.* 2017;34(1):34–41.

2 Meredith PJ. Has undergraduate education prepared occupational therapy students for possible practice in palliative care? *Aust Occup Ther J.* 2010;57(4):224–232. doi:10.1111/j.1440-1630.2009.00836.x.

3 Duthie E. *Virtual Patient Case #2: Mrs. Dubois - Chief Diagnosis: Breast Cancer.* [CD-ROM]. Milwaukee: Medical College of Wisconsin; 2009.

4 Briggs RW. Clinical decision making for physical therapists in patient-centered end-of-life care. *Top Geriatr Rehabil.* 2011;27(1):10–17.

5 Wilson CM, Mueller MK, Briggs RM. Physical therapists' contribution to the hospice and palliative care interdisciplinary team: A clinical summary. *J Hosp Palliat Nurs.* 2017;19(6):588–596. doi:10.1097/NJH.0000000000000394.

6 Kumar SP, Jim A, Sisodia V. Effects of palliative care training program on knowledge, attitudes, beliefs and experiences among student physiotherapists: A preliminary quasi-experimental study. *Indian J Palliat Care.* 2011;17(1):47.

7 World Health Organization. WHO definition of palliative care. https://www.who.int/cancer/palliative/definition/en/. Accessed June 28, 2020.

8 World Health Organization. *Framework for Action on Interprofessional Education and Collaborative Practice.* Geneva, Switzerland: WHO; 2010. https://www.who.int/hrh/resources/framework_action/en/. Accessed August 16, 2020.

9 Gilbert JH, Yan J, Hoffman SJ. A WHO report: Framework for action on interprofessional education and collaborative practice. *J Allied Health.* 2010;39(3):196–197.

10 Campbell D, Trojanowski S, Smith LM. An interprofessional end-of-life simulation to improve knowledge and attitudes of end-of-life care amongst nursing and physical therapy students. *Rehabil Oncol.* 2020;38(1): 45–51. doi: 10.1097/01.REO.0000000000000192.

11 Dame L, Hoebeke R. Effects of a simulation exercise on nursing students' end-of-life care attitudes. *J Nurs Educ.* 2016;55(12):701–705.

22 Policy Issues and Clinical Documentation

Christopher M. Wilson and Amy J. Litterini

Introduction

Practice guidelines, institutional policies, payment structures, research, and clinical documentation are critical concepts for therapists in this area of care. Research has demonstrated that, as compared to traditional physical activity or rehabilitation, there is an outsized external influence of policy and governmental factors as well as social and cultural issues influencing the therapist's role in caring for the individual with a terminal illness. Challenges include access and payment, governmental priorities for funding, clinical documentation to reflect patient care provision and skilled services, as well as proactive advocacy for the patient, and the therapist's role in this care setting.

Institutional Policies and Regulations on End-of-Life and Palliative Care

Therapist provision of services in palliative care (PC), or at the end of life, are heavily influenced by a variety of external factors.[1-3] These can occur at the institutional level,[4,5] the governmental/legislative level,[6] and are also influenced by the payment system (e.g. private versus public payers).[2] In some healthcare institutions or jurisdictions, PC services may not be established as a high priority for therapist interactions. There may be several reasons for this decreased prioritization, including competing priorities of other patient care diagnoses or service lines. For example, in some institutions the population of patients in PC may be relatively small compared to other service lines such as orthopedics or neurology. In situations like this, there may be political influences within a healthcare institution that may result in patients with life-threatening illnesses being prioritized less highly than more "emergent" or urgent conditions. For example, if an acute care hospital has an extremely high volume of orthopedic surgeries such as joint replacements, this may result in prioritization of these patients on a therapist's schedule as opposed to patients at the end of life. Hospital systems may rely quite heavily on elective procedures because they are depending on them to meet budgetary or volume-related goals.[7] With these competing political and influential interests, patients without a clear anticipation of recovery or a slower rehabilitation process, who do not require daily intensive therapy, may be prioritized lower than an elective orthopedic surgery.

In addition, institutional scheduling systems for therapists may not be conducive to non-traditional practice and scheduling models. Some outpatient or ambulatory therapy facilities may only be used to scheduling patients for series visits such as two times a week or three times a week. Less frequent or sporadic treatment schedules may not "fit in" to the traditional scheduling model. When a therapist feels that a patient would benefit from a decreased frequency of visits (e.g. once every two weeks or once a month),[8] there may be administrative resistance to this treatment model (especially in busy clinics), as it may not be an "easy fit" for scheduling systems. This scenario will require the advocacy skills of the therapist to justify to the manager or supervisor why the service is warranted, beneficial, and medically necessary. In addition, prevention services may not consistently be prioritized as highly on a busy therapist's schedule if there is an exceptionally long waiting list to see a therapist. An example of this is if there is a patient with early stage COPD who requires an exercise prescription and health behavior/maintenance advice waiting for therapy at the same time as a patient who has recently sustained a cerebrovascular accident requiring neurologic rehabilitation, historically, the patient with the cerebrovascular accident might be prioritized higher on the therapist's schedule before the individual with COPD.[9]

Professional Associations and Advocacy

Part of the professional role of the therapist and physical activity professional is to align with and advocate for their patients/clients via professional associations (aka societies) to best establish services, research, and policies in PC.[10,11] While therapists are often represented by their own professional association to their local or national government, these organizations may not consistently advocate for the therapist's role in PC.[3,6] As most therapy professional associations represent a diverse and varied scope of practice, there are frequent limitations of time and resources to specifically and consistently advocate for appropriate policy and legislation for therapists in PC. In addition, therapist involvement within PC is a relatively new concept; the associated policies and payment structures have not evolved as rapidly as the patient care demands. This leaves professional association leaders with the dilemma of focusing efforts and resources toward large issues that affect a significant number of therapists and their patients/clients (e.g. fair co-pays for private insurance, scope of practice issues, adequate staffing ratios) or lobbying for adequate patient access and payment for terminally ill individuals, a relatively small patient population. Although the authors of this textbook feel strongly that involvement in membership with a discipline's specific professional association/society (e.g. physical therapist membership in their nation's physical therapy association) is critical, limited advocacy for PC policy requires therapists to ALSO proactively seek involvement in professional associations and organizations that represent best practices for terminally ill individuals. Examples of these organizations include the Center to Advance Palliative Care (www.capc.org), European Association for Palliative Care (www.eapcnet.eu), and the African Palliative Care Association (www.africanpalliativecare.org). It is by this means that policy, accreditation standards, and governmental legislation will be advanced. In addition, through PC professional organizations, therapists can improve their involvement in integration into PC, hospices, and end-of-life care. A useful example of how this was effectively employed was reflected by therapist engagement and involvement in a variety of national cancer organizations in the United States.

Within cancer care, a similar conundrum is encountered where therapists are not consistently part of the care team. Through active therapist engagement and representation in the relevant accrediting agencies, the American College of Surgeons' Commission on Cancer amended their 2020 Accreditation Standards with two important revisions that involve therapists.[12] In order to achieve accreditation standards, cancer healthcare systems must now demonstrate evidence of rehabilitation involvement as access to these services are now a standard for Commission on Cancer accreditation. Prior to 2020, a cancer center had to identify 'sources' for rehabilitation referrals in order to become accredited. Now, the new standard requires that a cancer center has policies and procedures documented for the use of rehabilitation services. The standard describes the relevant members of the rehabilitation team and gives guidance on the necessary components and guidelines as to what should be included in rehabilitation. In addition, as of 2020, there is a revised survivorship standard that requires a cancer center to develop a Survivorship Program which requires a designated survivorship team. The standard now outlines guidance on who should be part of that team and the rehabilitation professionals are noted as a preferred service to be integrated. The Commission on Cancer accredits over 1,500 cancer centers in the United States, so there is broad relevance.

In this specific case, the therapists who were key in representing the profession (and interests of patients) were generally not explicitly invited to represent their profession at these committees; instead, these therapists proactively pursued involvement in this specific organization. In addition to advocacy, they provided scientific evidence that therapists' services were integral to care. Based on these regulatory changes, as part of pursuing or renewing accreditation as a cancer center, the accreditation body will be looking for substantial evidence of rehabilitation professionals' involvement in these various cancer activities and the associated policies and procedures. A similar model can be employed by therapists involved with PC organizations. As you have already expressed an interest in this topic (as evidenced by reading this book), it is hoped that you now have the confidence and inspiration to represent your respective profession at your professional PC organization. Finally, although some therapist professional organizations may not be able to consistently lobby for "niche" issues, they can officially appoint a person to represent their interests among PC organizations.

Advocacy for Public Research Funding

An additional important component of engagement with scientific professional organizations includes the establishment of policy, research agenda, and focus for public and private research grant funders.[13] As research studies are critical in demonstrating the evidence of the effectiveness of therapist services in PC, external funding remains a primary source to facilitate research projects in this area.[6] Historically, grant funding has been targeted for specific initiatives or critical issues as identified by research agendas and establishment of documented priority areas. Even if PC services are a focused area of funding, this does not automatically follow that *therapist services within PC* will be the priority funding issue. In addition, if PC therapist services become a funding priority issue and no investigators apply for this research funding, it is likely that future funding will not be dedicated toward this important topic. Researchers should also be cognizant that PC entails a variety of diagnoses and conditions and there may be grant resources available within those diagnosis-specific organizations (e.g. United Kingdom Multipe Sclerosis Society, American Brain Tumor Association, Singapore Cancer Society). Within these organizations research is often supported, and end-stage disease management with therapy would also likely be within the purview of these organizations.

Governmental Legislation and Payment Advocacy

Payment and finances are a barrier to administration of therapist services, which is especially significant in PC. In most nations, there is some level of public or governmental funding for therapist services, but these vary widely by nation. This may be through direct reimbursement for services rendered (such as Center for Medicare and Medicaid Services by the United States federal government) or through allocation of funding for therapist positions in publicly funded health systems (e.g. the National Health System of the United Kingdom). As these resources are often directly affected by the political climate, depending on which party controls governments, elections, support for healthcare in general, and therapy services specifically, such resources may be affected by unpredictable political shifts. Although this may be a challenge for therapist services in general, the rapid growth of PC services presents a unique opportunity for therapists. Many nations and jurisdictions are in the process of writing or updating their policies for PC. If therapists proactively advocate their services to these legislative bodies, it will facilitate further integration which will result in sustainable, equitable payment for therapist services. Conversely, as therapists are not consistently members of the core PC team, it is extremely likely that without this advocacy, these regulations will be written without adequate representation or allocation of resources for therapists, thereby leaving the patients without these valued services. Even if individual therapists do not have the time or resources to lobby their local governmental representatives, they can certainly achieve this representation via membership in their professional associations. This may also require these therapists to encourage these organizations to specifically lobby for therapist integration into PC services.

Lower- and Middle-Income Nations and Growth of PC

In some nations, PC has not reached full integration. There, therapists may identify suffering and other issues that can be managed with improved PC services; however, this requires a unique approach as PC in these nations may not yet have the infrastructure or critical mass of skilled PC professionals to provide these services.[14] In these nations, therapists may be able to affect change by using their skills and societal standing to improve PC integration.[14] The World Health Organization (WHO) "estimated that of the 20 million people needing palliative care at the end of their life, around 80% live in low- and middle-income countries; some 67% are elderly (more than 60 years of age), whereas about 6% are children."[15] The WHO identified four domains in their public health approach to PC: (1) Development of health system policies to ensure the integration of PC services into the structure and financing of national healthcare systems at all levels of care; (2) Establishment of policies for improving education and training of healthcare professionals and volunteers as well as education of the public; (3) Policies to ensure the availability of essential medicines for the management of symptoms (e.g. pain, psychological distress), specifically opioid medications for pain and dyspnea; and (4) Policies to research and establish best practices for PC, especially in areas with limited resources.[15]

In order for therapists to best advocate for their services within PC in lower- and middle-income nations (LMIN), a clear understanding of the barriers to adequate PC services is essential as the delivery of therapist PC services is not likely to be successful without a robust PC system to practice within.[14]

Health System Policies and Finances

In order to best support health systems in LMIN, therapists may be called upon to provide basic PC services as the volume of individuals who require PC may be outweighed by the numbers of PC physicians, nurses, and social workers.[15] In these circumstances, other providers such as trained community carers or volunteers can assist in providing PC in coordination with healthcare professionals.[15] A PC-focused therapist can utilize their skills by providing direct care or training caregivers in the various skills needed to help those with a terminal illness. As some PC services (e.g. medication administration) may be outside of the therapists' scope of practice, a coordinated division of tasks among providers is warranted for effective delivery of PC services.

In a strong statement of accessibility, the WHO noted that:

"Palliative care services need to be provided in accordance with the principles of universal health coverage. All people, without discrimination, should have access to nationally determined sets of basic health promotion, preventive, curative, rehabilitative, and palliative health services, and essential, safe, affordable, effective, and good-quality medicines and diagnostics. Furthermore, the use of these services must not lead to financial hardship, especially among poor people and populations living in vulnerable situations."[15]

Education and Training of Healthcare Professionals, Volunteers, and Public

In order to ensure that healthcare providers achieve adequate training in PC, basic education must be offered to medical students, nursing students, and all healthcare providers in the concepts of PC.[15] This includes aspects such as ethical issues, pain management, supporting caregivers, communication skills, managing gaps in care, and preventing crises.[16]

Availability of Medicines for Symptom Management

Some 80% of the world's population lack adequate access to medication needed for PC.[15] In 2017, the International Narcotics Control Board reported that 84.4% of the world's population, (mainly in LMIN), consumed only 13.6% of total morphine used for pain and suffering. Nonetheless, this is an improvement from 2014 when 80% of the world's population only used 9.5% of the morphine intended to manage pain and suffering.[17] They noted that "the disparity in the consumption of narcotic drugs for palliative care continues to be a matter of concern."[17] In order to best advocate for appropriate and beneficial PC, supporting policies for appropriate opioid availability near the end of life is warranted, especially in some nations where opioid abuse and misuse have reached epidemic proportions (e.g. the United States) and appropriate and warranted use may be stigmatized by media coverage and social perceptions (see Chapter 16).[18] This may result in some situations where individuals who need opioids may feel pressure not to accept them, thereby increasing their pain and suffering at the end of life.[19] As therapists often establish trusting relationships with these individuals, particularly as it relates to the topic of pain, advice on the appropriate use of opioids to optimize quality of life may be meaningful and effective.[19]

Policies to Research and Establish Best Practices for PC

The WHO noted that, in relation to PC, "research and training are often nonexistent or limited" in LMIN.[15] Although PC research is generally focused in higher-income nations, preliminary research into PC services in LMIN often demonstrates similar findings of improved quality of life, reduced readmissions, and subsequent reduction in pain and suffering.[15] In order to be effective, the PC services must be culturally appropriate and in conjunction with the local community.[15] Due to their integration into the medical community, focus on optimizing quality of life, and ability to provide culturally affirming care, therapists are well suited to be advocates for research and clinical care for those facing a life-threatening illness.[20]

Clinical Documentation

In addition to patient and family care, clinical documentation is one of the largest components of therapist provision.[3] Despite variability in customs and regulations in specific locales, there are some general principles that remain universal regardless of practice setting or type of therapy, one being that documentation is the:

> "process of recording of all aspects of patient/client care/management, including the results of the initial examination/assessment and evaluation, diagnosis, prognosis, plan of care/intervention/treatment, interventions/ treatment, response to interventions/treatment, changes in patient/ client status relative to the interventions/treatment, re-examination, and discharge/discontinuation of intervention and other patient/client management activities."[21]

Despite these commonalities, some key differences will be encountered during the therapists' clinical documentation for the individual with a life-threatening illness. Beyond just proof that an intervention was performed, this documentation also carries added weight when it is closely tied to billing or payment for therapist services. Many healthcare systems and disciplines utilize therapy documentation and functional outcome measures to demonstrate that therapy services were effective. This "effectiveness" has historically hinged on an objective demonstration that the person measurably improved in body structure and function performance, ability to perform an activity, or documented improvement in participation restrictions.

With an individual with a life-threatening or degenerative condition, although the therapist may be providing high-quality, state-of-the-art, value-added care, the person's physical function may continue to decline. If the clinical documentation does not clearly reflect that the therapist's services were medically necessary and improved clinical outcomes, they may be at risk for insurance denials or further scrutiny. For example, in the United States, and other nations with some form of privatized healthcare, insurance companies may request a review of therapist clinical documentation to establish that services were skilled, medically necessary, and within normal standards of practice.[22] One of the easiest mechanisms private insurance companies utilize to evaluate therapy effectiveness is via clear demonstration that the individual receiving therapy care "got better."[23] In traditional (non-PC) therapy, this may include things like improved range of motion and strength, better cardiopulmonary function, improvement in a six-minute walk test, improvement in the number of activities of daily living (ADLs) performed independently, or documentation that the person has been able to return to work. Unfortunately, in PC, these initial objective findings are not often readily available or apparent to reviewers. Therefore, the therapist must further contextualize or employ less commonplace measures of improvement or value.

Within each documentation format there are some commonalities, such as a *subjective* or *history* component, where the provider documents the patient/client's current status, continued impairments, and other contextual facilitators and barriers. After the subjective history, there is some form of objective information such as tests and measures, interventions performed on that date, and/or response to treatment. After this data collection, there is an *assessment* or *evaluation* where the provider documents their clinical judgment for the continued need for therapist services, as well as updating the plan of care or establishing other required services. Depending on the documentation format for an individual institution, goals may also be documented in the assessment or evaluation section of a note to establish milestones, as well as how and when this individual will achieve these milestones. Finally, there is generally an establishment of an overall *plan of care* with ongoing treatment modifications and adaptations. For this overall plan of care documentation, there are some unique characteristics for patients or individuals within PC or facing an end-of-life disease process, including conveying the anticipated disease progression (and related functional decline) and what therapeutic interventions will best mitigate them.

Subjective History

Although the actual history-taking and related documentation may be less conventional in PC as compared to non-PC subjective history, the clinical documentation and its organization remain a critical component. Within PC, it is encouraged that a patient be allowed to 'tell their story' and history-taking principles such as active listening, paraphrasing, reflection, and open-ended questioning are exceptionally valuable.[24] Although challenging to document concisely and effectively, this contextual information is extremely relevant to provide readers with a clear picture of the intent and focus of physical activity procedures. Important additional information within the subjective history includes the patient's goals, and their understanding of the disease process and their current situation. Although important in almost all therapy situations, within PC, documentation related to family and social support is key, including who will be the primary individuals charged with assisting the patient with mobility. These items will be invaluable in conveying these messages to other providers in order to ensure continuity of care. A thorough depiction of the patient and family's understanding of their medical situation and current overall goals of care will assist in developing a patient-centered plan of care while working to enkindle hope, while still maintaining realistic outcomes. Finally, in order to achieve a holistic, complete picture, clinical documentation may benefit from the inclusion of a spiritual history, values, and beliefs, to best align the therapist's care with the individual's belief systems.[25]

Objective Data and Tests and Measures

Within the objective section of a clinical note, (depending on the treatment set-ting) a thorough catalog of objective, impairment-level measurements (e.g. range of motion, manual muscle test) is generally expected. Within PC, intricate im-pairment-level measurements may not be the best use of a therapist's time based on the priorities and life goals of the patient. Traditional objective clinical doc-umentation is aimed to demonstrate improvement in these impairment-level findings, which will logically translate to improved functional performance and participation in activities. Although selected and strategic documentation of impairment-level measurements may be required by institutional policies or as a part of insurance payment expectations, they may be comparatively de-em-phasized as they may not consistently demonstrate the skill of a PC therapist or the medical necessity of therapist services.[2] One of the confounding variables with focusing on impairment-level objective measurements is that there is a substantial chance that they will decline or not show improvement. If these declines or lack of improvement are the only objective measurements provided (or they substantially outweigh the number of activity or participation objective measures), clinical documentation may not clearly establish the skill and med-ical necessity required for quantifying the overall value that therapists provide in this practice setting. Within the documentation, it behooves the therapist to clearly state when declining values are evidence of an advancing disease pro-cess and can justify the *Rehab in Reverse* care philosophy or adjustments to the current rehabilitation regimen that require the skills of a therapist. In order to convey these nuances, a thorough and detailed clinical note may be necessary; however, excessive elaboration may be detrimental as this may deter the reader from understanding the core facts of the clinical situation.

As the overall emphasis of PC is for expert pain and symptom management, optimizing quality of life, safe discharge home, and anxiety reduction, ther-apists should strive to quantify these domains objectively within the clinical note. These domains should be quantified via valid, reliable, and sensitive measures. See Chapter 18 for applicable and clinically relevant outcome measures. Looney et al.[26] described some of their challenges in an inpatient setting to utilizing traditional functional outcome measures, especially at or near the end of life when a person's physical functioning is progressively impaired and physical status was highly variable.

Evaluation, Assessment, and Clinical Judgment

The evaluation/assessment portion of therapists' documentation generally contains the clinical judgments and interpretation of subjective history and tests and measures. This section of documentation reflects the need for these skilled services and provides justification as to why these services are medi-cally necessary and warranted. In the authors' experience, this is often the most underutilized, challenging area for therapists to complete as it is not as straightforward as other components of the documentation where data are simply being collected or a factual treatment plan is being established or updated. In PC, this is probably the most important section of documentation where the therapist should spend significant effort. Things that would be beneficial to include in the assessment component include the therapists' care approach (i.e. Briggs' rehabilitation philosophy as described in Chapter 4), the anticipated disease trajectory, and a depiction of what the patient will "look like" in two future scenarios: without the therapist involvement and with the therapist involvement. When discussing the limitations and impairments that may be worsened more quickly without a therapist's involvement, it is also important to discuss the medical or safety-related events that are more likely to occur without therapist services. These may include falls, fractures, caregiver injuries, hospitalizations, readmissions, and the need for more pain medications, among others. Illustrative of this documentation is the case of a 57-year-old male with amyotrophic lateral sclerosis:

> "Therapist services are medically necessary to maintain or slow the decline of important functional tasks. Without therapist services, the patient would likely demonstrate worsening of balance, strength, range of motion, and increased pain. These symptoms would increase likelihood of hospitalization or falls and their associated costs. With therapist services, the patient is anticipated to maintain strength which would otherwise decline without these services. This maintenance of strength will keep the patient independent in key tasks such as transfers, ambulation, and ADLs for a longer duration, thereby reducing the risk of institutionalization or additional care costs."

In addition, a clear depiction of facilitators and barriers as they relate to contextual factors and participation in rehabilitation should be included in this section of documentation. Although there may be a concern that thorough documentation of the facilitators may "weaken the therapist's case" for justifying continued services, this does provide the opportunity for a therapist to have a strong understanding of what the individual's life circumstances are that can help facilitate successful therapeutic outcomes. For example, if the individual has strong, competent family support, this can facilitate having family members assist with ADLs to best achieve the therapist's goals of reducing readmissions, avoiding falls, and maintaining comfort. An astute therapist should leverage this information to provide education-based interventions to train the family and caregivers in caring for the patient. When identifying and listing contextual factors which are barriers in the clinical documentation, an equally thorough list is justified and valued. These may include things like pain, an inaccessible living situation or home environment, family disagreements, or lack of clarity of care goals considering the disease trajectory.

Goal Writing

Often within the assessment/evaluation/clinical judgment section of a note is the development of patient-centered goals. Within PC, the art of goal writing achieves a new level of complexity and stakes. Traditionally, therapists might write a goal for improving someone's ADL performance, cardiac status, number of repetitions performed of an exercise, or ability to perform a new task. As the patient's disease trajectory is generally expected to decline, it is often futile and not good clinical practice to write goals that continue to anticipate progress or strength that is not likely to happen. Conversely, if progression was anticipated, what magnitude of improvement would be expected? Based on the patient's disease burden and progression, it will likely be a lesser magnitude of improvement than a similar individual without this life-limiting disease process. Within the context of goal writing, most therapists will write short-term and long-term goals which may convey different tasks; a therapist may consider a positive outcome of a short-term goal to demonstrate a modest improvement in performance or function while establishing a long-term goal to be a safe, incident-free decline in function.

This prompts the ever-present question of *how do I know?* How will a therapist predict the future functional decline without therapy, in order to quantify the value of services in maintaining current status or slowing the decline? Admittedly this is a substantial conundrum for science-driven healthcare professions. As with many other conditions and disease states, the therapist will generally establish goals based on their prior experience with individuals with the same or similar conditions. Unfortunately, the current state of research as it relates to therapists' involvement in PC remains extremely limited and anecdotal. Despite this fact, there is value in accessing the currently available literature in this area via means of the concept of triangulation. For example, if an exercise physiologist is evaluating an individual with stage IV lung cancer with brain metastases, the clinician may not be able to find a specific article for exercise physiology interventions for late-stage lung cancer with brain metastases. The clinician may be required to "triangulate" their clinical approach based on the research that is out there.

When assessing the available evidence for therapist management of late-stage life-threatening or chronic disease, the concept of triangulation is a useful practice. It is not likely that a clinician will find a clinical practice guideline or other clinical protocol that will encapsulate all the unique clinical, psychosocial, emotional, and disease trajectory aspects of their client/patient. Instead, the provider may be required to seek literature or research on certain components of the diagnosis or the individual's clinical presentation (Figure 22.1).

Useful questions to examine or articles to identify include:

> What clinical diagnoses present similarly to this specific diagnosis? What interventions are successful for the symptoms that the patient is presenting with? What is a typical or anticipated disease trajectory for this diagnosis? What symptoms is this patient most affected by that are impacting the quality of life? What psychosocial issues or emotional issues is this patient experiencing or expected to experience and how are they mitigated?

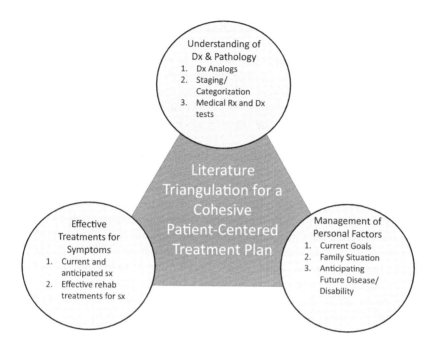

Figure 22.1 Using Triangulation to Establish a Plan of Care.

More experienced clinicians may not rely as heavily on this triangulation technique when establishing their plan of care, as they already have a relatively robust body of clinical experience to draw from in order to build their plan of care. The skill of triangulating around a diagnosis to build a therapeutic plan may be especially valuable for newer clinicians or a therapist who does not regularly care for those with life-threatening illnesses.

After a reasonable and achievable patient-centered plan of care is established, clinicians will generally establish goals or benchmarks to determine the effectiveness of their therapeutic interventions based on measurable and achievable goals. When establishing goals for individuals with a life-threatening illness, additional components may be warranted. This may include additional contextual information such as the immediate clinical rationale for this goal; what safety issues may occur if this goal is not accomplished; or what impairment or functional limitation or participation restriction may be experienced if the service is not administered. Examples of goals will be presented using each of Briggs' patient management models for PC that were outlined in Chapter 4 (Box 22.1).

Box 22.1   Therapists' Goal-setting in Palliative Care

Rehabilitation Light: Within four visits, the patient will be able to ascend a flight of stairs twice a day in order to access the upper level of his home while using the rating of perceived exertion scale to determine if he has enough strength to attempt the stairs. (Without this advanced disease process, the patient would be able to perform this task six to eight times a day).

Rehabilitation in Reverse: Within two visits the patient will demonstrate proper use of a rolling walker for ambulation in the household despite currently needing to use a standard cane for functional ambulation in anticipation of physical decline from his advancing disease process.

Skilled Maintenance: With the therapist's close supervision and the manual and verbal cues, the patient will be able to ambulate 100 feet with a standard walker while maintaining 5% partial weight-bearing due to bone metastases to be able to safely perform household ambulation.

Case Management: On next visit in one month, the patient will demonstrate the ability to perform her aerobic exercise routine as prescribed by the therapist 30 minutes a day for 3 to 5 days per week.

Supportive Care: Within two visits, the patient's family caregivers will demonstrate independence in lower-body dressing and passive range of motion to assist with ADL during the time when the patient is confined to bed.

Finally, a key approach to goal setting is conveying measurable knowledge and skills that the patient's family caregivers are now able to accomplish that they were not able to accomplish previously. These should convey skills and information that are essential for families and caregivers to understand and perform at home. Goals that begin *Patient/Family/Caregiver (will be knowledgeable) (will understand) (can recall)* would be followed by the skill or task that the specified party would achieve. This allows for increased independence and safety and reduces caregiver burden and stress which may lead to a reduced risk of emergencies, falls, or hospitalizations.

Treatment Planning

In providing clinical documentation for establishing a therapeutic treatment plan, in addition to the current interventions that will be administered and required, it is encouraged that providers also document relevant and necessary screenings including assessments for emerging disorders such as decubitus ulcers, peripheral neuropathy, or blood clots. Consideration should also be established for the procurement of future equipment needs and training that are not currently necessary. For example, if the patient is using a standard cane to ambulate to the bathroom but is expected to physically decline further, a walker, wheelchair, and bedside commode may be beneficial pieces of equipment to obtain and proficiently utilize. This anticipatory provision of equipment may be easier to facilitate under a hospice benefit, rather than a traditional medical plan. If the patient is at high risk of falls, establishing an intervention program for teaching fall prevention strategies is warranted as well as fall recovery activities are strongly recommended. If a patient has experienced a fall and does not know what to do after the fall, they may immediately resort to calling emergency services when it was not necessary. If the therapist can teach fall recovery techniques such as assessing themselves for an injury and biomechanically safe and effective techniques to return to an upright position, this issue may be mitigated.

Summary

Therapists have a unique skill set that can help prevent downstream issues and help contain healthcare costs. These include reducing readmissions, fall prevention activities, uncontrolled pain and anxiety, as well as providing interventions to optimize quality of life. In order to be able to provide patient access to these skills and knowledge, there are many external influences that must be overcome for those with a life-threatening illness. As therapists are not commonly considered to be core team members in PC and within hospices, the policies and procedures that influence care may be developed by others, without the input of therapists. In addition, within many healthcare systems or hospitals, palliative care services may only be one component of the overall depth and breadth of patient care activities that a department oversees. This may result in internal department conflict for disbursement of resources to different diagnostic service lines (e.g. orthopedics versus PC), resulting in palliative therapy services being less frequently or less highly prioritized. It behooves therapists to be strong and consistent advocates for equitable and unfettered access to their services.

Financial support and payment for therapy services as well as funding PC research often occur at the governmental level. In addition to individual therapist advocacy and lobbying to local governmental agents or elected officials, therapists would also benefit from engagement with professional associations to advocate for improved PC as well as improve therapist involvement within PC. As with institutional policies, therapist professional associations often must represent and advocate for a diverse depth and breadth of services, which may limit prioritization of PC services. Therapist involvement and engagement within palliative care organizations, where these regulations and legislation efforts originate, may be further enhanced. This will facilitate therapists being able to provide their skilled services to these patients to improve their quality of life.

References

1 Mueller K, Wilson CM, Briggs R. Chapter 27: Hospice and end of life. In: Avers D, Wong R, eds. *Guccione's Geriatric Physical Therapy.* St. Louis, MO: Mosby; 2019:612–645.

2 Wilson CM, Boright L. Documenting medical necessity for palliative care and degenerative or chronic conditions. *Rehabil Oncol.* 2017;35(3):153–156. doi:10.1097/01.REO.0000000000000663.

3 Wilson CM, Stiller CH, Doherty DJ, Thompson KA. The role of physical therapists within hospice and palliative care in the United States and Canada. *Am J Hosp Palliat Med.* 2017;34(1):34–41.

4 Wilson C, Roy D. Relationship between physical therapy, occupational therapy, palliative care consultations, and hospital length of stay. *J Acute Care Phys Ther.* 2017;8(3):106–112. doi:10.1097/JAT.0000000000000059.

5 Wilson CM, Barnes C. Physical therapy in interdisciplinary palliative care and hospice teams. *Rehabil Oncol.* 2018;36(2):143–145. doi:10.1097/01.REO.0000000000000109.

6 Baldwin A, Wilson C. Best practices for public policies for palliative care physical therapy. *Rehabil Oncol.* 2018;36(2):106–116. doi:10.1097/01.REO.0000000000000090.

7 Sharfstein JM. Global budgets for rural hospitals. *Milbank Q.* 2016;94(2):255.

8 Barawid E, Covarrubias N, Tribuzio B, Liao S. The benefits of rehabilitation for palliative care patients. *Am J Hosp Palliat Care.* 2015;32(1):34–43. doi:10.1177/1049909113514474.

9 Hand C, Law M, McColl MA. Occupational therapy interventions for chronic diseases: A scoping review. *Am J Occup Ther.* 2011;65(4):428–436.

10 Orlin MN, Cicirello NA, O'Donnell AE, Doty AK. The continuum of care for individuals with lifelong disabilities: Role of the physical therapist. *Phys Ther.* 2014;94(7):1043–1053. doi:10.2522/ptj.20130168.

11 Dhillon SK, Wilkins S, Law MC, Stewart DA, Tremblay M. Advocacy in occupational therapy: Exploring clinicians' reasons and experiences of advocacy. *Can J Occup Ther.* 2010;77(4):241–248.

12 American College of Surgeons. Optimal resources for cancer care (2020 standards). https://www.facs.org/quality-programs/cancer/coc/2020-standards. Updated 2019. Accessed August 16, 2020.

13 Morrison RS, Meier DE. The National Palliative Care Research Center and the Center to Advance Palliative Care: A partnership to improve care for persons with serious illness and their families. *J Pediatr Hematol Oncol.* 2011;33 (Supplement 2):S126–S131. doi: 10.1097/MPH.0b013e318230dfa0.

14 Fawcett L. Integration of palliative and hospice care in physical therapy: A much needed professional paradigm shift. *Rehabil Oncol.* 2020; 38(1):E7–E9. doi: 10.1097/01.REO.0000000000000187.

15 World Health Organization. Strengthening of palliative care as a component of integrated treatment throughout the life course. *J Pain Palliat Care Pharmacother.* 2014;28(2):130–134. doi:10.3109/15360288.2014.911801.

16 Center to Advance Palliative Care. Online clinical training courses for all clinicians. https://www.capc.org/training/. Accessed August 16, 2020.

17 International Narcotics Control Board. Estimated World Requirements of Narcotic Drugs for 2020. International Narcotics Control Board website. https://www.incb.org/incb/en/narcotic-drugs/estimates/narcotic-drugs-estimates.html. Updated May 2020. Accessed August 16, 2020.

18 Wilson CM. Opioid campaigns' impact on advanced cancer and hospice and palliative care. *Rehabil Oncol.* 2017;35(2):94–98. doi:10.1097/01.REO.0000000000000055.

19 Wilson CM, Briggs R. Physical therapy's role in opioid use and management during palliative and hospice care. *Phys Ther.* 2018;98(2):83–85. doi:10.1093/ptj/pzx108.

20 Barnes C, Mueller K, Fawcett L, Wagner B. Living and dying in a disparate healthcare system: Strategies to promote culturally affirming palliative and hospice care physical therapy. *Rehabil Oncol.* 2020;38(1): 30–38. doi:10.1097/01.REO.0000000000000199.

21 World Confederation for Physical Therapy. Documentation. https://www.wcpt.org/node/47877#1. Updated 2012. Accessed Nov 23, 2019.

22 Stover AD. Client-centered advocacy: Every occupational therapy practitioner's responsibility to understand medical necessity. *Am J Occup Ther.* 2016;70(5):7005090010p1-7005090010p6.

23 Granger CV, Carlin M, Diaz P, et al. Medical necessity: Is current documentation practice and payment denial limiting access to inpatient rehabilitation? *Am J PM&R.* 2009 Sep 1;88(9):755–765.

24 Donnelly M, Martin D. History taking and physical assessment in holistic palliative care. *Brit J Nurs.* 2016;25(22):1250. doi:10.12968/bjon.2016.25.22.1250.

25 Vermandere M, Warmenhoven F, Van Severen E, De Lepeleire J, Aertgeerts B. Spiritual history taking in palliative home care: A cluster randomized controlled trial. *Palliat Med.* 2016;30(4):338–350. doi:10.1177/0269216315601953.

26 Looney F, Cobbe S, Ryan A, Barriscale I, McMahon A. The search for a functional outcome measure for physical therapy in specialist palliative care: An ongoing journey. *Rehabil Oncol.* 2020;38(1): 22–29. doi:10.1097/01.REO.0000000000000194.

23 The Future of Physical Activity, Rehabilitation, and End-of-Life Care

Christopher M. Wilson and Amy J. Litterini

Introduction

As technology has allowed for a prolonged duration of life in the presence of ongoing disease, physical activity and therapist services play a key role in the quality of the remaining lifespan. The value of maintaining physical health is being increasingly recognized, and access to care is imperative. This includes telehealth/telemedicine concepts, health and technological literacy, remote monitoring, and creative care planning. Research is needed to advance the standard of practice, and advocacy for access and care team participation is critical.

Trends and Opportunities

Although palliative care (PC) as a clinical approach and therapist involvement within PC remains as works in progress, an astute and visionary clinician can seek to position themselves in the early stages of leveraging technology and recognizing future trends in this practice area. In addition to understanding regulatory and legislative opportunities, there are other areas where therapists can assist with integration into rapidly growing and evolving trends in pilot studies to provide patient-centered health care.

One of the major limitations to many of these technical innovations is the concept of technological literacy, especially among older adults and those with low incomes.[1,2] Similar to the concept of health literacy, some individuals may not be fluent or comfortable with utilizing even the most intuitive or user-friendly devices, including the internet as a resource for health information and informed decision-making.[3] Evidence shows that with coaching, support, and guidance, even those with limited technical literacy can apply and benefit from the use of these technologies.[4-6] As many of these technological innovations may involve physical activity, the therapist working with those with chronic conditions or life-threatening illnesses should strive to familiarize themselves with these beneficial technologies. In addition to the challenge of technical literacy, financial issues may arise as well. Many technological innovations are often expensive and of limited utility because of concepts like planned obsolescence. Some individuals are not able to even afford their prescription medications or transportation to doctors' appointments so it may not be the best use of that person's financial resources to procure a wearable activity monitor when life-sustaining medications cannot be procured. This is further limited by the concept of *planned obsolescence* where many technological corporations will only support an electronic device for a certain period of time in order to encourage replacement.[7] Anyone who has had a computer or a smartphone has likely experienced the effect of this planned obsolescence when the device that they purchased a year or two ago has already been superseded by a newer version with more features (and associated cost). With this increased support of the newer version of the device, there is less support and less ability to repair or recalibrate these older devices. This may add to frustration felt by an individual who has just spent valuable time and money purchasing a device that was designed to help them maintain their long-term health and function.

Telehealth and Digital Healthcare Practice

While around the globe there are population centers with significant and relatively convenient availability of PC practitioners, there will always be those individuals who have life-limiting or chronic, advanced health conditions that live in a rural area.[8,9] These individuals are often limited in their ability to manage their condition because of the distance required to travel to obtain health and physical activity services. With new technologies evolving and easier ways to connect over long distances, this leverages the ability to utilize digital technology for PC and therapy services; however, there are some nuances to consider with this treatment approach.[10] Telehealth is generally a means of connecting a patient with a healthcare provider using telecommunications or social networking services. Generally, these services are more than just a telephone call or voice communication; most commonly this is often video conferencing and may be a replacement for, or an adjunct to, in-person healthcare visits.[11] Healthcare systems have begun to utilize this technological support to assist with activities such as medication management and compliance, distance consultation, office visits, or even when triaging for emergency services.[11]

Although not traditionally employed by therapists or physical activity professionals, telehealth was thrust into the forefront of care during the social distancing and quarantine procedures as a result of the COVID-19 novel coronavirus pandemic of 2020.[12] Therapist professional associations quickly provided support and guidance for providers when needing to provide telehealth or digital practice services. The World Confederation for Physical Therapy (aka World Physiotherapy) published a joint report with the International Network of Physical Therapy Regulatory Authorities (INPTRA) to describe the various nuances and practice implications of *digital physiotherapy practice* (the preferred term over telehealth).[13] As this area of practice is new and rapidly evolving with the global pandemic, a variety of considerations must be taken into account and explored further, including privacy and cultural considerations. Instinctively, providers might wish to simply Skype or Facetime their clients; however, this transmittal of sensitive and private health information over an unsecured network may not be advisable and may violate regulations on healthcare privacy. In addition, currently, there are uncertain payment or reimbursement implications for the provision of these services, especially for therapist services. This is rapidly changing as therapists and their professional associations are proactively advocating for these services after COVID-19, resulting in close collaboration with insurance companies and governmental agencies to provide health services in the era of COVID-19.

One example of telehealth includes utilizing video conferencing or smartphone video conferencing applications in emergency services.[14] In PC, anxiety-producing health events occur with relative frequency and in the absence of qualified medical input, patients and families often resort to consulting emergency services and subsequent transportation to a local emergency room. This may result in a hospital admission even if the initial symptoms have resolved as unrelated sequelae of the disease process and may prompt a diagnostic workup which would result in treatment requiring an otherwise unwarranted admission. Many PC or home health agencies have embraced telecommunications and the 24-hour availability of a healthcare professional like a nurse. This nurse can help patients with their decision-making and assist in determining whether a health event warrants calling emergency services or to identify if another remedy can be administered in the home environment.[15] For example, if an older adult sustained a fall and was unable to determine whether they were injured enough to call emergency services or wait until the next day to go to their general practitioner, the patient or family could video conference with the home care nurse. The nurse could ask a series of triage questions and observe the patient's body structure and range of motion to determine whether there was a superficial soft tissue injury or whether a fracture was likely. This critical assistance may result in having the individual put ice on their traumatized body part and take some previously supplied medication with a follow-up to the physician the next day. This improved access and communication with the healthcare team might avoid unnecessary admission to the hospital (see Chapter 5).

In certain scenarios, physical activity and therapy services may be able to be delivered via telehealth through a live or pre-recorded exercise coaching session; these have already been implemented in conditions like congestive heart failure and pulmonary disorders.[16,17] Although there has been very little substantive research on the safety or efficacy of this intervention as compared to a one-on-one, in-person physical activity or therapy session, with the previous successes and proliferation of telehealth in light of COVID-19, it is inevitable that healthcare systems or therapists will begin to integrate telehealth physical activity or rehabilitation.[18]

When considering telehealth during physical activity, patient safety considerations are paramount. In cases where the patient is unsteady or has poor balance and the therapist's intent is to perform standing or balancing exercises, it is likely that a telehealth visit would not be appropriate. In this case the interventions delivered via telehealth may expose the individual to a higher fall risk when performing activities that challenge his or her balance without the close and direct personal supervision of a therapist.[19] Much of the opportunity for telehealth with rehabilitation may be with the more physically able, less symptomatic, or more medically stable individuals where the physical presence of the therapist is less necessary. At the other end of the spectrum, there is a role for a therapist in telehealth to provide consultative services in the home to assist with coaching families, caregivers, or other healthcare personnel in safe movement patterns or proper performance of techniques for an individual with advanced disease.[20] This may include coaching a patient and family through a mechanical lift transfer via video conferencing, reinforcing proper performance of manual lymphatic drainage or wrapping, or virtual coaching in lower extremity passive range of motion near the end of life.

Virtual Reality

As telehealth is an evolving area of practice that leverages new technology, the concept of virtual reality devices presents another extremely unique opportunity for therapists to assist in facilitating safe movement patterns and coaching in proper performance. Virtual reality is being examined for rehabilitation of individuals post stroke or brain injury and is demonstrating exciting findings as it relates to motor learning and motor planning.[21–26] Virtual reality is often experienced by wearing specialized goggles and a headset (see Figure 21.2). There are some consumer devices for virtual reality including the PlayStation VR by Sony Entertainment System, the HTC Vive, and the Oculus Rift, but these have been mainly utilized for entertainment purposes in the video game arena. Although the healthcare applications are currently limited, the use of these consumer products for entertainment purposes has resulted in the technology advancing at an extremely rapid rate as well as lowering the cost.

With this rapid acceleration and initial applications in healthcare, opportunities for utility in chronic disease, life-limiting illness, and end-of-life care may arise. Some examples of opportunities for the application of virtual reality include a virtual visit to an individual's favorite geographic location that they might want to visit one more time before they pass away.[27] With nearly the entire globe being mapped via satellite (e.g. Google Earth) and street-view cameras (e.g. Google Street View), a person may have the opportunity to wear goggles and "visit" their childhood home thousands of miles away and reminisce on some of the positive experiences. This person may have the opportunity to "visit" a favorite vacation destination virtually when their body may be too frail or medically unstable to be able to tolerate a physical journey.[27] These endeavors may assist in coping with death via distraction and adapting to a physical loss of function. As the authors are not aware of any scholarly investigations of this specific type of application, the utility and implications of this are academic and theoretical at this time.

Certainly, the potential applications for this technology are there to be leveraged appropriately; however, virtual reality may be recommended to be used with caution as overuse of some devices have been known to cause nausea. This motion sickness occurs because the visual system perceives motion in three dimensions, but this same motion is not perceived by the vestibular system, thereby causing symptoms similar to seasickness. In addition, the effects of virtual reality are unknown in the developing nervous systems of children, and virtual reality is generally contraindicated for use in children. However, if a child has a terminal illness, the therapeutic benefit of using virtual reality may be a more feasible option as the long-term concerns related to normal nervous system development may not be a primary consideration. Finally, distraction and guided meditation activities may also have applicability via virtual reality in end-of-life care to alleviate distress and anxiety.[28,29]

Other opportunities for virtual reality include utilizing virtual reality goggles and handsets to assist in virtual coaching of certain psychomotor tasks such as training a family caregiver on proper bed mobility and transfer technique. Again, this is generally theoretical as this would require an extensive amount of computer programming and force feedback mechanisms to assist the virtual reality participant to not just see and position themselves correctly but to also feel the appropriate forces and tactile effects of these activities. As virtual reality applications in health are advancing rapidly, there are inevitably a variety of uses that cannot even be conceptualized at this time.

Integrated Medical Record Systems

One of the most useful technological advances is the concept of a universal medical record system. Although initially challenging to adopt for many healthcare systems, electronic medical records (EMRs) have been integral in assisting healthcare providers with navigating the increasingly complex healthcare system. With this new technology, a physician, from their home or smartphone, can securely and promptly access their patients' lab tests, medications, imaging studies, and interdisciplinary care team notes and take immediate action.[30]

One of the major limitations to the integrated medical record is that it is generally isolated to one healthcare system. Because of the isolation of this valuable information, if an individual receives healthcare at several different institutions, some healthcare providers may not be aware of what other providers' prescriptions, orders, or medical opinions are; this challenge might be acutely encountered in emergency situations. For example, travel may not be an issue if an individual generally receives care at the healthcare institution of their choice and that institution is located farther away from their house, under convenient and normal circumstances. Some individuals have been known to pass two or three other competing healthcare systems to get to their healthcare system of choice. In emergency transport situations (e.g. ambulance), the individual may not have a choice or the luxury to be transported to their preferred healthcare system and are generally transported immediately to the nearest emergency department. If the medical records are not integrated, this emergency department may not have all the relevant information related to this person's chronic illness and more importantly, may not have documentation of the advance care directives. In the absence of a documented advanced care directive or valid do not resuscitate (DNR) order, the healthcare institution may have no choice but to attempt life-saving measures such as cardiopulmonary resuscitation even though it is against the patient's documented wishes.[31]

Another area where this may be a challenge is that some physicians in private practice may not participate in an integrated medical record with the healthcare system with which they are affiliated.[32] Some physicians may be affiliated with several different hospitals through their independent private practice office. Although for each individual health system, it would be more beneficial to have the physician document their office notes and diagnostic test results within the hospital system's medical record, this may not be a feasible or a financially viable option for the physician in private practice.

These examples illustrate the critical need for a universally integrated health network that connects all healthcare systems, physicians, and therapy providers into one integrated system. Although this is a relatively easily understood and logical concept, the realities of inter-operability of different computerized medical record systems require technical protocols and a concerted effort to achieve these goals. Health Information Exchange (HIE) – which is defined by Healthcare Information and Management Systems Society (HIMSS) as "providing the capability to electronically move clinical information among disparate healthcare information systems and maintain the meaning of the information being exchanged."[33] Many EMR developers are for-profit businesses that do not consistently have an immediate incentive to focus time, resources, and manpower toward achieving integration with the medical record systems of its competitors. In the technical programming and computer world, consumers (and therefore developers) often value EMR features such as availability of resources, rapid system navigation, and effective documentation. Based on this, EMR developers prioritize these aspects much higher than interoperability with their competitors' EMRs. This elicits the question - *how do we get there?* In most situations, it may require legislation or governmental assistance or incentive/penalties as the private, for-profit market has not consistently prioritized inter-operability. For example, within the United States, regulatory agencies have established a framework for exchanging health data in a structured way (e.g. HL-7, C-CDAs, FHIR) and the US federal government has facilitated adoption of these standards through *meaningful use* legislation and regulations.[34] In nations where EMR systems and paper records are still being utilized, if these institutions dedicate resources to investing in an integrated medical record system at a governmental level, these nations may actually be able to achieve a national integrated medical record system more rapidly than those nations that have already approached saturation of EMRs as the medical records have already been firmly entrenched in these nations.

Finally, therapy clinical documentation is a unique, specialized, and complex component of therapist practice. With this unique complexity has arisen specialized therapy-focused EMRs. As with office medical records of some private physicians, many therapists and physical activity professionals' records may not be consistently integrated into overall healthcare systems' EMRs. A further challenge is the fact that some prevention and wellness professionals who are not working in a traditional healthcare or medical model may not have the same documentation, billing, and coding requirements that other professionals like physical therapists or occupational therapists have. As these wellness and health promotion activities are exceptionally important in the overall maintenance of the health and behaviors of an individual with a chronic illness, it would behoove the entire interdisciplinary healthcare team to have access to this valuable information. As of this time, there is limited integration of wellness and health promotion and practitioner integration into medical record systems unless affiliated with a large hospital or healthcare system.

Activity Monitoring Devices

Another technological opportunity may involve the use and leveraging of consumer-focused wearable technologies such as activity monitors. As with virtual reality, this domain has advanced extremely rapidly providing many opportunities for innovation but leaving very little in the way of systematic, scientific application, or clear evidence of when, where, how, and which device is recommended for certain conditions or issues. It has been established that the accuracy of some of these movement trackers is not amenable to certain populations. For example, wrist-worn activity monitors may not accurately detect the physical mobility of individuals who use walkers or wheelchairs as their primary means of mobility.[35] In addition, if an individual walks slowly, does not generate sufficient arm swing, or step impact, steps might not be recorded on some activity trackers. Some activity monitors also utilize global positioning systems (GPS) to assist with tracking movement and activity though many GPS-enabled devices have limited accuracy, especially, in indoor environments. This is due to device limitations of syncing with a satellite signal, such as in large apartment buildings; this technology has limited utility especially for those with mobility limitations or those who may be homebound.[36] These more sophisticated wearable activity monitors tend to be more costly which may also limit the accessibility for those who are on a fixed income.

Besides, some individuals are generally suspicious of personal technology and how much information about themselves and their health behaviors is available or being transmitted, including those with sensitive diagnoses such as human immunodeficiency virus (HIV).[37] As there continues to be negative media stories almost daily of data breaches of private information, there is rationality and logic to this concern. Unfortunately, this may be limiting an individual's ability to utilize technology to assist with their own health and physical activity changes.

Certain activity monitors have features that may be beneficial for assisting in the provision of care of those with a life-threatening illness or frailty. These may include step trackers to determine how many steps a person has taken.[38] Trends could be identified if gait speed slows or daily ambulation distance decreases. This could potentially indicate the exacerbation of an illness or onset of an injury. In addition, some wearable activity monitors or smart watches also have accelerometers built into them to assist with fall detection.[39] In the event of a fall, the accelerometers would detect a rapid change in speed with an abrupt deceleration in a characteristic fashion.[39] If the device detects a fall, the device can notify family, caregivers, or emergency personnel who can then contact or go visit the individual to see if medical assistance is necessary. Finally, even a simple pedometer or low-tech activity monitor may have useful features to assist in coaching and healthy behaviors. Some wearable activity monitors will vibrate or make a tone to remind an individual to get out of their seat and walk or remind an individual to take medications or drink water.[40] As these features come and go from different wearable activity monitors, the therapist should be an educated health coach in the utility and applicability of these devices.

Meta-data and Predictive Algorithms

When considering some of the care models outlined in Chapters 1 and 4, such as *palliative prehabilitation* and *skilled maintenance*, some of the challenges entail the therapist's limited ability to predict the time and progression of varying disease processes. If the therapist's contention that physical activity interventions would help to slow or maintain a progressive disorder, this contention should be confirmed by some data or evidence. Currently there are no valid or robust data sets to quantify this predictable functional decline or disease progression.

A useful analogy would be from normal childhood development. Pediatric specialists generally have fairly accurate physical milestones that are predictable and achievable as a child matures and grows. For example, pediatric physical therapists can reasonably expect children to be able to sit up unsupported at approximately six months and be able to stand with support at one year.[41] If a child is not able to achieve these milestones, therapeutic services are generally warranted to assist the child in achieving these milestones. Unfortunately, analogous functional decline milestones are not available but would be extremely beneficial for therapists to predict at what point certain assistive devices or therapeutic interventions would be beneficial based on disease stages or biomarkers. In addition, should a therapist have a valid, data-driven, predictive model for their patient's functional decline, and they were then able to provide interventions to delay or slow physical decline, this would provide substantive evidence that the physical activity services are warranted and medically necessary.

Likely the best means to accomplish this predictive modeling and robust data set is through de-identified meta-data.[42]

> "Increasingly researchers have access to 'big' data, as evident by meta-analyses using individual participant data (IPD) from multiple studies, and by analyses of registry databases containing electronic health (e-health) records for thousands or even millions of patients from multiple practices, hospitals, or countries."[42]

This conglomeration of de-identified meta-data may be another substantial benefit of an integrated EMR system. Currently, there are privacy regulations that restrict or control the release and use of identifiable medical information that often restricts the use of most health data (including de-identified meta-data). This meta-data, if utilized properly and ethically, may provide a robust and valid data set to establish when certain types of patients in certain demographic categories, and with certain diagnoses, may experience health events or declines.[42] There will always be individual patient circumstances and unforeseen events; however, this information may have potential utility and assist in the predictive care of those with life-threatening illnesses.

This concept of the use of meta-data is not without controversy and ethical dilemmas.[43] It has been long discussed that this information may potentially be used for nefarious purposes. For example, if a predictive model has established that a person with rapidly advancing multiple sclerosis will succumb to the disease in three months, there may be certain parties or organizations that may be reluctant to provide care services or surgical interventions to this individual because of this anticipated outcome. Certainly, these immediate and long-term ethical issues must be worked out and discussed; however, this data may be able to assist in establishing best practices for therapists working with individuals with life-threatening illnesses to determine when resources are best applied or when screenings or interventions would be most beneficial.[43]

Genomics, Genetics, and Personalized Healthcare and Medicine

Since the discovery of DNA and mapping of the human set of genes via the Human Genome Project, the application of knowledge of genetics and genomics in identifying disease risk and progression has revolutionized healthcare and spawned the field of personalized medicine. The overarching concept of personalized medicine is utilizing a person's genetic makeup and genome to be able to best develop medications and treatments based on the specific nuances of an individual and their exact disease process.[44] Although this concept is in its infancy, it has the potential to theoretically cure or control many diseases that may have otherwise been fatal, turning them into manageable chronic conditions. Another benefit of this personalized medicine is that a person's genetic profile can be utilized to individually select or tailor medications to reduce the side effect profile or optimize the efficacy of an individual's medications.

A related topic is the concept of targeted therapies and immune checkpoint inhibitors in cancer care. One of the challenges with cancer chemotherapy is that it is systemic and often negatively affects nearly all tissues in the body if administered through the bloodstream.[45] Chemotherapy intends to disrupt the replication of rapidly dividing cells, such as cancer cells, but it can also impact the replication of other rapidly dividing cells, characteristically cells within the gastrointestinal system or hair follicles, and often cause some of the common side effects such as nausea and vomiting or alopecia. With the ongoing advent of targeted therapies and immune checkpoint inhibitors for cancer care, the necessity for systemic broad-spectrum chemotherapy may be reduced. This has the potential to further refine the effectiveness of cancer treatment, again potentially turning some previously fatal cancers into chronic or slow-growing conditions.[45]

An increasingly common immunotherapy treatment for hematologic cancers is chimeric antigen receptor T-cell therapy (CAR-T), which results in modification of T-cells that can identify and attack the cancer cells. This process is depicted in Figure 23.1. First, T-cells are extracted from the patient's bloodstream via IV access. After extraction, genetic information for the specific antigen of the cancer cells is encoded into the T-cells. These new CAR receptors found on the surface of the T-cells will help the T-cells to recognize and fight hematologic cancer. Once coding is successful, the new antigen-specific T-cells are replicated and infused into the patient's bloodstream in order to attack the cancer cells.

One recent example of this is the use of targeted therapies in non-small cell lung cancer (NSCLC). As lung cancer is frequently asymptomatic until it is at an advanced stage, palliative chemotherapy was one of the few treatment

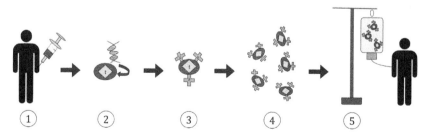

Figure 23.1 Chimeric Antigen Receptor T-cell Therapy (CAR-T). By Reyasingh56-Own work, CC BY-SA 4.0, https://commons.wikimedia.org/w/index.php?curid=69702021.

options available to treat stage IV cancer. Recently, there have been advancements in biomarker testing for specific genetic mutations in the lungs such as epidermal growth factor receptors (EGFR), anaplastic lymphoma kinase (ALK), ROS-1, neurotrophic receptor tyrosine kinase (NTRK), and the V600E mutation of the BRAF gene.[46] The United States Food and Drug Administration has approved targeted therapies for cancer with these biomarkers which may have a significant impact on longevity or quality of life.[46]

Medication classes such as immune checkpoint inhibitors aim to utilize a person's own immune system to attack cancer cells without attacking healthy non-cancerous cells. One of the challenges with cancer is that the cancerous cells are genetically closely related to non-cancer cells, thereby causing no clear immune response to fight the cancer cells. In general, immune checkpoint inhibitors upregulate or disinhibit an immune response. In the case of lung cancer, a commonly used mechanism is the engagement of T lymphocyte cells. Lee et al.[47] performed a meta-analysis of three studies that compared immune checkpoint inhibitors (nivolumab, pembrolizumab, and atezolizumab) against docetaxel in individuals with NSCLC. It was found that immune checkpoint inhibitors significantly prolonged overall survival as compared to docetaxel. This is one example of an aggressive, often lethal disease that is being morphed into a longer-term chronic illness that will require physical activity to assist in the management.

Social Networking for Palliative Therapists

One of the most basic but potentially most significant innovations for the future of therapist care when dealing with a life-threatening illness is the opportunity for collaboration and mentorship among therapists in diverse geographic regions. Recently, therapists have reported that they do not consistently get much training or education for the care of those with life-threatening illnesses or PC concepts, and much of their PC training has been from continuing education and direct mentoring.[48] Unfortunately, this means that if continuing education or mentoring is not available in one's immediate geographical practice area, the therapist's services or skills may not be fully developed and therefore terminally ill individuals may not receive optimum care. With the advent of robust social networking and nationwide alliances of like-minded health professionals such as special interest groups or networks, these geographical barriers to education and mentoring are no longer as problematic as they once were. For example, in Australia, a group of allied health professionals have established a network called the Australian Allied Health in PC network (AAHPC) (https://www.caresearch.com.au/caresearch/tabid/2939/Default.aspx). As Australia is a broad continent with significant geographical distances between population centers, there is limited opportunity for easy collaboration and coordination of care. The AAHPC assists in facilitating allied health professionals, including therapists, as far away from each other as Perth and Sydney (4,000 km) to share ideas, resources, and compare best practices for patients. In addition to the social networking and individual therapist collaboration, these organic social networks can ally with established professional associations or organizations to advocate for legislation or regulatory reform to best meet PC patient and client needs.

Finally, with the advent of online learning and distance learning, there are substantial opportunities for the education of therapists and other healthcare providers in the unique intervention models and communication skills. Video modules, podcasts, and online certifications are all readily available via technology to improve the provision of patient-centered care without the need to attend an in-person course. A recent example of this is the rapid, global dissemination of reputable health information related to the management of individuals infected with the COVID-19 novel coronavirus. During this global pandemic, a therapist had a wide variety of resources including webinars, online meetings, and peer-reviewed articles to help facilitate the rapidly changing clinical roles and treatment approaches that were required during the evolution of this health crisis. Although the actual number of individual lives that were saved due to this rapid availability of healthcare provider education will never be known, the authors can confidently state that without this online availability of reputable continuing education, many more lives would have been lost.

Summary

There are a variety of emerging opportunities for an innovative and technologically minded therapist to facilitate patient-centered care. These technological innovations may include researching the impact of virtual reality, telemedicine, or wearable activity monitors; however, technical hurdles, health literacy, and technology literacy issues must also be addressed. There is also a significant opportunity for establishing predictive models to assist therapists in providing individualized, and effective care via predictive modeling and meta-data, although this must be carefully examined within the context of healthcare ethics. Finally, for all therapists, there is an immediate and beneficial opportunity to network with colleagues in their local jurisdictions, nations, or even globally through social networks. These networking opportunities will likely grow as these technological networks become more robust and can offer continuing education via online modules or certifications.

References

1 Levy H, Janke AT, Langa KM. Health literacy and the digital divide among older Americans. *J Gen Internet Med.* 2015;30(3):284–289.
2 Jensen JD, King AJ, Davis LA, Guntzviller LM. Utilization of internet technology by low-income adults: The role of health literacy, health numeracy, and computer assistance. *J Aging Health.* 2010;22(6):804–826.
3 Jordan-Marsh M. *Health Technology Literacy: A Transdisciplinary Framework for Consumer-Oriented Practice.* Burlington, MA: Jones & Bartlett Publishers; 2010.

4   Xie B. Effects of an eHealth literacy intervention for older adults. *J Med Internet Res.* 2011;13(4):e90.
5   Xie B. Older adults, e-health literacy, and collaborative learning: An experimental study. *J Am Soc Inf Sci Technol.* 2011;62(5):933–946.
6   Xie B. Experimenting on the impact of learning methods and information presentation channels on older adults' e-health literacy. *J Am Soc Inf Sci Technol.* 2011;62(9):1797–1807.
7   Zallio M, Berry D. Design and planned obsolescence. Theories and approaches for designing enabling technologies. *Des J.* 2017;20(Supplement 1):S3749-S3761.
8   Robinson CA, Pesut B, Bottorff JL. Issues in rural PC: Views from the countryside. *J Rural Health.* 2010;26(1):78–84.
9   Bradford NK, Caffery LJ, Smith AC. Telehealth services in rural and remote Australia: A systematic review of models of care and factors influencing success and sustainability. *Rural Remote Health.* 2016;16(4):3808.
10 Watanabe SM, Fairchild A, Pituskin E, Borgersen P, Hanson J, Fassbender K. Improving access to specialist multidisciplinary PC consultation for rural cancer patients by videoconferencing: Report of a pilot project. *Support Care Cancer.* 2013;21(4):1201–1207.
11 Kidd L, Cayless S, Johnston B, Wengstrom Y. Telehealth in PC in the UK: A review of the evidence. *J Telemed Telecare.* 2010;16(7):394–402.
12 Hollander JE, Carr BG. Virtually perfect? Telemedicine for COVID-19. *N Engl J Med.* 2020. doi:10.1056/NEJMp2003539.
13 World Confederation for Physical Therapy and International Network of Physiotherapy Regulatory Authorities. *Report of the WCPT/INPTRA Digital Physical Therapy Practice Task Force.* Geneva, Switzerland: World Confederation for Physical Therapy; 2019.
14 Langabeer JR, II MG, Alqusairi D, et al. Telehealth-enabled emergency medical services program reduces ambulance transport to urban emergency departments. *West J Emerg Med.* 2016;17(6): 713–720. doi:10.5811/westjem. 2016.8.30660.
15 Johnston B, Kidd L, Wengstrom Y, Kearney N. An evaluation of the use of telehealth within PC settings across Scotland. *Palliat Med.* 2012;26(2):152–161.
16 Stickland MK, Jourdain T, Wong EY, Rodgers WM, Jendzjowsky NG, MacDonald GF. Using telehealth technology to deliver pulmonary rehabilitation to patients with chronic obstructive pulmonary disease. *Can Respir J.* 2011;18(4):216–220.
17 Rawstorn JC, Gant N, Direito A, Beckmann C, Maddison R. Telehealth exercise-based cardiac rehabilitation: A systematic review and meta-analysis. *Heart.* 2016;102(15):1183–1192.
18 Tenforde AS, Hefner JE, Kodish-Wachs JE, Iaccarino MA, Paganoni S. Telehealth in physical medicine and rehabilitation: A narrative review. *PM&R.* 2017;9(5):S51-S58.
19 Cason J, Hartmann Kim, Jacobs K, Richmond T. Telehealth. *Am J Occup Ther.* 2013;67(6):S69-S90.
20 Forducey PG, Glueckauf RL, Bergquist TF, Maheu MM, Yutsis M. Telehealth for persons with severe functional disabilities and their caregivers: Facilitating self-care management in the home setting. *Psychol Serv.* 2012;9(2): 144–162. doi:10.1037/a0028112.
21 McEwen D, Taillon-Hobson A, Bilodeau M, Sveistrup H, Finestone H. Virtual reality exercise improves mobility after stroke: An inpatient randomized controlled trial. *Stroke.* 2014;45(6):1853–1855.
22 Singh DK, Rajaratnam BS, Palaniswamy V, Pearson H, Raman VP, Bong PS. Participating in a virtual reality balance exercise program can reduce risk and fear of falls. *Maturitas.* 2012;73(3):239–243.

23 Laver KE, Lange B, George S, Deutsch JE, Saposnik G, Crotty M. Virtual reality for stroke rehabilitation. *Cochrane Database Syst Rev.* 2017;11(11):CD008349.

24 Saposnik G, Levin M, Stroke Outcome Research Canada (SORCan) Working Group. Virtual reality in stroke rehabilitation: A meta-analysis and implications for clinicians. *Stroke.* 2011;42(5):1380–1386.

25 Glegg SM, Holsti L, Velikonja D, Ansley B, Brum C, Sartor D. Factors influencing therapists' adoption of virtual reality for brain injury rehabilitation. *Cyberpsychol Behav Soc Netw.* 2013;16(5):385–401.

26 Pietrzak E, Pullman S, McGuire A. Using virtual reality and videogames for traumatic brain injury rehabilitation: A structured literature review. *Games Health J.* 2014;3(4):202–214.

27 Pabla K, Knight J, Motley M. O-24 virtual reality transforming the lives of terminally ill patients. *BMJ Support Palliat Care.* 2017;(7):A9–A10.

28 Popert S, Riat H, Hodges E. P-35 can virtual reality (VR) guided meditation reduce pain? A feasibility and acceptability study. *BMJ Support Palliat Care.* 2017;7:A22.

29 Mills M, Roughneen S, Mason S, Chapman L, Khodabukus A, Nwosu A. O-18 virtual reality distraction therapy in PC: A feasibility study. *BMJ Support Palliat Care.* 2018; 8(Suppl. 2):A7.2–A7.

30 Menachemi N, Collum TH. Benefits and drawbacks of electronic health record systems. *Risk Manag Healthc Policy.* 2011;4:47.

31 Lamba S, Nagurka R, Zielinski A, Scott SR. PC provision in the emergency department: Barriers reported by emergency physicians. *J Palliat Med.* 2013;16(2):143–147.

32 Lau F, Price M, Boyd J, Partridge C, Bell H, Raworth R. Impact of EMR on physician practice in office settings: A systematic review. *BMC Med Inform Decis Mak.* 2012;12(1):10. doi:10.1186/1472-6947-12-10.

33 Marchant M, Rubin J. Navigating the interoperability landscape with the HIMSS environmental scan. https://www.himss.org/resources/navigating-interoperability-landscape-himss-environmental-scan. Updated 2018. Accessed Nov 2, 2019.

34 Tippett PS. The year of universal medical record sharing. https://www.himss.org/news/year-universal-medical-record-sharing. Updated 2018. Accessed Nov 2, 2019.

35 Godfrey A. Wearables for independent living in older adults: Gait and falls. *Maturitas.* 2017;100:16–26. doi:10.1016/j.maturitas.2017.03.317.

36 Mahoney EL, Mahoney DF. Acceptance of wearable technology by people with Alzheimer's disease: Issues and accommodations. *Am J Alzheimer's Dis.* 2010;25(6):527–531. doi:10.1177/1533317510376944.

37 Schnall R, Higgins T, Brown W, Carballo-Dieguez A, Bakken S. Trust, perceived risk, perceived ease of use and perceived usefulness as factors related to mHealth technology use. *Stud Health Technol Inform.* 2015;216:467–471.

38 Mercer K, Giangregorio L, Schneider E, Chilana P, Li M, Grindrod K. Acceptance of commercially available wearable activity trackers among adults aged over 50 and with chronic illness: A mixed-methods evaluation. *JMIR Mhealth Uhealth.* 2016;4(1):e7. doi:10.2196/mhealth.4225.

39 Delahoz SY, Labrador AM. Survey on fall detection and fall prevention using wearable and external sensors. *Sensors.* 2014;14(10). doi:10.3390/s141019806.

40 Reeder B, David A. Health at hand: A systematic review of smart watch uses for health and wellness. *J Biomed Inform.* 2016;63:269–276. doi:10.1016/j.jbi.2016.09.001.

41 Centers for Disease Control and Prevention. Developmental milestones. https://www.cdc.gov/ncbddd/actearly/milestones/index.html. Updated 2018. Accessed Nov 3, 2019.

42 Riley RD, Ensor J, Snell KIE, et al. External validation of clinical prediction models using big datasets from e-health records or IPD meta-analysis: Opportunities and challenges. *BMJ*. 2016;353:i3140. doi:10.1136/bmj.i3140.

43 Mittelstadt BD, Floridi L. The ethics of big data: Current and foreseeable issues in biomedical contexts. *Sci Eng Ethics*. 2016;22(2):303–341. doi:10.1007/s11948-015-9652-2.

44 Hamburg MA, Collins FS. The path to personalized medicine. *N Engl J Med*. 2010;363(4):301–304. doi:10.1056/NEJMp1006304.

45 Schilsky RL. Personalized medicine in oncology: The future is now. *Nat Rev Drug Discov*. 2010;9(5):363–366. doi:10.1038/nrd3181.

46 American Lung Association. Targeted therapies for lung cancer. https://www.lung.org/lung-health-diseases/lung-disease-lookup/lung-cancer/patients/treatment/types-of-treatment/targeted-therapies. Updated 2020. Accessed April 30, 2020.

47 Lee CK, Man J, Lord S, et al. Checkpoint inhibitors in metastatic EGFR-mutated Non–Small cell lung Cancer—A meta-analysis. *J Thorac Oncol*. 2017;12(2):403–407. doi:10.1016/j.jtho.2016.10.007.

48 Wilson CM, Stiller CH, Doherty DJ, Thompson KA. The role of physical therapists within hospice and PC in the United States and Canada. *Am J Hosp Palliat Med*. 2017;34(1):34–41. doi:10.1177/1049909115604668.

Afterword

Richard Briggs

In some ways, the technical knowledge and skills to provide end-of-life care to those with a terminal illness is the easy part. While the extensive information in this textbook will be useful to develop your clinical acumen for evidence-based practice in this field, a question remains. A question that may have occurred to you, or may yet be unvoiced but still present. Certainly, it will arise in time, or be posed when a friend or colleague learns of your work: 'How can you be with all of the loss, suffering, and dying?'. This Afterword is offered not to answer this question, but to provide some direction and resources to further your understanding, should you be interested in exploring the experience of end-of-life issues. Consider how you might enhance your emotional health, spiritual awareness, and understanding of such events while your practice evolves in end-of-life care.

Let's examine each of these aspects individually. *Loss* is inherent to healthcare, and most certainly to rehabilitation. It is what brings people to us for care, and we use the aforementioned skills to help resolve or manage their issues as well as possible. Whether that be to recover from an accident, injury, or acute illness, or live well with a developmental or chronic condition, therapy or activity is beneficial. Life-threatening conditions tend to be more complex, by their nature. At the very least, they are disruptive to one's regular activity, life plans, or goals; at the most, they put one's very existence into question. Dying is the ultimate disability.

Suffering is more of an existential issue, of not having what one needs or wants, or having an undeniably difficult experience. Experiencing pain and the associated angst or desire to be rid of it, magnifies the pain and evokes suffering. The example of having a thorny rose stem in your open hand is instructive. Rather than just observe and acknowledge its presence and associated discomfort, to grasp it more tightly, only worsens the sensation. Suffering comes from our reactions and the attachment to the life we live and all of the pleasures and activities it affords us, when that is brought into question. We can be attached to our possessions; attached to a job; attached to our family; attached to this life; and, thus, need to mourn all of these losses. There is an abundance of literature that explores the practice of non-attachment, a skill that helps deal with the inevitable losses in life, and the suffering we are prone to experience over its course.

Which leads us to dying. At some level we have an awareness that we ourselves, and all beings, have a mortal existence; we are born, and we will die. The expression goes "no one gets out of here alive". But, most of all our culture turns away from this, and in my experience, bringing up the topic of death or dying in a social context is often met with averted eyes and avoidance. There are people who regularly face this reality in their work, and they are commonly found in the hospice and palliative care community. The questions raised and the seeking of understanding deepen the awareness of life, its processes, and its inevitable ending, and are worthy of exploration.

Working with individuals facing death demands that we examine our *selves* and our *souls*. Sitting with someone who is facing the end of his or her life is often akin to sitting in front of a mirror. If we truly see the loss, we cannot help but reflect on the possibility that this person could be our parent, sibling, friend, partner, child, or our self. An array of emotion is likely to arise and be expressed through our body language, facial expressions, and language. We all have continuous work to do in exploring our own relationship with life and death, to become clearer and more at peace with the process for ourselves, and, thus, for others.

I have found the following books useful as guides in exploring this part of living and dying. It can be helpful to read the words of others, and experiencing their conversations secondhand can be beneficial. Take some quiet time to reflect with them. Some may speak to you, some may elicit strong emotions and tears, others warmth and a knowing smile. These are signs of the work that we all need to do in the course of our living and dying. It is a personal practice, not dissimilar from our professional practice, which needs regular attention. It helps one live with a more open and richer human experience and it can make working with the dying deeply rewarding. The words of Christine Longaker are instructive: *The path of life is already a journey towards death, and once you decide to make that path a spiritual one, then every aspect of your life, including your caregiving work, gives a positive momentum to your spiritual path.*

Suggested Readings

Bauby J. *The Diving Bell and the Butterfly.* New York, NY: Vintage International; 1997.

Byock I. *Dying Well.* New York, NY: Riverhead Books; 1997.

Byock I. *The Four Things that Matter Most.* New York, NY: Simon and Schuster; 2004.

Callanan M, Kelley P. *Final Gifts.* New York, NY: Poseidon Press; 1992.

Chochinov MH. *Dignity Therapy: Final Words for Final Days.* New York, NY: Oxford University Press; 2012.

Frankl V. *Man's Search for Meaning.* New York, NY: Washington Square Press; 1959.

Gawande A. *Being Mortal.* New York, NY: Metropolitan Books, Henry Holt and Company; 2014.

Halifax J. *Being with Dying: Cultivating Compassion and Fearlessness in the Presence of Death.* Boulder, CO: Shambhala Press; 2008.

Hennezen M. *Intimate Death: How the Dying Teach Us to Live.* New York, NY: Vintage Books; 1998.

Kabat-Zinn J. *Full Catastrophe Living: Using the Wisdom of Your Body and Mind to Face Stress, Pain, and Illness.* New York, NY: Bantam Doubleday Dell; 1990.

Kalanithi P. *When Breath Becomes Air.* New York, NY: Random House; 2016.

Kramer H, Kramer K. *Conversations at Midnight.* New York, NY: William Morrow and Company; 1993.

Kubler-Ross E. *On Death and Dying.* New York, NY: Macmillan; 1969.

Kubler-Ross E. *Death is of Vital Importance.* Barrytown, NY: Station Hill Press; 1995.

Levine S. *Who Dies.* Garden City, NY: Anchor Press; 1982.

Levine S. *Meetings at the Edge.* Garden City, NY: Anchor Press; 1984.

Levine S. *A Year to Live: How to Live This Year as If It Were Your Last.* New York, NY: Bell Tower; 1993.

Longaker C. *Facing Death and Finding Hope.* New York, NY: Doubleday; 1997.

Martin W, Martin N. *The Caregiver's Tao Te Ching.* Novato, CA: New World Library; 2011.

Muller W. *How, then, Shall We Live.* New York, NY: Bantam Books; 1996.

Nuland S. *How We Die.* New York, NY: Alfred A. Knopf; 1994.

Ostaseski F. *The Five Invitations: Discovering What Death Can Teach Us about Living Fully.* New York, NY: Flatiron Books; 2017.

Pausch R, Zaslow J. *The Last Lecture.* New York, NY: Hyperion; 2008.

Remen RN. *My Grandfather's Blessings: Stories of Strength, Refuge, and Belonging.* New York, NY: Riverhead Books; 2000.

Remen R. *Kitchen Table Wisdom.* New York, NY: Riverhead Books; 1996.

Rimpoche S. *The Tibetan Book of Living and Dying.* New York, NY: HarperCollins; 2020.

Sharp J. *Living Our Dying.* New York, NY: Hyperion; 1996.

Singh KD. *The Grace in Dying.* New York, NY: HarperCollins; 1998.

Stoddard S. *The Hospice Movement; A Better Way to Care for the Dying.* New York, NY: Vintage Books; 1992.

Wiman C. *My Bright Abyss: Meditation of a Modern Believer.* New York, NY: Farrar, Straus, and Giroux; 2013.

Part V

Appendix and Resources

Appendix 1
Advanced Care Planning

When caring for individuals with life-limiting illnesses, it is imperative for the clinician to be aware of completed components of advance care planning (ACP), or the lack thereof. ACP has several elements that are useful throughout the process of planning for future medical needs, and in exploring values and goals that can be documented. ACP may include practical planning aspects such as financial/legal affairs, final gifts (e.g. bequests, organ donations), autopsies, burial/cremation wishes, funeral/memorial services, or guardianship. In addition, ACP often details procedures and preferences related to the final hours of life, such as personal choices, desired settings, and proxy decision makers. For more background on ACP, see Chapter 1.

The process of ACP includes: the introduction of the topic; engagement in structured discussions; documentation of patient preferences; regular review and updates as necessary; and the application of directives when the need arises. It also includes professional and legal responsibilities to determine a proxy decision maker in the event of the patient's lost capacity. ACP is also a way to reduce uncertainty, avoid confusion and conflict, and allow for peace of mind and trust between the patient-family unit and their healthcare providers. An *advance directive* includes the components of a living will and a durable power of attorney. It may also include portable medical orders (e.g. POLST [see next]). A *living will* is the documentation of the patient's wishes regarding their care. Such specifications often include withholding or withdrawing of artificial feeding, hydration, mechanical ventilation, or cardiopulmonary resuscitation (CPR). Additionally, wishes pertaining to initiating life-sustaining treatments are often also included such as elective intubation, surgery, dialysis, blood transfusions or products, artificial nutrition, antibiotics, or future hospital admissions. A *durable power of attorney* (DPOA) is a designated, competent adult who acts as an agent for financial or healthcare decision-making on behalf of the patient when they are no longer able to make their own decisions. When specified, particularly for the purpose of healthcare-related decision-making, the proxy is referred to as DPOA-HC. Ideally, the patient would also designate an alternate proxy in the event that the primary was unavailable, or unable, to participate in end-of-life decision-making for any reason.

Honoring a patient's known wishes, such as a do-not-resuscitate (DNR) order, is not only critical for maintaining the patient's autonomy and quality of life, but is also legally binding and ethically important. For example, a clinician might witness a patient experience sudden cardiac arrest and proceed to perform CPR, despite the patient's advance directive specifying a DNR order which would restrict this lifesaving measure. Under these circumstances, the clinician and their employer may be held liable for unnecessary life-sustaining measures that are counter to the patient's documented wishes. For this reason, medical record review and/or orientation to core ACP documents will appropriately orient the clinician prior to providing care to the individual with a life-limiting illness. In the homecare setting, ACP documents may be posted within a patient's home (often next to the front door or on the refrigerator). In the United States, there are particular legal criteria that need to be met in order to have a legally binding advance directive; importantly, these regulations vary by state or jurisdiction. The National Hospice and Palliative Care Organization (NHPCO) provides links to advance directives formatted for each state in the United States (see Table A1.1).

For individuals with dementia, there are specific advance directives aimed at documenting patient choices prior to the loss of cognitive capabilities. Decision-making capacity includes one's ability to understand information,

Table A1.1 Advance Care Planning Resources

National Institute of Health/ National Institute on Aging: Advance Care Planning: Healthcare Directives	https://www.nia.nih.gov/health/advance-care-planning-healthcare-directives
NHPCO Advance Directives by State	https://www.nhpco.org/patients-and-caregivers/advance-care-planning/advance-directives/downloading-your-states-advance-directive/
Advance Health Care Directives: Towards a Coordinated European Policy?	https://www.academia.edu/457880/Advance_Health_Care_Directives_Towards_a_Coordinated_European_Policy_with_N._Biller-Andorno_and_S._Brauer_
Advance Directive for Individuals with Dementia	https://dementia-directive.org/
Aging with Dignity (Five Wishes): Advance Directive available in 27 languages	www.agingwithdignity.org
The Conversation Project (see Appendix 4)	www.theconversationproject.org
Caring Info	http://www.caringinfo.org/i4a/pages/index.cfm?pageid=3277
Compassion & Choices Advance Care Planning Toolkit	https://compassionandchoices.org/wp-content/uploads/2018/09/My-End-of-Life-Decisions-Guide-Toolkit-FINAL-8-28-18.pdf
The National POLST Paradigm	https://polst.org/

the ability to make decisions based on information, and the ability to communicate this choice. For individuals with evolving cognitive impairments (e.g. dementia), there is uncertainty associated with the loss of capacity in their own decision-making. Therefore, proactive, timely documentation of wishes is particularly critical with these individuals (see Table A1.1).

Physician orders for life-sustaining treatment (POLST) are portable medical orders, also known by several different acronyms (e.g. POST, MOST, MOLST). These orders are written and signed by the medical provider and are designed specifically for individuals with advanced diseases, frailty, and/ or terminal conditions. The intention is that these medical orders travel with the individual from setting to setting (e.g. hospital to home, nursing home to hospital), and take effect immediately upon inability to communicate wishes. Portable medical orders typically include specifications such as DNR, do not intubate (DNI), and do not transfer (e.g. to emergency room, hospital, or intensive care unit). Additionally, they are designed to specify the level of aggressiveness one wishes to pursue with their medical care (e.g. full treatments or medical interventions, selected/limited treatments or medical interventions, comfort care). Specific interventions such as the use of antibiotics, medically-assisted nutrition and hydration, as well as resuscitation procedures and attempts (e.g. CPR, intubation) are outlined with specific timelines and goals in mind.

Appendix 2
End of Life Option Act/Medical Aid in Dying

With the current climate of respecting patient choice and autonomy at the end of life, opportunities have arisen for individuals and their families facing a terminal illness to be able to choose the time, method, and circumstances of death. Medical Aid in Dying (MAiD) is now an available option for patients in several United States jurisdictions, as well as internationally. First passed in the United States in Oregon in 1994, the *Death With Dignity Act* (ORS 127.8) was upheld by the US Supreme Court in 1997. This act has now been officially titled *The End of Life Options Act* (H. 1926) and similar legislation has been passed in other states including Washington (2008), Vermont (2013), California (2015), Colorado (2016), the District of Columbia (2017), Hawaii (2018), and New Jersey and Maine (2019); other states have legislation pending.

In contrast to the often stigmatized and controversial concept of *physician-assisted suicide*, or euthanasia, the Death with Dignity movement (https://www.deathwithdignity.org/) has elevated MAiD to a viable clinical option for those eligible patients who choose it in jurisdictions where it is permitted. There are significant differences between physician-assisted suicide and MAiD, including the process that the patient then self-determines the timing of their deliberate, conscious ingestion of the necessary medications prescribed to end their life. Even for those individuals who receive the necessary medications via prescription, many ultimately do not use the medication. However, knowing it is available allows them peace of mind to control at least the potential aspect of timing at the end of life when so much control and dignity has often already been lost.

There are several safeguards in place to protect vulnerable, seriously ill patients, including eligibility criteria such as the inevitability of a terminal outcome (a prognosis of six or fewer months), mental evaluation for capacity to make informed decisions, as well as screening for coercion or abuse of the process. Unfortunately, some state regulations are so cumbersome that they actually present significant barriers to timely access for patients choosing the MAiD option including a waiting period, as well as requiring two physician's opinions on the anticipated timeframe of death before issuing the relevant prescriptions. In some communities, even though MAiD is legal, the stigma remains substantial. Some physicians experience significant pressure not to participate, causing patients to seek out 'specialist' physicians who do not have a personal relationship, but are willing to assist in this process.

For patients initiating the conversation about their end-of-life options, and/or experiencing decisional conflict, allowing for an open, honest dialogue is ideal. It is critical to listen intently, keep personal biases in check and approach the topic from a safe place of caring and appropriate concern. Refer the individual to their medical provider for a discussion of their options, to further explore the process, and their wishes. Honoring the patient's autonomy and validating their concerns with appropriate, supportive referrals, are the best approaches to this delicate but important topic.

Appendix 3
Grief and Bereavement

For individuals with terminal diagnoses and their loved ones, the journey toward the end of life elicits many emotions and experiences. From the initial diagnosis and transition to illness, through disease progression and followed by the ultimate realization that the end of life is approaching, emotions will ebb and flow. The feeling of grief and the process of bereavement are highly individualized experiences, yet many similarities exist between individuals. Likewise, the terms grief, bereavement, and mourning are frequently used interchangeably, while in fact, they have different meanings. A firm understanding of the concepts and processes can better prepare clinicians to support, and care for, individuals with life-limiting illnesses and their families.

Grief

Grief is an individual's personal response to loss, which includes several domains (e.g. behavioral, emotional, cognitive, physical, social, and spiritual).[1] Elisabeth Kübler-Ross, MD, psychiatrist and hospice pioneer, first described Five Stages of Grief[TM] in 1969 in her book *On Death and Dying*, including denial, anger, bargaining, depression, and acceptance (see Chapter 1 and Table A3.1).[2] The original concept of the stages was not intended to indicate that one moves along them in a linear fashion or step-by-step sequentially, but rather individuals often fluctuate between and/or remain in particular stages. Subsequently, enhancement of the original stages has included the precursor

Table A3.1 Original Five Stages of Grief with Additions[2,3]

		Shock	Awareness/Recognition of a Fatal Illness
Hope	1	*Denial*	"This can't be happening to me."
	2	*Anger*	"*Why* is this happening? Who is to blame?"
	3	*Bargaining*	"Make this not happen, and in return I will ____."
	4	*Depression*	"I'm too sad to do anything."
	5	*Acceptance*	"I'm at peace with what happened."
		Decathexis	Emotional withdrawal prior to death

Source: Elisabeth Kubler-Ross Foundation. Five stages of grief. https://www.ckrfoundation.org/5-stages-of-grief/5-stages-grief/. Published 2020. Accessed June 22, 2020.

of *shock* with the recognition of a fatal illness. The concept of *hope* has also been extended across the stages, with the realization that hope changes (e.g. hope for a cure, hope for more time, hope for less pain, hope for a peaceful death). The final stage is considered *decathexis*, or emotional withdrawal, which occurs prior to death. Additionally, emphasis has since been placed on the concepts of *preparatory* (anticipatory) *grief*, and *partial denial*.

Mourning and Bereavement

Stroebe et al.[4] defined bereavement as "*a state of loss, triggering a grief reaction that manifests in a set of behaviours known as mourning.*" *Mourning* is the outward expression of grief and the active reaction to suffering a loss through which grief is resolved.[5] *Bereavement* is considered a process, or an intense period of mourning, often also described in stages. The dual process model of coping with bereavement by Stroebe and Schut[6] includes both *loss-oriented processes* (e.g. grief work, breaking bonds/ties), and *restoration-oriented processes* (e.g. distraction from grief, establishing new rules). Worden[7] suggested that grief is work, and is resolved through active tasks of mourning including: (1) accepting the reality of loss; (2) working through and experiencing grief; (3) adjustment to the environment without the deceased person; and (4) withdrawing emotionally from the deceased person to move on.

Recognizing the need for referral to a professional for grief counseling and bereavement support throughout the end-of-life process is a critical role for the interdisciplinary team caring for individuals with terminal illnesses, as well as for their families. Timely referral by clinicians to specialists such as clinical social workers, bereavement counselors, death educators, chaplains, local and regional bereavement centers, and educational resources is essential

Table A3.2 Grief and Bereavement Resources

Mental Health America: Bereavement and Grief	https://www.mhanational.org/bereavement-and-grief
American Cancer Society: Grief and Bereavement	https://www.cancer.org/treatment/end-of-life-care/grief-and-loss/grieving-process.html
United Kingdom National Health Service: Grief after bereavement or loss	https://www.nhs.uk/conditions/stress-anxiety-depression/coping-with-bereavement/
Australian Centre for Grief and Bereavement	https://www.grief.org.au/
National Cancer Institute: Grief, Bereavement, and Coping With Loss (PDQ®)–Patient Version	https://www.cancer.gov/about-cancer/advanced-cancer/caregivers/planning/bereavement-pdq
Mayo Clinic: Grief: Coping with reminders after a loss	https://www.mayoclinic.org/healthy-lifestyle/end-of-life/in-depth/grief/art-20045340
Hospice Foundation of America: Grief Resources	https://hospicefoundation.org/Grief-(1)

(see Table A3.2). Dedicated peer bereavement support groups with individuals with similar, shared experiences (e.g. loss of a child, widow/widower, motherless daughters, suicide loss) can be helpful during the bereavement process. Significant dates, which can often be painful triggers (e.g. birthdays, anniversaries, holidays), are important to recognize especially in the early stages of bereavement such as the first thirteen months following a loss (to include the anniversary of a death).

References

1 Greenstreet W. Why nurses need to understand the principles of bereavement theory. *Br J Nurs.* 2004;13(10):590–593.
2 Kubler-Ross E. *On Death and Dying.* London, England: Macmillan; 1969.
3 Elisabeth Kubler-Ross Foundation. Five stages of grief. https://www.ekrfoundation.org/5-stages-of-grief/5-stages-grief/. Published 2020. Accessed June 22, 2020.
4 Stroebe MS, Stroebe W, Hansson RO (eds). *Handbook of Bereavement: Theory, Research, and Intervention.* New York, NY: Cambridge University Press; 1993.
5 Buglass E. Grief and bereavement theories. *Nurs Stand.* 2010;24(41):44–47.
6 Stroebe M, Schut H. The dual process model of coping with bereavement: Rationale and description. *Death Stud.* 1999;23(3):197–224.
7 Worden JW. *Grief Counseling and Grief Therapy: A Handbook for the Mental Health Practitioner.* 2nd ed. London, England: Routledge; 1991.

Appendix 4
Conversation Guides

Initiating difficult conversations can often be challenging for many health-care providers (see Chapter 7). The pressure to always know the right thing to say, and worrying about disclosing too much or not enough information, can be heavy when our patients/clients are facing a terminal illness. Having the appropriate resources, including evidence-based guides, can assist us with some structure for these tough topics. Practice with the format also increases the comfort level with which we are able to initiate these types of conversations. One of the most commonly used is Vital Talk (www.vitaltalk.org). This online resource has a wide variety of video vignettes and scenarios. In addition to a smartphone application (currently available on the Apple iOS store), this nonprofit organization has published several resource guides and one-page quick resources for having challenging conversations. Vital Talk offers a conversation structure when a provider has to deliver difficult or unwelcome news (Table A4.1).

When encountered, distinct and purposeful strategies will help a therapist to respond to emotion. Vital Talk again offers useful conversation strategies for facilitating an emotional or difficult conversation. An important component to responding to an emotional expression is to respect and acknowledge it. Vital Talk offers the NURSE conversation steps to help facilitate this as seen in Table A4.2 (https://www.vitaltalk.org/guides/responding-to-emotion-respecting/).

In addition to Vital Talk's GUIDE and NURSE models of communication, two additional examples include the *Serious Illness Conversation Guide* and the *Conversation Project*.

Serious Illness Conversation Guide

Developed by clinicians from the Dana-Farber Cancer Institute and Harvard Medical School through Ariadne Labs (https://www.ariadnelabs.org/), the Serious Illness Conversation Guide (SICG) was designed as a learning tool to help facilitate early person-centered communication between clinicians and their patients facing serious illnesses using best practices for conversation flow (i.e. *set up, assess, share, explore, and close*) and proven/patient-tested language (e.g. "I wish...", "I hope...", "I'm worried that..."). The goal of the tool is to discover their values, goals, and preferences within the context of their prognosis.

Table A4.1 GUIDE Steps for Disclosing Serious News

- Get ready: In this stage, the therapist should be preparing for this crucial conversation by having all the relevant information, key individuals, and privacy for the forthcoming discussion. This may include family members, diagnostic tests, and current knowledge of future care goals.
- Understand: Prior to conveying any information, the therapist should query to understand what the patient currently knows about their health condition or prognosis. "Please tell me what your doctors have told you about your health condition and what your hopes are for after the hospital."
- Inform: Deliver your opinion or findings clearly and concisely without jargon. Start with the most important piece of information first. After this delivery, stop and allow the individual to process this information. When they are ready, deliver the contextual information. "You have been working very hard in therapy but unfortunately your physical status is declining." STOP! This amount of shocking information will require time for the person to process and collect their thoughts.
- Demonstrate empathy: Anticipate and respond to emotion. Acknowledge this emotion overtly and clearly. "I can see that this news is upsetting. It is natural to feel this way in this situation."
- Equip: Prepare and facilitate the next steps. Avoid saying everything will be okay or avoiding the subject. Let the person know that you will be there to help them during this process. "I know this is not the news you were hoping for, but we will work on a plan together. Tell me how I can help you."

---

https://www.vitaltalk.org/guides/serious-news/

Table A4.2 NURSE: Respecting and Responding to Emotion

- Naming: Attempt to reduce the emotion and intensity of the situation by naming the emotion that you are observing. "I can see this is very upsetting to you."
- Understanding: Acknowledge that the emotional response helps to understand the response. Be careful not to say, "I understand" as this risks a response like "No, you don't." A better response may be "This helps me to understand what you are feeling."
- Respecting: Acknowledge efforts and steps the person has been taking or attempting to take. "I have seen how hard you are working to take care of your mother."
- Supporting: Verbalize your commitment to help as best you can. "I know these are difficult circumstances, but I am going to do my best to help out however I can."
- Exploring: Further facilitate the conversation more deeply without being perceived as 'psychoanalyzing' the person. A focused question will assist with this. For example, "You said you were worried about what you would do when you get home. Can you please tell me more about that?"

A qualitative study of 118 advanced cancer survivors and 41 clinicians revealed the SICG to be feasible, and associated with positive experiences for both the patients and the oncology clinicians.[1] The SICG can be accessed here: https://www.ariadnelabs.org/wp-content/uploads/sites/2/2017/05/SI-CG-2017-04-21_FINAL.pdf

From the Institute of Healthcare Improvement, there are several resources available for individuals with life-limiting illnesses to communicate with family members as well as their healthcare providers, and for family members to communicate with individuals with serious illnesses (https://theconversationproject.org/starter-kits/). Several resources are available, including: the Conversation Starter Kit (general); the Conversation Starter Kit for patients with Alzheimer's/dementia; Who will speak for you? (how to choose and be a healthcare proxy); How to talk to your doctor; and the Pediatric Starter Kit (having the conversation with your seriously ill child). Additionally, following the global COVID-19 pandemic, The Conversation Project also collaborated with Ariadne Labs to create a Conversation Starter Kit specifically for COVID-19 (https://theconversationproject.org/wp-content/uploads/2020/04/tcpcovid19guide.pdf). The Conversation Starter Kits are available in 13 different languages, as well as the availability of an audio version in English. (https://www.youtube.com/watch?v=v20Cz8NS5K8).

Reference

1 Paladino J, Koritsanszky L, Nisotel L, et al. Patient and clinician experience of a serious illness conversation guide in oncology: A descriptive analysis. *Cancer Med.* 2020;9(13):4550–4560. doi:10.1002/cam4.3102.

Index

For Product Safety Concerns and Information please contact our EU
representative GPSR@taylorandfrancis.com Taylor & Francis Verlag GmbH,
Kaufingerstraße 24, 80331 München, Germany

Printed and bound by CPI Group (UK) Ltd, Croydon, CR0 4YY

08/06/2025

01897002-0008